AF441832

Alzheimer's Disease and Related Disorders Annual

Edited by

Serge Gauthier MD FRCPC

Professor and Director
Alzheimer's Disease Research Unit
The McGill Centre for Studies in Aging
Douglas Hospital
Verdun PQ
Canada

Jeffrey L Cummings MD

Director, UCLA Alzheimer's Disease Center
Augustus S Rose Professor of Neurology
Professor of Psychiatry and Biobehavioral Sciences
UCLA School of Medicine
Los Angeles CA
USA

Martin Dunitz

© Martin Dunitz Ltd 2000

First published in the United Kingdom in 2000 by
Martin Dunitz Ltd
The Livery House
7–9 Pratt Street
London NW1 0AE

Tel:		+44-(0)20-7482-2202
Fax:		+44-(0)20-7267-0159
E-mail:		info@mdunitz.globalnet.co.uk
Website:	http://www.dunitz.co.uk

All rights reserved. No part of this publication may be reproduced, stored in a retrieval system, or transmitted, in any form or by any means, electronic, mechanical, photocopying, recording or otherwise, without the prior permission of the publisher or in accordance with the provisions of the Copyright Act 1988.

A CIP catalogue record for this book is available from the British Library

ISBN 1-85317-909-4

Distributed in the United States by:
Blackwell Science Inc.
Commerce Place, 350 Main Street
Malden, MA 02148, USA
Tel: 1-800-215-1000

Distributed in Canada by:
Login Brothers Book Company
324 Salteaux Crescent
Winnipeg, Manitoba, R3J 3T2
Canada
Tel: 1-204-224-4068

Distributed in Brazil by:
Ernesto Reichmann Distribuidora de Livros, Ltda
Rua Coronel Marques, 335,
Tatuape 03440-000
São Paulo
Brazil

Composition by Wearset, Boldon, Tyne and Wear
Printed and bound in Spain by Grafos, S.A. Arte sobre papel

Contents

Contributors

Paul S Aisen MD
Professor, Department of Neurology, Georgetown University Medical Center, Washington DC, USA.

Yuri L Bronstein MD
Department of Neurology, UCLA School of Medicine, Los Angeles CA, USA.

Jeffrey L Cummings MD
The Augustus S Rose Professor of Neurology, Professor of Psychiatry and Biobehavioural Sciences, UCLA Alzheimer's Disease Center, Reed Neurological Research Center, UCLA School of Medicine, Los Angeles CA, USA.

Timo Erkinjuntti MD PhD
Department of Clinical Neurosciences, Helsinki University Central Hospital, Helsinki, Finland.

Hellmut Erzigkeit PhD
Professor, Klinische Psychologie, Psychiatrische Klinik mit Poliklinik der Universität Erlangen-Nürnberg, Erlangen, Germany.

Serge Gauthier MD FRCPC
Professor and Director, Alzheimer's Disease Study Unit, McGill Centre for Studies in Aging, Verdun PQ, Canada.

Victor W Henderson MD MS
The Kenneth and Bette Volk Professor of Neurology, and Professor of Gerontology and Psychology, University of Southern California, Los Angeles CA, USA.

Hartmut Lehfeld PhD
Institut Methodenforum e.V. Theodor-Klippel-Str. 7 91052 Erlangen Germany.

Irene Litvan MD
Chief, Cognitive Neuropharmacology Unit, Defence & Veterans Head Injury Program, Henry M Jackson Foundation, Bethesda MD, USA.

Ian G McKeith MD BS FRCPsych
Professor, Department of Old Age Psychiatry, Institute for the Health of the Elderly, Wolfson Research Centre, Newcastle General Hospital, Newcastle-upon-Tyne, UK.

David MA Mann PhD
Professor of Neuropathology, Department of Medicine, University of Manchester, Manchester, UK.

Bruce L Miller MD
Department of Neurology, University of California at San Francisco, San Francisco CA, USA.

David Neary MB ChB FRCP
Professor of Neurology and Consultant
Neurologist, Department of Neurology,
Manchester Royal Infirmary,
Manchester, UK.

Leonardo Pantoni MD PhD
Department of Neurological and
Psychiatric Sciences, University of
Florence, Florence, Italy.

Florence Pasquier MD PhD
Department of Neurology–Memory
Clinic, University Hospital, Lille,
France.

Peter H St George-Hyslop MD FRCPC
Director, Centre for Research in
Neurodegenerative Disease,
Professor, Department of Medicine,
University of Toronto, Department of
Medicine (Neurology), University
Health Network, Toronto ON, Canada.

Julie S Snowden
Department of Neurology, Manchester
Royal Infirmary, Manchester, UK.

Preface

Owing to the rapid pace of research in the field of Alzheimer's disease (AD) and related disorders, we feel that it is appropriate to publish a yearbook which reviews the 'topics of the year' in the realms of pathology of dementia, diagnosis, natural history and treatment.

In *Alzheimer's Disease and Related Disorders Annual*, our focus ranges from genetics of AD and frontotemporal dementia to the diagnostic criteria for dementia with Lewy bodies, parkinsonism, and subcortical ischemia. Additionally, we discuss the natural history of minimal cognitive impairment as relevant to randomized clinical trials (RCT) which aim to delay conversion into dementia; whereas, structured functional and behavioural assessments are now very much part of RCT which focus on symptomatic treatment. Therapy with cholinesterase inhibitors, hormonal replacement and anti-inflammatory drugs is discussed with RCT and a clinical practice point of view.

We hope that readers will find these topics helpful in their clinical practices and that this yearbook will provide a platform for exciting discussion in future editions.

Serge Gauthier MD
Jeffrey Cummings MD
June 2000

1

Genetics of Alzheimer's disease

Peter H St George-Hyslop

Introduction

The clinical features and the classical neuropathological hallmarks of Alzheimer's disease (AD) can arise from several different genetic and non-genetic causes. In the past few years, a number of genetic epidemiology studies[1–7] have strongly argued that the familial aggregation of AD is not due simply to the high frequency of AD in the general population. These studies suggest that the age-dependent risk and the overall lifetime risk for AD in first-degree relatives of AD probands varies from 10 to 50%. The most comprehensive recent study suggests an age-dependent risk curve asymptotic to a final risk of 38% by age 85 years.[7] This study, as well as several other earlier studies, make it difficult to assign a pure Mendelian mode of transmission in the majority of AD cases. Instead, these studies imply that the majority of cases of familial aggregation of AD probably reflect a complex mode of transmission such as:

- one or more common independent, but incompletely penetrant, single autosomal gene defects;
- a multigenic trait; or
- a mode of transmission in which genetic and environmental factors interact.

Nevertheless, there is a small proportion of AD cases (about 10%) that are transmitted as a pure autosomal-dominant Mendelian trait with age-dependent (but high) penetrance. Analysis of these pedigrees has led to the discovery of four different genetic loci associated with inherited susceptibility to AD.

Genetic loci

Amyloid precursor protein

The β-amyloid precursor protein (APP) gene on chromosome 21 encodes an alternatively spliced transcript, which, in its longest isoform, encodes a single transmembrane-spanning polypeptide of 770 amino acids.[8-11] The β-APP precursor protein undergoes a series of endoproteolytic cleavages.[12] One of these cleavages results from the putative membrane-associated α-secretase, which cleaves β-APP between residues 16 and 17 of Aβ and liberates the extracellular *N*-terminus of β-APP, which was previously identified at protease nexin II (a protease inhibitor possibly involved in coagulation) and which has potential neurotrophic activity. This pathway precludes the formation of Aβ peptide. The other pathway involves cleavage by β- and γ-secretases, which gives rise to a series of peptides that contain the 40–42 amino acid Aβ peptide. Aβ ending at residue 40 is the predominant isoform produced during normal metabolism of β-APP.[13-18] Current evidence suggests that $A\beta_{40}$ is predominantly produced in endosomal–lysosomal systems.[19,20] Aβ peptides ending at residue 42 ($A\beta_{42}$, or long-tailed Aβ), on the other hand, are thought to be more fibrillogenic and more neurotoxic.[18] Substantial evidence suggests that these longer isoforms may be generated at intracellular sites such as the endoplasmic reticulum and cis-Golgi, which (in neurons at least) are distinct from the sites of $A\beta_{40}$ synthesis,[21-23] although other lipid-rich raft domains have also been suggested.[24]

Several different mis-sense mutations in exons 16 and 17 of the β-APP gene have been found in families with early-onset AD (Table 1.1). Although some of these mis-sense mutations are probably not pathogenic, the mis-sense mutations at codons 670–671 (Swedish mutation),[25] codon 692 (Flemish mutation),[26] codon 693,[27] codon 715, codon 716,[28] codon 717[29-33] and codon 723, are thought to be pathogenic. The mutations at codon 670–671 and at codon 692 are rare, having been seen only in single families. Mutations at codon 717 have been seen in approximately 20 unrelated pedigrees from different ethnic origins. Most of the codon 717 mutations have been seen in Anglo-Saxon, Italian and Japanese subjects.

All of the clearly pathogenic mutations cluster close to the β-secretase site (Lys670Asn–Met671Leu), the α-secretase site (Ala692Gly and Glu693Gln) or the γ-secretase site (codons 715, 716, 717 and 723). This led to the hypothesis that these mutations might influence the processing of β-APP.[25] Indeed, mutations at codons 715, 716, 717 and 723 cause selective increase in $A\beta_{42-43}$.[28,34-38] The Lys670Asn–Met671Leu mutation, on the other hand, appears to augment the production of both $A\beta_{40}$ and $A\beta_{42-43}$,[39] whereas the Ala692Gly mutation has a more complicated effect on β-APP processing and causes impaired α-secretase cleavage, increased heterogeneity of secreted Aβ species and increased hydrophobicity of the Aβ.[37] The Ala692Gly mutation also has clinical features that are, in some cases, similar to those of HCHWA-D and that are, in other cases, more similar to AD but with somewhat subtle differences in the size of the amyloid cores.[40] The Glu693Gln mutation causes an increased propensity for Aβ to form fibrils.[41]

The hypothesis that relative or absolute overproduction of Aβ peptide,

Table 1.1 Mis-sense mutations in the β-APP gene.

Codon	Mutation	Phenotype
665	Gln → Asp	Late-onset AD (no segregation)[160]
670/671	Lys–Met → Asn–Leu	Familial AD (increased Aβ production)[25]
673	Ala → Thr	No disease phenotype[161]
692	Ala → Gly	Familial AD plus cerebral haemorrhage (increased Aβ)[26]
693	Glu → Gly	Late-onset AD (no segregation)[162]
	Glu → Gln	HCHWA-D[27]
713	Ala → Val	Schizophrenia (no segregation)[163]
	Ala → Thr	AD (no segregation)[164]
715		Familial AD
716	Ile → Val	Familial AD[28]
717	Val → Ile	Familial AD (increased long Aβ isoforms)[29,32,33]
	Val → Phe	Familial AD[31]
	Val → Gly	Familial AD[30]
723		Familial AD

and in particular of $A\beta_{42}$, is an effect of β-APP mutations that leads to neurodegeneration is attractive. This hypothesis is supported by the observations that $A\beta_{42}$ peptides have an enhanced propensity to form fibrils[15,17,18] and that this conformational change is necessary to change the inert (or even marginally neurotrophic) soluble Aβ into toxic Aβ.[17,18] Multiple molecular mechanisms have been postulated to explain the neurotoxic effects of Aβ. These include induction of apoptosis by either direct effects on cell membranes or by indirect effects such as potentiation of neurotoxic effects of excitatory amino acids, oxidative stress, and increases in intracellular calcium and free radicals.[42-44] However, at least one experimental result has suggested that APP mutations could also induce apoptosis by a mechanism that is independent of Aβ peptide production.[45,46] In this regard, it is worth emphasizing that overproduction of Aβ peptide (as opposed to increased deposition or decreased clearance) is not a universal feature of all cases of sporadic AD.[47]

Apolipoprotein E

Analysis of pedigrees with predominantly late-onset familial aggregations of AD provided suggestive evidence ($z = +2.5$ at $\theta = 0.00$) for the existence of a second AD susceptibility locus on chromosome 19q12–q13 near the markers *BCL3* and *ATP1A3*.[48] Subsequent investigation of candidate genes revealed that the chromosome 19 AD locus was the apolipoprotein E (APOE) gene.[49] In humans, the APOE gene contains three common coding sequence polymorphisms:

- the most common coding sequence variant, ε3, reflects the presence of a cysteine at codon 112 and arginine at codon 158; this sequence is present in approximately 75% of Caucasians;

- the second coding sequence variant, ε4, reflects substitution of arginine for cysteine at codon 112; this sequence is present in approximately 15% of Caucasians;
- the third coding sequence variant, ε2, contains cysteine at codons 112 and 158; this sequence is present in approximately 10% of Caucasians.

Analysis of the frequency distributions of these three variants in normal control populations and in patients with AD has consistently shown that:

- there is an increase in the frequency of the ε4 allele in patients with AD (the ε4 allele frequency in AD is approximately 40%);[50] and
- there is a smaller reduction in the frequency of the ε2 allele (to about 2% in AD).[51]

More significantly, there is dose-dependent relationship between the number of copies of ε4 and the age of onset of AD, such that ε4/ε4 subjects have an earlier age of onset (mean age of onset is less than 70 years) than heterozygous ε4 subjects (mean age of onset for ε2/ε3 is over 90 years).[52] Subjects with an ε2 allele, on the other hand, have a later onset.[51] The association between ε4 and AD has been robustly confirmed in numerous studies and in several different ethnic groups.[53] The association is weaker with advanced age of onset, and the putative protective role of the ε2 allele is less clear at younger ages of onset (where ε2 may even be associated with a more aggressive course).[54,55] Currently, the major exceptions to the association of APOE ε4 with AD arises from studies in black Americans and Hispanics that have generated conflicting results.[56–58] It remains unclear whether these conflicting results reflect the effects of statistical confounders or whether there is a true lack of association between AD and APOE ε4 in subsets of these populations.

Although the association between APOE ε4 and AD is robust, it is not entirely specific. Thus, patients with head injury[59,60] patients with spontaneous intracerebral haemorrhage[61] and patients undergoing elective cardiac bypass surgery[62] all have a poorer outcome when they carry the ε4 allele. There is also evidence for synergistic effects of a history of head injury and APOE ε4 on risk of AD,[59] such that patients with APOE ε4 and a head injury have a 10-fold increase in risk of AD (compared with a two-fold increase with APOE ε4 alone and no increase for head injury alone). There is also a confirmed association between the ε4 allele and the Lewy body variant of AD, which has a subtly different clinical phenotype from classical AD (e.g. more frequent hallucinations, sensitivity to neuroleptics).[63]

The mechanisms by which the ε4 allele is associated with an earlier onset of AD and by which the ε2 allele is associated with a later onset are unclear. Nevertheless, a large body of biochemical evidence has been accumulated to support various hypotheses on how these APOE-coding sequence polymorphisms might promote or protect against AD. The most obvious hypothesis is that APOE ε4/ε2 polymorphisms influence the production, distribution or clearance of the Aβ peptide. This hypothesis is supported by observations that the genotype at APOE accounts for some of the variation in age of onset in subjects who carry the β-APP Val717Ile mutation (but not the APP$_{692}$ mutation); this suggests a direct biochemical interaction between APOE and β-APP or its metabolic products.[64–67] Secondly, subjects with one or more APOE ε4 alleles have a higher Aβ peptide plaque burden than subjects with no ε4 alleles.[68] In vitro studies suggest that delipidated APOE ε4 binds Aβ more avidly than APOE ε3 does.[49,69] Thirdly, there is evidence that both APOE and Aβ may be cleared through the lipoprotein-related receptor and that APOE ε4 and the Aβ peptide may compete for clearance through this receptor.[70] Finally, transgenic mice that have an intact endogenous APOE gene and that overexpress human β-APP with the Val717Phe mutant under the control of the PDGF β-subunit promoter develop profuse deposits of extracellular Aβ by 9 months of age. In contrast, when the same transgene is expressed in an APOE$^{-/-}$ background, there is a dramatic reduction in extracellular Aβ deposition, which supports the hypothetical role for APOE in sequestering extracellular Aβ.[71]

A relationship between APOE and neurofibrillary tangles and synaptic density has also been suggested. In vitro APOE isoform-specific binding experiments with tau and MAP2 suggests that ε3 binds to both tau and MAP2 better than the ε4 isoform does.[72–74] This suggests that ε2 and ε3 may protect and sequester microtubule-associated proteins better than ε4 does, thereby reducing the ability of tau to bind to itself, become hyperphosphorylated and form paired helical filaments.

Finally, APOE may be involved in synaptic plasticity during regeneration and repair, and the ε4 allele may be less efficient in this role. Thus, APOE knock-out mice also show an age-dependent decrease in synaptic density and spontaneous Aβ peptide aggregation within astrocytic processes.[75] Several types of neural tissue culture cells demonstrate decreased neurite outgrowth in the presence of APOE ε4 in the media rather than APOE ε3.[76,77] Perhaps, then, the APOE isoforms might differentially affect synapse formation in response to injury, learning and ageing.

In addition to the ε2/ε3/ε4 coding sequence polymorphisms, several polymorphisms have been discovered in the 5'-promoter of the APOE gene. In some studies,[78,79] these polymorphisms are suspected to increase risk for AD independently of APOE ε4 and to cause this increased risk of AD by altering the transcriptional activity of APOE (although direct proof of the latter in vivo has not yet been obtained). However, several other independent studies have been unable to replicate these findings, although they do confirm that the B491 A/T polymorphism at least, is in linkage disequilibrium with the APOE $\epsilon2/\epsilon3/\epsilon4$ polymorphism.[80,81]

Presenilin-1

A third familial AD locus that is associated with a very aggressive, early-onset AD has been mapped to chromosome 14q24.3 near the markers D14S43, D14S71, D14S77 and D14S53.[82–84] The chromosome 14 familial AD gene (presenilin-1, PS1) was isolated using a positional cloning strategy[85] and a homologue (presenilin-2) was then mapped to chromosome 1.

PS1 is highly conserved in evolution, being present in *Caenorhabditis elegans*[86] and *D. melanogaster*.[87] It encodes a polytopic integral membrane protein with between six and 10 possible transmembrane domains (see below). PS1 is transcribed at low levels in many different cell types, both within the central nervous system and also in non-neurological tissues.[85] In the central nervous system, PS1 transcripts can be detected by in situ hybridization in the neocortex (especially in cortical neurons in layers II and IV), the neurones of the CA1–CA3 fields of the hippocampus, the granule cell neurones of the dentate gyrus, the subiculum, the cerebellar Purkinje and granule cells and deep nuclei, as well as in lesser amounts in the olfactory bulb, the striatum, some brainstem nuclei and the thalamus.

Immunoblotting and immunohistochemical studies suggest that the PS1 protein is approximately 50 kDa in size and is predominantly located within intracellular membranes in the endoplasmic reticulum, perinuclear envelope, the Golgi apparatus and some (as yet uncharacterized) intracytoplasmic vesicles.[88,89] Studies of the topology of PS1 suggest that the *N*-terminus and the residues in the TM6–TM7 loop are both located in the cytoplasm.[88,90–92] The orientation of the *C*-terminus is not yet completely resolved.[88,90–92] However, the predominance of opinion suggests that it is oriented to the cytoplasm and that the preceding hydrophobic residues are either membrane-associated or represent two additional transmembrane domains (TM7 and TM8). Studies of the PS1 protein in brain tissue, as well as many other peripheral tissues, reveal that only very small amounts of the PS1 holoprotein exist within the cell at any given time.[93,94] Instead, the holoprotein is actively catabolized, possibly by at least two different proteolytic mechanisms. One of these mechanisms appears to involve the proteasome.[95] Another proteolytic mechanism involves a series of heterogeneous endoproteolytic cleavage near residue 290 within the TM6–TM7 loop domain.[93,94] This endoproteolytic cleavage generates a series of *N*-terminal heterogeneous fragments (NTFs) of approximately 35 kDa and *C*-terminal heterogeneous fragments (CTFs) of approximately 18–20 kDa. Remarkably, the stoichiometry of the NTFs and

CTFs is tightly maintained on a 1:1 ratio and the absolute abundance of NTFs and CTFs is also tightly regulated such that artificial overexpression of PS1 results in only a modest increase in NTFs and CTFs.[93]

Both the full-length PS1 and the NTFs and CTFs exist as components of independent high molecular weight, multimeric protein complexes. Thus, the holoprotein appears to be a component of a complex of approximately 180 kDa.[96–98] Both the NTF and the CTF associate with each other as heterodimeric components of a larger (approximately 250 kDa) multimeric protein complex.[24,96–98]

The identity of the other components of the presenilin complexes is currently under investigation. However, a variety of studies reveal that in peripheral tissues and in brain, the presenilins associate with β-catenin, a member of the armadillo protein superfamily.[98,99] In brain, the presenilins also associate with a novel armadillo protein termed neuronal plakophillin-related armadillo protein (NPRAP) or δ-catenin.[98,99] The functional significance of the presenilin–armadillo interactions is not entirely clear because the armadillo proteins have diverse functions that range from a structural role in stabilization of intercellular junctions (including synapses), intracellular transduction of receptor mediated signals (e.g. Wnt and certain growth factors), to participation in apoptotic cell death pathways. There is evidence from some laboratories that presenilins may also directly interact with a number of other proteins such as β-APP[100,101] and filamin-binding protein.[102] However, not all laboratories confirm these latter results.[97]

Ablation of functional PS1 expression by homozygous targeted disruption of the murine PS1 gene causes inhibition of proteolytic processing of β-APP and Notch, which argues that PS1 is involved in processing of a subclass of type I transmembrane proteins that undergo a intramembranous proteolytic cleavage.[103] Inhibition of Notch processing provides an explanation for the developmental abnormalities that arise from homozygous null mutations in PS1 (PS1$^{-/-}$) in both invertebrates and vertebrates. The loss of mammalian Notch processing causes severe abnormalities in the central nervous system and the caudal axial skeleton.[104,105] These abnormalities are similar to those seen in *Notch* and *Delta-like* knockouts.[106] In *C. elegans*, null mutations in the presenilin orthologue *sel12* exert a suppressor effect on abnormalities in vulva progenitor cell fate decisions induced by activated *Notch* mutants.[86] Absence of PS1 also causes the failure of γ-secretase cleavage of the *C*-terminal stubs of β-APP derived from α-secretase or β-secretase cleavage.[103,107] Failure of γ-secretase cleavage results in the accumulation of uncleaved α-secretase or β-secretase stubs in a variety of intracellular loci including the endoplasmic reticulum, Golgi and lysosomes.[103,108] It remains unclear, however, whether these effects are due to a direct catalytic role of the presenilins in proteolysis γ-secretase-mediated intramembranous cleavage of β-APP and Notch (perhaps as γ-secretase itself), or whether the presenilins have an indirect role (perhaps as an activator of γ-secretase, or trafficking components of the γ-secretase–substrate complex).

It has also been postulated that PS1 plays a role in the regulation of intercellular signal transduction in apoptosis and possibly in intracellular calcium ion homoeostasis. A role in the suppression of apoptosis has been suggested from studies in transfected cells. Overexpression of full-length, wild-type PS1 or wild type PS2 can cause apoptosis in transfected cells, and mutations further sensitize these cells to apoptosis, possibly through a mechanism that involves heterotrimeric G-coupled proteins that are sensitive to pertussis toxin.[109] It is of note that mutations in β-APP are also thought to cause constitutive activation of programmed cell death pathways that involve heterotrimeric G-coupled proteins.[45,46]

More than 40 different mutations have been discovered in the PS1 gene (Table 1.2), the majority of which are mis-sense mutations. These mutations are predominantly located:

- in highly conserved transmembrane domains;
- at or near putative membrane interfaces; or
- in the *N*-terminal hydrophobic or *C*-terminal hydrophobic residues of the putative TM6–TM7 loop domain.

Two splicing defect mutations have been identified. One involves a point mutation in the splice acceptor site at the 5' end of exon 10 (in some exon numbering systems, exon 10 is labelled exon 9).[110–112] The second splice site mutation arises from deletion of a G-nucleotide from the splice donor site at the 3' end of exon 5',[113] (Rogaeva, unpublished data). Both splicing mutations result in in-frame fusions of the resultant mutant protein.

The wide scattering of mis-sense mutations has led to speculation that the effect of most of the familial AD-related mutations is a 'gain of function' effect.[114] This is partially borne out by two observations in PS1 gene knock-out animals (PS1$^{-/-}$). First, these animals have a phenotype of early perinatal mortality without evidence of AD.[104,105] This loss of function phenotype in PS1$^{-/-}$ animals can be completely rescued by both wild-type and mutant PS1 transgenes.[115,116] Secondly, PS1$^{-/-}$ mice have a defect in β-APP processing that manifested by the failure of γ-secretase cleavage and the accumulation of the *C*-terminal stubs of β-APP following α- and β-secretase cleavage (α- and β-stubs).[104] This defect in β-APP processing is completely reversed by both wild-type and mutant PS1 transgenes. A gain of function is imparted by the mutant transgenes because it also induces an increase in Aβ$_{42}$, which (as described below) is a consistent biochemical effect of PS1 mutations.[115,116] However, studies that have used human PS1 transgenes in complementation assays of mutant sel12 in *C. elegans* suggest that the wild-type human PS1 transgenes, but not mutant human PS1 transgenes, are able to complement the loss-of-function sel12 mutants.[117,118] The latter result argues that the

Table 1.2 Mis-sense mutations in the presenilin genes.

| | Presenilin 1 (S182) | | |
Codon	Location	Mutation	Phenotype
79	*N*-term loop	Ala → ?	Familial AD, onset 64 years
82	TM1	Val → Leu	Familial AD, onset 55 years[165]
96	TM1	Val → Phe	Familial AD[166]
115	TM1 → TM2 loop	Tyr → His	Familial AD, onset 37 years[165]
117	TM1 → TM2 loop	Pro → Leu	Familial AD, onset 28 years[167]
120	TM1 → TM2 loop	Glu → Asp	Familial AD, onset 48 years
139	TM2	Met → Thr	Familial AD, onset 49 years[165]
139	TM2	Met → Val	Familial AD, onset 40 years[168]
143	TM2	Ile → Thr	Familial AD, onset 35 years[169]
146	TM2	Met → Leu	Familial AD, onset 45 years[85]
146	TM2	Met → Val	Familial AD, onset 38 years[168]
146	TM2	Met → Ile	Familial AD, onset 40 years
163	TM3 interface	His → Arg	Familial AD, onset 50 years[85]
163	TM3 interface	His → Tyr	Familial AD, onset 47 years[168]
171	TM3	Leu → Pro	Familial AD, onset 40 years[170]
209	TM4 interface	Gly → Val	Familial AD[166]
213	TM4 interface	Ile → Thr	Familial AD[166]
231	TM5	Ala → Thr	Familial AD, onset 52 years[165]
233	TM5	Met → Thr	Familial AD, onset 35 years[112]
235	TM5	Leu → Pro	Familial AD, onset 32 years[171]
246	TM6	Ala → Glu	Familial AD, onset 55 years[85]
260	TM6	Ala → Val	Familial AD, onset 40 years[127]
263	TM6 → TM7 loop	Cys → Arg	Familial AD, onset 47 years
264	TM6 → TM7 loop	Pro → Leu	Familial AD, onset 45 years[165]
267	TM6 → TM7 loop	Pro → Ser	Familial AD, onset 35 years[168]
280	TM6 → TM7 loop	Glu → Ala	Familial AD, onset 47 years[168]
280	TM6 → TM7 loop	Glu → Gly	Familial AD, onset 42 years[168]
285	TM6 → TM7 loop	Ala → Val	Familial AD, onset 50 years[127]
286	TM6 → TM7 loop	Leu → Val	Familial AD, onset 50 years[85]
del291–319	TM6 → TM7 loop	Short loop	Familial AD[110–112]
384	TM6 → TM7 loop	Gly → Ala	Familial AD, onset 35 years[169]
392	TM6 → TM7 loop	Leu → Val	Familial AD, onset 25–40 years[127]
410	TM7	Cys → Tyr	Familial AD, onset 48 years[85]

| | Presenilin 2 (E5–1) | | |
Codon	Location	Mutation	Phenotype
141	TM2	Asn → Ile	Familial AD, onset 50–65 years[127,128]
239	TM5	Met → Val	Familial AD, onset variable, 45–84 years[127]

human PS1 mutants may not be fully functional (but it does not preclude a gain-of-function effect as well).

One consistent effect of PS1 mutations is to alter the processing of β-APP by preferentially favouring the production of Aβ$_{42}$,[47,119–122] Fibroblasts

from heterozygous carriers of PS1 mutations, various cell lines transfected with β-APP and PS1 cDNAs, and the brain from transgenic mice
that overexpress mutant PS1 transgenes all contain or secrete increased
quantities of long Aβ peptide isoforms with only a variable but minor
increase in short-tailed Aβ peptides.[47,119–122] Direct measurements of Aβ
peptide isoforms in the post mortem brain tissue of patients dying with
PS1-linked familial AD also show marked increases in the amount of long-
tailed Aβ isoforms compared with both control brain tissue and brain
tissue from subjects with sporadic AD.[123]

PS1 and PS2 mutations may also modulate cellular sensitivity to apoptosis induced by a variety of factors, including staurosporine, Aβ peptide,
serum withdrawal and nerve growth factor withdrawal.[109,124–126] At the current time these data are still evolving; the apparent paradox of a putative
'apoptosis-promoting effect' for the presenilins and the existence of
viable transgenic mice that overexpress mutant or wild-type presenilin
cDNAs but lack widespread apoptosis remains to be explained.

Presenilin 2

During the cloning of the PS1 gene on chromosome 14, a homologous
gene on chromosome 1q42.1 was identified.[127,128] This gene, called presenilin 2 (PS2) encodes a polypeptide whose open reading frame contained 448 amino acids, with substantial amino acid sequence identity to
that of PS1 (overall identity is approximately 60%). However, in contrast
to PS1, which is expressed more or less homogeneously in the brain and
in peripheral tissues, PS2 is maximally expressed in cardiac muscle,
skeletal muscle and pancreas. Not surprisingly, the predicted topology of
PS2 is similar to that of PS1, and it also forms similar but independent
multimeric protein complexes which contain β-catenin.[96,98]

Three different mis-sense mutations have been found in the PS2 gene
in families segregating early-onset forms of AD. The first mutation
(Asn141Ile) was detected in a proportion of families of Volga German
ancestry, in which the familial AD locus had been independently mapped
by genetic linkage studies to chromosome 1.[127,128] The second mutation
(Met239Val) was discovered in an Italian pedigree.[127] A third mutation
has recently been found in a Spanish kindred. However, in contrast to the
frequency of PS1 mutations, screening of large data sets reveal that
PS22 mutations are likely to be rare.[129]

PS2 mutations differ from those in the β-APP and PS1 gene by virtue of
the fact that the phenotype associated with PS2 mutations is much more
variable.[129,130] The range of age of onset in heterozygous carriers of PS2
mutations is between 40 and 85 years, and there is at least one instance
of apparent non-penetrance in an asymptomatic octogenarian transmit-
ting the disease to affected offspring.[129,131,132]

It seems likely that PS1 and PS2 have similar or overlapping activities.

Thus, PS2 mutations, like PS1 mutations, increase the secretion of long-tailed Aβ peptides.[47,122] PS2 mutations may also cause increased sensitivity to apoptosis, but it is unclear whether this effect is independent of their ability to cause increased Aβ peptide secretion.[12,126] However, in contrast to knock-out of PS1, homozygous null mutations in PS2 (PS2$^{-/-}$) have little effect on development or β-APP processing (Donoviel, in preparation). This may arise because there is partial overlap of function between PS1 and PS2. Thus, overexpression of PS2 partly compensates for the absence of PS1 in PS1$^{-/-}$ mice (Chishti, in preparation). Conversely, PS2$^{-/-}$ mice on a PS1$^{-/+}$ background have a severe developmental defect similar to that of PS1$^{-/-}$ mice (Donoviel, in preparation).

The chromosome 12 locus

A novel AD locus has been tentatively mapped to the pericentromeric region of chromosome 12 between the markers D12S1042 and D12S390 ($z = 3.5$) in two independent data sets of late-onset AD pedigrees ($n = 16$; $n = 38$).[133] Follow-up studies in a data set of 53 independent pedigrees confirmed the presence of an AD susceptibility gene within a larger (approximately 60 cM) region of chromosome 12 in a subset of pedigrees.[134] The subset of pedigrees that do not show linkage to chromosome 12 presumably reflect the presence of one or more genetic susceptibility factors elsewhere in the genome.

Several candidate genes, including α-2-macroglobulin (A2M), low-density lipoprotein receptor-related protein (LRP1), and ARF2, map within or near the chromosome 12 interval. Some of these genes (e.g. ARF3, Wnt1, plakophilin 2, ITR2) have been excluded by the failure to find nucleotide sequence changes in their open reading frames that are either enriched in, or unique to, patients with the chromosome 12 form of AD (Song, in preparation). Some biochemical studies have suggested a role for A2M protein in AD (through its ability to bind Aβ and through competition with both Aβ and APOE for clearance through the LRP1 receptor), and this has led to speculation that A2M might be the site of mutations associated with AD.[135] Considerable support for this concept (which would link Aβ, APOE, A2M, and LRP1 in one biochemical cascade) was provided when a preliminary family-based association study detected an association between AD and an intronic insertion–deletion polymorphism at the 5'-splice site of exon 18 of A2M in a data set of 104 pedigrees collected by the National Institute of Mental Health.[135] However, follow-up studies in a larger data set of National Institute of Mental Health pedigrees ($n = 142$), in several data sets of independent pedigrees (more than 60 pedigrees each) and in several sporadic AD case-control data sets (more than 100 subjects each) failed to confirm an association between AD and this insertion–deletion polymorphism in

A2M.[136] Furthermore, no biological effect could be discerned for the A2M polymorphism. These results suggested that the original observation may have been an artefact. Another potential candidate gene on chromosome 12, LRP1, has also generated ambiguous results when studied with conventional allelic association (case-control) methods.[137–145]

Other genes

It is likely that there are several familial AD genes remaining to be found, because pedigrees that lack mutations in any of the four known AD genes and that fail to co-segregate with chromosome 12 markers do not display a singular phenotype, but instead comprise a mix of early-onset autosomal-dominant pedigrees and late-onset multiplex pedigrees. Some of these familial AD loci will probably be found to be associated with rather rare but highly penetrant defects similar to those seen with mutations in PS1 and β-APP. Other genes may result in incompletely penetrant autosomal-dominant traits such as those associated with PS2. However, it is likely that a significant proportion of the remaining genes have effects similar to those of APOE, in which the ultimate phenotype is influenced by the presence or absence of other genetic and environmental risk factors.

Attempts to identify novel AD susceptibility genes have followed two strategies. One strategy, a continuation of the conventional positional cloning strategy, has attempted to show cosegregation of marker alleles with the disease phenotype (identity by descent) in pedigrees that are multiply affected by AD. These studies have assessed co-segregation using both conventional parametric lod score methods and newer non-parametric methods.[146] However, because these methods work best for pedigrees that are multiply affected with AD, increasing emphasis has been placed on the use of simple case-control studies (such as those that were very effectively used to discover the association between AD and APOE). More recently, the case-control method for discovering allelic associations has been supplemented by novel statistical methods (family-based association methods), which allow the examination of allele sharing between affected siblings compared with unaffected siblings, such as the sibship disequilibrium transmission test (SDT) and the sib-transmission disequilibrium test (S-TDT).[135,147] These family-based association methods examine the parental alleles transmitted to unaffected siblings as a source of control chromosome information that is theoretically better matched for ethnicity and genetic background.

The conventional case-control allelic association tests have yielded positive results for a significant number of genes, many of which are plausible biochemical candidate genes. However, most of these studies have not received the same robust replication as the association between AD and the ε4 allele of APOE. As a result, it has been difficult to discern whether the reported associations are true but perhaps limited to particular subsets of AD, or whether they represent statistically significant but biologically incorrect results. The possibility of biologically false-positive results in allelic association studies is a well-recognized problem in human genetics, which can arise when the test and control populations are not drawn from identical genetic backgrounds (which occurs because of population stratification). Recently, in an attempt to rectify the high false-positive rate for simple allelic association studies, some studies have begun to use the family-based association methods even though they have not yet been fully validated.[135]

A partial list of candidate genes that have been provisionally identified as putative AD susceptibility loci include:

- homozygosity for the AA allele of an intronic polymorphism α1-chymotrypsin;[148]
- A5 repeat allele of an intronic insertion–deletion polymorphism in the very low density lipoprotein receptor;[149]
- neutral coding sequence and intronic polymorphisms in LRP1;[140]
- homozygosity for the common A1 allele of an intronic polymorphism in presenilin 1;[150]
- presenilin 2;
- K-variant of butyrylcholinesterase;[151] and
- homozygosity for the val–val variant of the Val443Ile polymorphism in bleomycin hydroxylase.[152]

However, most of these candidate genes have not received the same widespread confirmation as APOE ϵ4 when they have been tested in independent but comparable data sets.[80,81,153–157]

Clinical implications

Physicians are being asked with increasing frequency to consider the merits of genetic counselling and genetic testing. At the current time, in the absence of clearly effective preventative or curative treatments that do not have significant side effects, the main reason for genetic counselling and genetic testing is for the provision of information only. Obviously, once an effective preventative or curative treatment becomes available, there will be a greater need to undertake genetic testing so that at-risk people can be treated before the onset of potentially irreversible neurodegeneration. Nevertheless, even at the current time, the provision of information about a person's risk of developing inherited forms of AD can be empowering to that person and may therefore have significant benefit. Thus, for instance, knowing his or her genetic status, at-risk family members may be able to organize their affairs to ensure that if they are carriers of a disease-causing mutation, then their financial affairs are placed in order and appropriate legal vehicles are put in place so that they will not be a burden upon their family when they develop clinical illness. Such information can also be empowering in terms of decisions about child-rearing, career paths, and so on. On the other hand, it is clear that such information has the potential to be misused to the subject's disadvantage (e.g. the denial of health-care insurance, long-term disability insurance or job promotion). Consequently, it is vitally important that any form of genetic counselling and genetic testing should be undertaken in an appropriately certified institution by qualified practitioners.

There is currently relatively little practical experience with genetic counselling of members of families that multiply affected with AD. Consequently, most of the paradigms used for genetic counselling of members of AD families are based on paradigms similar to those used in the counselling of subjects with Huntington's disease.[158] The Huntington's disease model is quite useful for counselling of members of families with early-onset familial AD associated with mutations in PS1, PS2 or β-APP because the age of onset is often similar (30–65 years) and there is a similar pattern of transmission (highly penetrant, age-dependent penetrance, autosomal-dominant segregation). Thus, in members of families with mutations in the β-APP and PS1 genes, it is possible to screen at-risk family members for the presence of mutations detected in affected subjects and to counsel these family members based upon the concept that β-APP and PS1 mutations are highly penetrant (approximately 95%) with a typical age at symptom onset of 35–65 years. PS2 mutations, on the other hand, have a lower penetrance and a more variable age of onset (45–85 years). Using the Huntington's disease paradigm, the author's group and several other groups have had the opportunity of counselling a small number of members of families with PS1 and β-APP mutations without significant problems.

Although the use of the Huntington's disease paradigm will probably work well for PS1, PS2 and β-APP mutations, it should be noted that mutations in these genes are a comparatively rare cause of familial AD, cumulatively accounting for about 50% of early-onset familial AD. A much more common clinical experience is the presence of two or three affected family members with late-onset AD in a small nuclear pedigree. Frequently, in these 'multiplex' late-onset AD pedigrees, the disease does not inherit as a classic autosomal-dominant trait. As a result, in any given family, it is frequently unclear whether the multiplex pedigree structure reflects an incompletely penetrant autosomal-dominant trait or a more complex mode of transmission that involves either the additive effects of several genes or the interaction of genes and environment. Empirical counselling of pedigrees of this type is difficult and must be largely based on recent epidemiological studies such as those of Lautenschlager *et al.* Although the use of molecular genetic studies would clearly facilitate counselling in such pedigrees, the only locus that has shown robust association with late-onset AD is the APOE gene. Retrospective studies, in both autopsy and clinical series, have suggested that the cumulative lifetime risk for AD in subjects who are homozygous for APOE ϵ4 may be as high as 90% by the age of 90 years. However, even from these retrospective studies, it is apparent that there is a huge variation in the age of onset of AD even in subjects who are homozygous for APOE ϵ4 (50–90 years). To confound matters further, a small number of limited prospective studies suggest that the APOE genotype is a relatively poor predictor of the onset of AD even in high-risk groups such as those with age-associated memory loss. Consequently, a number of research groups have recommended that the APOE genotype not be used for presymptomatic testing.[159] The question of whether the APOE genotype may be of assistance in establishing the diagnosis of AD in demented patients who undergo diagnostic work-up is currently a matter of some discussion. Most experts agree that, although the APOE genotype studies might form a part of the diagnostic armamentarium, they are unlikely to be the only test that should be done even in subjects with classical clinical features of AD.

Another role of genetic testing is in the design of a therapeutic programme for subjects who are affected with AD. Given the obvious genetic heterogeneity of AD, it would not be unreasonable to suspect that this aetiological heterogeneity would be reflected in different biochemical pathogenic pathways, which might lead to differences in response to specific treatments. It is conceivable, therefore, that some subtypes of AD might respond better to specific therapeutic agents than others. There is some provisional evidence that the APOE genotype may be associated with differences in response to the cholinesterase inhibitor tacrine. Obviously, as additional drugs are developed, it will be important to ascertain whether there are differential responses among different subtypes of AD.

It is likely that additional AD susceptibility genes will be identified in the next few years. However, until most or all of the AD genes are identified and their relative frequencies as a cause of AD in specific populations can be defined, genetic testing of at-risk family members can only be reasonably performed if there is a testable, clinically affected member available. If an affected pedigree member is available, that person's DNA can be screened for mutations in the known AD susceptibility genes. If mutations are found, this information can then be used for the testing in at-risk family members. When no mutations in the affected subject's DNA are found, it can be reasonably assumed that the disease is caused by mutations or polymorphisms in other AD genes that are not yet identified, and mutation screening studies in at-risk family members would not be indicated. In the absence of a living affected member who can be tested, the screening for mutations in the DNA of at-risk family members is likely to be a fruitless task, because failure to discover disease-related polymorphisms or mutations in the four known AD genes can give no reassurance that the at-risk family member is not a carrier of a mutation in another AD susceptibility gene.

References

1. Heyman A, Wilkinson WE, Stafford JA, Helms MJ, Sigmon AH, Weinberg T. Alzheimer's disease: a study of epidemiological aspects. Ann Neurol 1984;15:335–341.

2. Rocca WA, Amaducci LA, Schoenberg BS. Epidemiology of clinically diagnosed Alzheimer's disease. Ann Neurol 1986;19: 415–424.

3. Breitner JC, Silverman JM, Mohs RC, Davis KL. Familial aggregation in Alzheimer disease: comparison of risk among relatives of early- and late-onset cases, and among male and female relatives in successive generations. Neurology 1988;38: 207–212.

4. Farrer LA, Myers RH, Connor L, Cupples LA, Growdon JH. Segregation analysis reveals evidence of a major gene for Alzheimer disease. Am J Hum Genet 1991;48:1026–1033.

5. Bergem ALM, Engedal K, Kringlen E. Twin concordance and discordance for vascular dementia and dementia of the Alzheimer type. Neurobiol Aging 1992;13(suppl 1):66.

6. Katzman R, Kawas C. The epidemiology of dementia and Alzheimer disease. In: Terry RD, Katzman R, Bick KL, eds. Alzheimer disease. New York: Raven Press; 1994:105–122.

7. Lautenschlager NT, Cupples LA, Rao VS, et al. Risk of dementia among relatives of Alzheimer disease patients in the MIRAGE study: what is in store for the oldest old? Neurology 1996;46: 641–650.

8. Kang J, Lemaire HG, Unterbeck A, et al. The precursor of Alzheimer disease amyloid A4 protein resembles a cell surface receptor. Nature 1987;325: 733–736.

9. Goldgaber D, Lerman MI, McBride OW, et al. Characterization and chromosomal localization of a cDNA encoding brain amyloid of Alzheimer's disease. Science 1987;235: 877–880.

10. Robakis NK Lahiri, DK, Brown, HR et al. Expression studies of the gene encoding the Alzheimer's disease and Down syndrome amyloid peptide. In: Swann JW, ed. Disorders of the developing nervous system: changing views on their origins, diagnoses and treatments. New York: Alan R Liss; 1988: 183–193.

11. Tanzi RF, Gusella JF, Watkins PC, Bruns GAP, St George-Hyslop PH, Van Keuren ML. Amyloid β-protein gene: cDNA, mRNA distribution and genetic linkage near the Alzheimer locus. Science 1987;235:880–884.

12. Selkoe DJ. Normal and abnormal biology of β-amyloid precursor protein. Ann Rev Neurosci 1994;17:489–517.

13. Shoji M, Golde T, Ghiso J, et al. Production of the Alzheimer amyloid β protein by normal proteolytic processing. Science 1992;258:126–129.

14. Haass C, Schlossmacher MG,

Hung AY, *et al.* Amyloid β-peptide is produced by cultured cells during normal metabolism. Nature 1992;359:322–325.

15. Jarrett JT, Lansbury PT. Seeding one-dimensional crystallization of amyloid: a pathogenic mechanism in Alzheimer's disease and scrapie? Cell 1993;73: 1055–1058.

16. Yankner BA, Duffy LK, Kirschner DA. Neurotrophic and neurotoxic effects of amyloid β protein: reversal by tachykinin neuropeptides. Science 1990; 250:279–282.

17. Pike CJ, Burdick D, Walencewicz AJ, Glabe CG, Cotman CW. Neurodegeneration induced by beta-amyloid peptides in vitro: the role of peptide assembly state. J Neurosci 1993;13: 1676–1678.

18. Lorenzo A, Yanker BA. β-Amyloid neurotoxicity requires fibril formation and is inhibited by Congo red. Proc Natl Acad Sci U S A 1994;91:12243–12247.

19. Golde TE, Estus S, Younkin LH, Selkoe DJ, Younkin SG. Processing of the amyloid protein precursor to potentially amyloidogenic derivatives. Science 1992;255:728–730.

20 Haass C, Koo EH, Mellon A, Hung AY, Selkoe DJ. Targelting of cell surface β-amyloid precursor protein to lysosomes: alternative processing into amyloid bearing fragments. Nature 1992; 357:500–503.

21. Wild-Bode C, Capell A, Yamazaki T, *et al.* Intracellular generation and accumulation of amyloid beta-peptide terminating at amino acid 42. J Biol Chem 1997;272:16085–16088.

22. Cook DG, Forman M, Sung JC, *et al.* Alzheimer amyloid β(1–42) peptide is generated in the endoplasmic reticulum/intermediate compartment of NT2N cells. Nature Med 1997;3: 1021–1023.

23. Hartmann T, Beiger S, Bruhl B, *et al.* Distinct sites of intracellular production for Alzheimer's disease AB40/42-amyloid peptides. Nature Med 1997;3: 1016–1020.

24. Lee SJ, Liyanage U, Bickel P, Xia W, Lansbury PT, Kosik K. A detergent-insoluble membrane compartment contains Abeta in vivo. Nature Med 1998;4: 730–734.

25. Mullan MJ, Crawford F, Axelman K, *et al.* A pathogenic mutation for probable Alzheimer's disease in the APP gene at the *N*-terminus of β-amyloid. Nature Genet 1992;1:345–347.

26. Hendricks M, van Duijn CM, Cras P, *et al.* Presenile dementia and cerebral hemorrhage linked to a mutation at codon 692 of the β-amyloid precursor protein gene. Nature Genet 1992;1: 218–221.

27. Levy E, Carman MD, Fernandez-Madrid IJ, *et al.* Mutation of the Alzheimer's disease amyloid gene in hereditary cerebral hemorrhage: Dutch type. Science 1990;248:1124–1126.

28. Eckman CB, Mehta ND, Crook R, *et al.* A new pathogenic mutation in the APP gene (I716V) increases the relative production of Abeta(42/43). Hum Mol Genet 1997;6:2087–2089.

29. Goate AM, Chartier-Harlin MC, Mullan M, *et al.* Segregation of a missense mutation in the amyloid precursor protein gene with familial Alzheimer disease. Nature 1991;349:704–706.

30. Chartier-Harlin MC, Crawford F, Holden H, *et al.* Early onset Alzheimer's disease caused by mutations at codon 717 of the β-amyloid gene. Nature 1991;353: 844–846.

31. Murrell J, Farlow M, Ghetti B, Benson MD. A mutation in the amyloid precursor protein associated with hereditary Alzheimer's disease. Science 1991;254:97–99.

32. Karlinsky H, Vaula G, Haines JL, *et al*. Molecular and prospective phenotypic characterization of a pedigree with familial Alzheimer disease and a missense mutation in codon 717 of the β-amyloid precursor protein (APP) gene. Neurology 1992;42: 1445–1453.

33. Naruse S, Igarashi S, Kobyashi H, *et al*. Missense mutation (Val to Ile) in exon 17 of the amyloid precursor protein gene in Japanese familial Alzheimer disease. Lancet 1991;337:978–979.

34. Citron M, Oltersdorf T, Haass C, *et al*. Mutation of the β-amyloid precursor protein in familial Alzheimer's disease increases β-protein production. Nature 1992;360:672–674.

35. Cai XD, Golde TE, Younkin SG. Release of excess amyloid beta protein from a mutant beta protein precursor. Science 1992; 259:514–516.

36. Susuki N, Cheung TT, Cai XD, *et al*. An increased percentage of long amyloid β protein secreted by familial amyloid β protein precursor (BAPP717) mutants. Science 1994;264:1336–1340.

37. Haass C, Hung AY, Selkoe DJ, Teplow DB. Mutations associated with a locus for familial Alzheimer's disease result in alternative processing of amyloid β-protein precursor. J Biol Chem 1994;269:17741–17748.

38. Haas C, Lemere C, Capell A, Citron M, Selkoe D. The Swedish mutation causes early onset Alzheimer's disease by β-secretase cleavage within the secretory pathway. Nature Med 1995; 1:1291–1296.

39. Citron M, Vigo-Pelfrey C, Teplow DB, *et al*. Excessive production of amyloid β-protein by peripheral cells of symptomatic and presymptomatic patients carrying the Swedish familial Alzheimer's disease mutation. Proc Natl Acad Sci U S A 1994; 91:11993–11997.

40. Crass P, Van Harskamp F, Hendriks L, *et al*. Presenile Alzheimer's dementia characterized by amyloid angiopathy and large amyloid core type senile plaques in the APP 692 Ala to Gly mutation. Acta Neuropathol 1998;1996:253–260.

41. Wisniewski T, Frangione B. Peptides homologous to the amyloid protein of Alzheimer's disease containing a glutamine for a glutamic acid substitution have accelerated amyloid fibril formation. Biochem Biophys Res Commun 1991;180:1528–1529.

42. Arispe N, Pollard HB, Rojas E. Giant multilevel cation channels formed by Alzheimer disease amyloid β protein in a bilayer membrane. Proc Natl Acad Sci U S A 1993;90:10573–10577.

43. Mattson MP, Cheng B, Davis D, Bryant K, Lieberburg I, Rydel R. Beta-amyloid peptides destabilize calcium homeostasis and render human cortical neurons vulnerable to excitotoxicity. J Neurosci 1992;12:376–389.

44. Mattson MP, Goodman Y. Different amyloidogenic peptides share a similar mechanism of neurotoxicity involving reactive oxygen species and calcium. Brain Res 1995;676:219–224.

45. Okamoto T, Takeda S, Murayama Y, Ogata E, Nishimoto I. Ligand-dependent G protein coupling function of amyloid transmembrane precursor. J Biol. Chem 1995;270: 4205–4208.

46. Yamatsuji T, Nishimoto I. G protein-mediated neuronal DNA fragmentation induced by familial Alzheimer's disease associated mutants of APP. Science 1996;272:1349–1352.

47. Scheuner D, Eckman L, Jensen M, *et al.* Secreted amyloid-β protein similar to that in the senile plaques of Alzheimer disease is increased in vivo by presenilin 1 and 2 and APP mutations linked to FAD. Nature Med 1996;2:864–870.

48. Pericak-Vance MA, Bedout JL, Gaskell PC, Roses AD. Linkage studies in familial Alzheimer disease: evidence for chromosome 19 linkage. Am J Hum Genet 1991;48:1034–1050.

49. Strittmatter WJ, Saunders AM, Schmechel D, *et al.* Apolipoprotein E: high affinity binding to B/A4 amyloid and increased frequency of type 4 allele in familial Alzheimers disease. Proc Natl Acad Sci U S A 1993;90: 1977–1981.

50. Saunders A, Strittmatter WJ, Schmechel S, *et al.* Association of apoliprotein E allele ε4 with the late-onset familial and sporadic Alzheimer disease. Neurology 1993;43:1467–1472.

51. Corder EH, Saunders AM, Risch NJ, *et al.* Apolipoprotein E type 2 allele decreases the risk of late-onset Alzheimer disease. Nature Genet 1994;7:180–184.

52. Corder EH, Saunders AM, Srittmatter WJ, *et al.* Gene dosage of apolipoprotein E type 4 allele and the risk for Alzheimer's disease in late onset families. Science 1993;261: 921–923.

53. Roses AD. Apolipoprotein E alleles as risk factors in Alzheimer disease. Annu Rev Med 1996; 47:387–400.

54. Rebeck GW, Perls T, West H, Sodhi P, Lipsitz LA, Hyman BT. Reduced apolipoprotein ε4 allele in the oldest old Alzheimer's patients and cognitively normal individuals. Neurology 1994;175:46–48.

55. Van Duijn CM, de Knijff P, Cruts M, *et al.* Apolipoprotein E4 allele in a population based study of early onset Alzheimer disease. Nature Genet. 1994;7:74–78.

56. Maestre G, Ottman R, Stern Y, Mayeux R. Apolipoprotein E and Alzheimer disease: ethnic variation in genotype risks. Ann Neurol 1995;37:254–259.

57. Hendrie HC, Hall KS, Hui S. Apolipoprotein E genotypes and Alzheimer's disease in a community study of elderly African Americans. Ann Neurol 1995;37:118–121.

58. Tang MX, Stern Y, Marder K, *et al.* The APOE ε4 and the risk of Alzheimer disease among African Americans, whites, and Hispanics. JAMA 1998;279: 751–755.

59. Mayeux R, Ottman R. Synergistic effects of traumatic head injury and ApoE ε4 in patients with Alzheimer's disease. Neurology 1995;45:555–557.

60. Roses AD, Saunders AM. Head injury, amyloid β and Alzheimer's disease. Nature Med 1995;1:603–604.

61. Alberts MJ, Graffagnino C. ApoE genotype and survival from intracerebral haemorrhage. Lancet 1995;346:575.

62. Newman MF, Croughwell ND. Predictors of cognitive decline after cardiac operation. Ann Thorac Surg 1995;59:1326–1330.

63. Olichney JM, Hansen LA, Galasko D, *et al.* The ApoE ε4 allele is associated with increased neuritic plaques and cerebral amyloid angiopathy in AD and in Lewy body variant.

Neurology 1996;47:190–196.

64. St George-Hyslop PH, Tsuda T, Crapper McLachlan DR, Karlinsky H, Pollen D, Lippa C. Alzheimer's disease and possible gene interaction. Science 1994;263:536–537.

65. Sorbi S, Nacmias B, Forleo P, Amaducci L. Epistatic effect of APP717 mutation and apolipoprotein E genotype in familial Alzheimer disease. Ann Neurol 1995;38:124–128.

66. Nacmias B, Latteraga S, Tulen P, et al. ApoE genotype and familial Alzheimer's disease: a possible influence on age-of-onset in APP717Val to Ile mutated families. Neurosci Lett 1995;183:1–3.

67. van Broeckhoven C, Backhovens H, Cruts M, et al. APOE genotype does not modulate age of onset in families with chromosome 14 encoded Alzheimer's disease. Neurosci Lett 1994;169:179–180.

68. Schmechel DE, Saunders AM, Strittmatter WJ, et al. Increased amyloid beta-peptide deposition in cerebral cortex as a consequence of apolipoprotein E genotype in late-onset Alzheimer's disease. Proc Natl Acad Sci U S A 1993;90:9649–9653.

69. Strittmatter WJ, Weisgraber KH, Huang DY, Schemechel D, Saunders AM, Roses AD. Binding of human lipoprotein E to synthetic amyloid beta peptide: isoform-specific effects and implications for late onset AD. Proc Natl Acad Sci U S A 1993;90:8098–8102.

70. Kounnas MZ, Moir RD, Rebeck GW, et al. LDL Receptor related protein, a multifunctional ApoE receptor binds secreted βAPP and mediates its degradation. Cell 1995;82:331–340.

71. Bales KR, Verina T, Dodel RC, et al. Lack of apolipoprotein E dramatically reduces amyloid beta-peptide deposition. Nature Genet 1997;17:254–256.

72. Strittmater WJ, Saunders AM, Goedert M, et al. Isoform specific interactions of ApoE with microtubule associated protein tau: implications for Alzheimer disease. Proc Natl Acad Sci U S A 1994;91:11183–11186.

73. Huang DY, Goedert M, Strittmatter W, Schmechel D, Weisgraber K, Roses AD. Isoform-specific interactions of apolipoprotein E with microtubule associated protein MAP2c: implications for Alzheimer disease. Neurosci Lett 1995;182:55–58.

74. Huang DK, Weisgraber KH, Strittmatter D, Goldgaber D, Roses AD. ApoE3 binding to tau tandem repeat I is abolished by tau serine262 phosphorylation. Neurosci Lett 1995;192:209–212.

75. Masliah E, Mallory M. Neurodegeneration in the central nervous system of ApoE deficient mice. Exp Neurol 1995;136:107–122.

76. Nathan BP, Bellosta S, Sanan DA, Weisgraber KH, Mahley RW, Pitas RE. Differential effects of apolipoproteins E3 and E4 on neuronal growth in vitro. Science 1994;264:850–852.

77. Nathan BP, Bellosta S. The inhibitory effect of apolipoprotein E ε4 on neurite outgrowth is associated with microtubule depolymerization. J Biol Chem 1995;270:19791–19799.

78. Bullido MJ, Artiga MJ, Recuero M, et al. A polymorphism in the regulatory region of APOE associated with risk for Alzheimer's disease. Nature Genet 1998;18:69–71.

79. Lambert JC, Pasquier F, Cottel

D, Frigard B, Amyouel P, Chartier-Harlin JC. A new polymorphism in the APOE promoter associated with risk of developing Alzheimer's disease. Hum Mol Genet 1998;7:533–540.

80. Town T, Paris D, Fallin D, *et al.* The -491 A/T apolioprotein E promoter poylymorphism association with Alzheimer's disease: independent risk and linkage disequilibrium with the known APOE polymorphism. Neurosci Lett 1998;252:95–98.

81. Song YQ, Rogaeva E, Premkumar S, *et al.* Absence of association between Alzheimer disease and the -491 regulatory polymorphisms of APOE. Neurosci Lett 1998;250:189–192.

82. Schellenberg GD, Bird TD, Wijsman EM, *et al.* Genetic linkage evidence for a familial Alzheimer's disease locus on chr 14. Science 1992;258: 668–670.

83. St George-Hyslop P, Haines J, Rogaev E, *et al.* Genetic evidence for a novel familial Alzheimer disease gene on chromosome 14. Nature Genet 1992;2:330–334.

84. Van Broeckhoven C, Backhovens H, Cruts M, *et al.* Mapping of a gene predisposing to early-onset Alzheimer's disease to chromosome 14q24.3. Nature Genet 1992;2:335–339.

85. Sherrington R, Rogaev E, Liang Y, *et al.* Cloning of a gene bearing missense mutations in early onset familial Alzheimer's disease. Nature 1995;375:754–760.

86. Levitan D, Greenwald I. Facilitation of lin-12-mediated signalling by sel-12, a *Caenorhabditis elegans* S182 Alzheimer's disease gene. Nature 1995;377: 351–354.

87. Boulianne G, Livne-Bar I, Humphreys JM, Rogaev E, St George-Hyslop P. Cloning and mapping of a close homologue of human presenilins in *D. melanogaster.* NeuroReport 1997;8:1025–1029.

88. De Strooper B, Beullens M, Contreras B, *et al.* Postranslational modification, subcellular localization and membrane orientation of the Alzheimer's disease associated presenilins. J Biol Chem 1997;272:3590–3598.

89. Walter J, Capell A, Grunberg J, *et al.* The Alzheimer's disease associated presenilins are differentially phosphorylated proteins located predominantly within the endoplasmic reticulum. Mol Med 1996;2:673–691.

90. Lehmann S, Chiesa R, Harris DA. Evidence for a six transmembrane domain structure for PS1. J Biol Chem 1997;272: 12047–12051.

91. Li X, Greenwald I. Membrane topology of the *C. elegans* sel12 presenilin. Neuron 1996;17: 1015–1021.

92. Doan A, Thinakaran G, Borchelt DR, *et al.* Protein topology of presenilin 1. Neuron 1996;17: 1023–1030.

93. Thinakaran G, Borchelt DR, Lee MK, *et al.* Endoproteolysis of presenilin 1 and accumulation of processed derivatives in vivo. Neuron 1996;17:181–190.

94. Podlisny M, Citron M, Amarante P, *et al.* Presenilin proteins undergo heterogeneous endoproteolysis between Thr291 and Ala299 and occur as stable *N*- and *C*-terminal fragments in normal brain tissue. Neurobiol Dis 1997;3:325–337.

95. Fraser PE, Levesque G, Yu G, *et al.* Presenilin 1 is actively degraded by the 26S proteasome. Neurobiol Aging 1998; 19(Suppl 1):S19–21.

96. Capell A, Grunberg J, Pesold B,

et al. The proteolytic fragments of the Alzheimer's disease associated presenilin-1 form heterodimers and occur as a 100–150 kDa molecular mass complex. J Biol Chem 1998; 273:3205–3211.

97. Thinakaran G, Regard JB, Bouton CML, *et al.* Stable association of the presenilin derivatives and absence of presenilin interactions with APP. Neurobiol Dis 1998;4:438–453.

98. Yu G, Chen F, Levesque G, *et al.* The presenilin 1 protein is a component of a high molecular weight intracellular complex that contains β-catenin. J Biol Chem 1998;273:16470–16475.

99. Zhou J, Liyanage U, Medina M, *et al.* Presenilin 1 interacts with a novel member of the armadillo family. NeuroReport 1997;8: 2085–2090.

100. Weidemann A, Paliga K, Durrwang U, *et al.* Formation of stable complexes between two Alzheimer's disease gene products: presenilin-2 and β-amyloid precursor protein. Nature Med 1997;3:328–332.

101. Xia W, Zhang J, Perez R, Koo EH, Selkoe DJ. Interaction between amyloid precursor protein and presenilins in mammalian cells: implications for the pathogenesis of Alzheimer disease. Proc Natl Acad Sci U S A 1997;94:8208–8213.

102. Zhang W, Han SW, McKeel DW, Goate A, Wu JY. Interaction of presenilins with the filamin family of actin binding proteins. J Neurosci 1998;18:914–922.

103. De Strooper B, Saftig P, Craessaerts K, *et al.* Deficiency of presenilin 1 inhibits the normal cleavage of amyloid precursor protein. Nature 1998;391: 387–390.

104. Shen J, Bronson RT, Chen DF, Xia W, Selkoe DS, Tonegawa S. Skeletal and CNS defects in presenilin-1 deficient mice. Cell 1997;89:629–639.

105. Wong PC, Zheng H, Chen H, *et al.* Presenilin 1 is required for Notch and Dll1 expression in the paraxial mesoderm. Nature 1997;387:288–292.

106. Conlon RA, Reaume AG, Rossant J. Notch1 is required for the coordinate segmentation of somites. Development 1995; 121:1533–1545.

107. De Strooper B, Annert W, Cupers P, *et al.* A presenilin dependent gamma-secretase-like protease mediates release of Notch intracellular domain. Nature 1999;398:518–522.

108. Chen F, Rozmahel R, St George-Hyslop P, *et al.* 1998.

109. Wolozin B, Iwasaki K, Vito P, *et al.* Participation of presenilin 2 in apoptosis: enhanced basal activity conferred by an Alzheimer mutation. Science 1996;274:1710–1713.

110. Sato S, Kamino K, Miki T, *et al.* Splicing mutation of presenilin 1 gene for early onset familial Alzheimer's disease. Hum Mutation 1998;Suppl 1:591–594.

111. Perez-Tur J, Froelich S, Prihar G, *et al.* A mutation in Alzheimer's disease destroying a splice acceptor site in the presenilin 1 gene. NeuroReport 1996;7: 297–301.

112. Kwok JB, Tadder K, Fisher C, *et al.* Sequence analysis of presenilin genes in early-onset Alzheimer disease reveals a novel (Met233Thr) presenilin 1 mutation. 1997 (submitted).

113. Tysoe C, Whittaker J, Xuereb J, *et al.* A presenilin-1 truncating mutation is present in two cases with autopsy confirmed early-onset Alzheimer disease. Am J Hum Genet 1998;62:70–76.

114. Van Broeckhoven C. Presenilins and Alzheimer disease. Nature Genet 1995;11:230–232.

115. Davis JA, Naruse S, Chen H, *et al*. An Alzheimer's disease-linked PS1 variant rescues the developmental abnormalities of PS1 deficient embryos. Neuron 1998;20:603–609.

116. Qian S, Jiang P, Guan XO, *et al*. Mutant human presenilin protects presenilin 1 null mouse against embryonic lethality and elevates Abeta1–42/43 expression. Neuron 1998;20:611–617.

117. Levitan D, Doyle T, Brousseau D, *et al*. Assessment of normal and mutant human presenilin function in *Caenorhabditis elegans*. Proc Natl Acad Sci U S A 1996;93:14940–14944.

118. Baumeister R, Leimer U, Zweckbronner I, Jakubek C, Grunberg J, Haass C. Human presenilin-1, but not familial Alzheimer's disease (FAD) mutants, facilitate *Caenorhabditis elegans* Notch signalling independently of proteolytic processing. Genes Function 1997;1:149.

119. Martins RN, Turner BA, Carroll RT, *et al*. High levels of amyloid beta-protein from S182 (Glu246) familial Alzheimer's cells. NeuroReport 1995;7:217–220.

120. Duff K, Eckman C, Zehr C, *et al*. Increased amyloid beta 42(43) in brains of mice expressing mutant presenilin 1. Nature 1996;383:710–713.

121. Borchelt DR, Thinakaran G, Eckman CB, *et al*. Familial Alzheimer's disease linked presenilin 1 variants elevate Abeta1–42/1–40 ration in vitro and in vivo. Neuron 1996;17:1005–1013.

122. Citron M, Westaway D, Xia W, *et al*. Mutant presenilins of Alzheimer's disease increase production of 42 residue amyloid β-protein in both transfected cells and transgenic mice. Nature Med 1997;3:67–72.

123. Tamaoka A, Fraser PE, Ishii K, *et al*. Amyloid beta-protein isoforms in brain of subjects with PS1 linked, β-APP linked, and sporadic Alzheimer disease. Brain Res Mol Brain Res 1998;56:178–185.

124. Vito P, Lacana E, D'Adamio L. Interfering with apoptosis: Ca(2+)-binding protein ALG-2 and Alzheimer's disease gene ALG-3. Science 1996;271:521–525.

125. Gou Q, Sopher BL, Furukawa K, *et al*. Alzheimer's presenilin mutation sensitizes neural cells to apoptosis induced by trophic factor withdrawal and amyloid β-peptide: involvement of calcium and oxyradicals. J Neurosci 1997;17:4212–4222.

126. Deng G, Pike CJ, Cotman CW. Alzheimer-associated presenilin 2 confers increased sensitivity to apoptosis in PC12 cells. FEBS Lett 1996;397:50–54.

127. Rogaev EI, Sherrington R, Rogaeva EA, *et al*. Familial Alzheimer's disease in kindreds with missense mutations in a novel gene on chromosome 1 related to the Alzheimer's disease type 3 gene. Nature 1995;376:775–778.

128. Levy-Lahad E, Wijsman EM, Nemens E, *et al*. A familial Alzheimer's disease locus on chromosome 1. Science 1995;269:970–973.

129. Sherrington R, Froelich S, Sorbi S, *et al*. Alzheimer's disease associated with mutations in presenilin-2 are rare and variably penetrant. Hum Mol Genet 1996;5:985–988.

130. Bird TD, Levy-Lehad E, Poorkaj J, *et al*. Wide range in age of onset for chromosome 1 related

familial AD. Ann Neurol 1997; 40:932–936.

131. Bird TD. Familial Alzheimer's disease in American descendents of the Volga Germans: probable genetic founder effect. Ann Neurol 1988;23:25.

132. Bird TD, Sumi SM, Nemens EJ, *et al*. Phenotypic heterogenity in familial Alzheimer's disease: a study of 24 kindreds. Ann Neurol 1989;25:12–25.

133. Pericak-Vance MA, Bass MP, Yamaoka LH, *et al*. Complete genomic screen in late-onset familial Alzheimer disease. Evidence for a new locus on chromosome 12. JAMA 1997;278: 1282–1283.

134. Rogaeva E, Premkumar S, Song Y, *et al*. Evidence for an Alzheimer disease susceptibility locus on chr 12, and for further locus heterogeneity. JAMA 1998;280:614–618.

135. Blacker D, Wilcox MA, Laird NM, *et al*. Alpha-2-macroglobulin is genetically associated with AD. Nature Genet 1998;19:357–360.

136. Rogaeva E, Premkumar S, Grubber J, *et al*. Re-analysis of the association of alpha-2-macroglobulin and Alzheimer's disease. Nature Genet 1999; 22:19–22.

137. Lendon CL, Talbot CJ, Craddock NJ, *et al*. Genetic association studies between dementia of the Alzheimer's type and three receptors for apolipoprotein E in a Caucasian population. Neurosci Lett 1997;222: 187–190.

138. Wavrant-DeVrieze F, Perez-Tur J, Lambert JC, *et al*. Association between the low density lipoprotein receptor-related protein (LRP) and Alzheimer's disease. Neurosci Lett 1997;227:68–70.

139. Clatworthy AE, Gomez-Isla T, Rebeck GW, Wallace RB, Hyman BT. Lack of association of a polymorphism in the low density lipoprotein receptor related protein gene with Alzheimer's disease. Arch Neurol 1997;54:1289–1292.

140. Kang DE, Saitoh T, Chen X, *et al*. Genetic association of the low density lipoprotein receptor-related protein gene (LRP), an apolipoprotein E receptor with late onset Alzheimer's disease. Neurology 1997;49:56–61.

141. Kamboh MI, Ferrell RE, DeKosky ST. Genetic association studies between Alzheimer's disease and two polymorphisms in the low density lipoprotein receptor related protein gene. Neurosci Lett 1998;244:65–68.

142. Hollenbach E, Ackerman S, Hyman BT, Rebeck GW. Confirmation of an association between a polymorphisms in exon 3 of the low density lipoprotein receptor related protein gene and Alzheimer's disease. Neurology 1998;50: 1905–1907.

143. Fallin D, Kundtz A, Town T, *et al*. No association between the low density lipoprotein receptor related protein (LRP) gene and late onset Alzheimer's disease in a community based sample. Neurosci Lett 1997;233: 145–147.

144. Baum L, Chen L, Ng HK, *et al*. Low density lipoprotein receptor related gene exon 3 polymorphism association with Alzheimer disease in Chinese. Neurosci Lett 1998;247:33–36.

145. Woodward R, Singleton AB, Gibson AM, Edwardson JA, Morris CM. LRP gene and late onset Alzheimer's disease. Lancet 1998;352:239–240.

146. Kruglyak L, Daly MJ, Reeve-Daly MP, Lander ES. Parametric and non-parametric linkage

analysis: a unified multipoint approach. Am J Hum Genet 1996;58:1347–1363.

147. Spielman RS, Ewens WJ. A sibship test for linkage in the presence of association: the sib transmission/disequilibrium. Am J Hum Genet 1998;62:450–458.

148. Kamboh MI, Sanghera DK, Ferrell RE, DeKosky ST. ApoE e4 associated Alzheimer's disease risk is modified by alpha 1 antichymotrypsin polymorphism. Nature Genet 1995;10:486–488.

149. Okuizumi K, Onodera O, Namba Y, *et al.* Genetic association of the very low density lipoprotein (VLDL) receptor gene with sporadic AD. Nature Genet 1995;11:207–209.

150. Wragg M, Hutton M, Talbot C, *et al.* Genetic association between and intronic polymorphism in presenilin 1 gene and late onset Alzheimer disease. Lancet 1996;347:509–512.

151. Lehmann DJ, Johnston C, Smith AD. Synergy between the genes for butyrylcholinesterase K variant and apolipoprotein E4 in late onset confirmed Alzheimer disease. Hum Mol Genet 1997; 6:1933–1936.

152. Montoya SE, Aston CE, DeKosky ST, Kamboh MI, Lazo JS, Ferrell RE. Bleomycin hydrolase is associated with risk of sporadic Alzheimer's disease. Nature Genet 1998;18:211–212.

153. Haines JL, Pritchard ML, Saunders AM, *et al.* No genetic effect of alpha-1 antichymotrypsin in Alzheimer disease. Genomics 1996;33:53–56.

154. Brindle N, Song Y, Rogaeva E, *et al.* Analysis of the butrylcholinesterase gene and nearby chromosome 3 markers in Alzheimer disease and aging. Hum Mol Genet 1998;7: 933–935.

155. Crawford F, Fallin D, Suo Z, *et al.* The butyrylcholinesterase gene is neither independently nor synergistically associated with late-onset AD in clinic and community based populations. Neurosci Lett 1998;249: 115–118.

156. Farrer LA, Pericak-Vance MA, Haines JL, *et al.* Analysis of the association between bleomycin hydrolase and Alzheimer disease in Caucasians. Ann Neurol 1998;44:808–811.

157. Scott WK, Growdon JH, Roses AD, Haines JL, Pericak-Vance M. Presenilin 1 polymorphism and Alzheimer disease. Lancet 1996;347:1186–1187.

158. Copley TT, Wiggins S, Dufrasne S, *et al.* Are we all of one mind? Canadian collaborative study for predictive testing for Huntington disease. Am J Med Genet 1995;58:59–69.

159. Relkin N, Breitner J, Farrer L, *et al.* Apolipoprotein E genotyping in AD. Lancet 1996;347: 1091–1095.

160. Peacock ML, Murman DL, Sima AAF, Warren JT, Roses AD, Fink JK. Novel amyloid precursor protein gene mutation (codon 665Asp) in a patient with late-onset Alzheimer disease. Ann Neurol 1994;35:432–438.

161. Peacock M, Warren JT, Roses AD, Fink JK. Novel polymorphism in the A4-region of the amyloid precursor protein gene in a patient without Alzheimer's disease. Neurology 1992;43: 1254–1256.

162. Kamino K, Orr HT, Payami H, *et al.* Linkage and mutational analysis of FAD kindreds for the APP region. Am J Hum Genet 1992;51:998–1014.

163. Jones CT, Morris S, Yates CM, *et al.* Mutation in codon 713 of the beta amyloid precursor pro-

tein gene presenting with schizophrenia. Nature Genet 1992;1: 306–309.

164. Carter D, Desmerais E, Bellis M, *et al*. More missense in amyloid gene. Nature Genet 1992;2: 255–256.

165. Campion D, Flaman JM, Brice A, *et al*. Mutations of the presenilin-1 gene in families with early onset Alzheimer's disease. Hum Mol Genet 1995;4:2373–2377.

166. Kamino K, Sato S, Sakaki Y, *et al*. Three different mutations of the presenilin 1 gene in early onset Alzheimer's disease families. Neurosci Lett 1996;208: 195–198.

167. Wisniewski T, Dowjat WK, Buxbaum JD, *et al*. A novel Polish presenilin-1 mutation (P117L) is associated with familial Alzheimer's disease and leads to death as early as the age of 28 years. NeuroReport 1998;9:217–221.

168. The Alzheimer's Disease Collaborative Group. The structure of the presenilin I gene and the identification of six mutations in early onset AD pedigrees. Nature Genet 1995;11:219–222.

169. Cruts M, Martin JJ, Van Broeckhoven C. Molecular genetic analysis of familial early-onset Alzheimer's disease linked to chromosome 14q24.3. Hum Mol Genet 1995;4:2363–2371.

170. Ramirez-Duenas MG, Rogaeva E, Leal CA, *et al*. A novel mutation in presenilin 1 gene in a Mexican family with early onset Alzheimer disease. Ann Genet 1997;41:149–153.

171. Campion D, Brice A, Dumanchin C, *et al*. A novel presenilin 1 mutation in familial Alzheimers disease with onset age of 29 years. NeuroReport 1996;7: 1582–1584.

2
Chromosome 17 and frontotemporal dementia

David MA Mann, David Neary and Julie S Snowden

Introduction

Frontotemporal lobar degeneration (FTLD) refers to a group of non-Alzheimer forms of dementia. Cases that can be classified under FTLD are characterized by behavioural and personality changes that involve disinhibition, stereotypy, antisocial acts and language disorders, which lead relentlessly to apathy, mutism and late neurological (frontal release or extra-pyramidal) signs.[1] Frontotemporal dementia (FTD) is the most common of these clinical syndromes that arise from a progressive and regionally variable atrophy of the frontal, anterior temporal and anterior parietal lobes of the brain.

First descriptions of a progressive behavioural disorder associated with an atrophy of the frontal lobes were given by Arnold Pick.[2,3] Emphasis was given to the focal frontal lobe atrophy in several subsequent reports to which Pick's name was ascribed.[4-7] However, despite these early studies, reports of focal cerebral atrophy had dramatically diminished by the second half of the 20th century. The prevailing wisdom at the time was that dementia was a generalized and non-selective impairment of mental function. This has been challenged in the past two decades, largely by the longitudinal studies of patients based in Lund, Sweden[8-10] and Manchester, UK.[1,11-13] These studies identified a form of dementia caused by a degeneration of the frontal and anterior temporal lobes of the brain with clinical characteristics that are indicative of dysfunction of the frontal lobes. The histological changes that underlie the atrophy are distinct from those of Alzheimer's disease.[14-18] The Swedish and British workers[19] reached consensus on the term 'frontotemporal dementia' (FTD) to refer to the behavioural disorder. Refined and internationally accepted clinical diagnostic criteria for FTD and related syndromes have recently been published.[20]

Although the great majority of cases conform clinically to the FTD prototype, the spectrum of illness extends far wider and involves cases in which a movement disorder, with relatively mild dementia, is the major disabling feature.[21–23] Hence, diverse clinical presentations, revelling under titles such as hereditary frontotemporal dementia (HFTD),[24] disinhibition, dementia, parkinson with amyotrophy complex (DDPAC),[23] hereditary dysphasic disinhibition dementia (HDDD),[25,26] rapidly progressive autosomal-dominant parkinsonism and dementia with pallidopontonigral degeneration (PPND),[21,22] familial multiple system tauopathy with presenile dementia (MSTD),[27] dementia lacking distinctive histology (DLDH)[28] and progressive subcortical gliosis (PSG),[29] have been coined to describe some of these clinical variants, according to their overriding symptomatology.

The shared genetic linkage of some cases to the long arm of chromosome 17[24,26,27,30–39] led to the identification of causative mutations in the tau gene,[40–42] and the term frontotemporal dementia and parkinsonism linked to chromosome 17 (FTDP-17)[37] was adopted to describe such cases.

Nonetheless, it is important to recognize that FTD is clinically, pathologically and neurochemically distinct from Alzheimer's disease (AD). This is reflected in their differing patterns of atrophy, their different underlying pathologies and their differing genetic basis. Despite recent genetic insights into the cause of FTD, classification of the disease still remains largely the province of clinical observation and pathological findings.

In this chapter the clinical, pathological and molecular characteristics of FTDP-17 are described, with reference to how conditions that fall under this heading might relate to, or provide insight into, the wider constellation of FTLD.

Demographic features of FTD

FTD may account for up to one-quarter of patients who present before the age of 65 years with dementia due to primary cerebral atrophy.[12–14] Reports of FTD from other parts of the world[28,43–49] suggest that the disorder is widespread. It is evident that FTD has been significantly underdiagnosed; increased understanding of the disorder will lead to its proper recognition.

Onset of disease occurs most commonly between the ages of 45 and 65 years, although the range is wide; it may occasionally occur in the elderly, and the youngest recorded onset is at age 21 years. There is equal incidence in men and women. The length of illness is highly variable, ranging from 2 to 20 years, with a mean duration of about 8 years.

A family history of dementia in a first-degree relative has been identified in about one-half of patients, and the pattern of inheritance in some families indicates the action of an autosomal-dominant gene.[1,50] In other cases with family history, however, the mode of inheritance is less clearly defined, and there are many patients in whom no apparent family history of disease exists. There are no obvious socioeconomic determinants of FTD. Patients come from all social classes and a wide range of occupational backgrounds.

Clinical and behavioural characteristics of FTD

FTD is characterized by profound character changes and alterations in personal and social conduct sufficient to render sufferers incapable of managing their own affairs.[1] The onset of FTD is insidious. Affective disorder and transient psychiatric symptoms may herald the onset of behavioural and cognitive decline, and subtle mood disturbances are often the precursor to the major alterations in personality and social conduct that characterize the disease. Symptoms of anxiety and depression and rapid shifts of mood give way, however, to loss of emotions. Affect becomes bland, shallow and indifferent, and there is a loss of feelings of sympathy and empathy. Patients become unconcerned, lacking in initiative, judgement and foresight, and they neglect personal responsibilities. Patients can be overactive, restless, distractible and overtly disinhibited, or else apathetic, inert and lacking in spontaneity. Overactive patients may become increasingly inert as the disease progresses. Lack of conformity to social conventions, with reduction in courtesy and general manners, is a common early symptom. Social *faux pas* become gradually more glaring and patients lose personal modesty and may wander naked. Typically, patients neglect personal hygiene and need to be encouraged, if not forced, to wash and change their clothes. Incontinence is associated with lack of concern rather than neurological deficit.

Changes in eating and drinking patterns are common. Overeating, especially a relish for sweet foods, may lead relatives to ration food to prevent obesity. Excessive and indiscriminate eating may be superseded later in the disease by selective food fads, usually involving favoured sweet foods. Hyperorality, involving the mouthing of inedible objects, is observed in some patients. Repetitive eating and drinking may constitute one aspect of utilization phenomena.

Changes in sleep pattern may occur, particularly in apathetic patients who may display increased somnolence.

Altered sexual behaviour is common. There is usually a loss of libido, although some patients may make inappropriate sexual advances, which are presumably attributable to their behavioural disinhibition and lack of awareness of social mores.

Patients become increasingly inflexible and may adopt a fixed daily routine in which activities acquire a marked stereotypic quality. They may clock-watch, carrying out a particular activity at precisely the same time each day. Wandering may involve completion of an identical route on each occasion. Patients may constantly repeat a phrase or sentence, or even recount verbatim a complete repertoire of phrases. Overactive, disinhibited patients may repeatedly sing the same ditty, dance the same steps, produce the same puns or clap a favoured rhythm. Repetitive motor actions, such as rubbing the hands, may occur in more inert patients. On formal neuropsychological testing repetitive behaviours are manifested by response perseverations, both in a verbal and motor domain.

Speech output is characteristically reduced. Patients do not initiate conversation, and responses to questions are brief and unelaborated. Concreteness of thought, echolalia and verbal perseveration are common. There may be increased reliance on stereotyped words or phrases. Nevertheless, primary linguistic competence is relatively preserved and patients speak without grammatical or phonological error. This reduction in propositional speech contrasts with the relative preservation of overlearnt aspects of language. Patients may repeat phrases, recite series such as the months of the year, complete nursery rhymes and join in songs at a time when spontaneous utterances are virtually absent. They also may read aloud notices and advertising hoardings. However, mutism occurs towards the final stages of the disease.

Symptoms of visuospatial disorientation are notably absent. Patients have no difficulty localizing objects, and they can manipulate and orientate clothing correctly and negotiate their environment without becoming lost. Even when patients become formally untestable and mute, they may fixate and reach for objects without difficulty, and they may show behaviours that demonstrate preserved spatial skills, such as repeated folding of a handkerchief or aligning of papers

Memory is inefficient but there is no dense amnesia. Patients typically perform poorly on formal tests of memory. However, they are typically oriented for time and place and test performance can be improved by the use of directed questions rather than open-ended questions and by the provision of multiple-choice alternative responses. These features suggest failure to implement effective retrieval strategies. This 'frontal'-type of memory impairment contrasts with the classical amnesia typical of AD.

Performance on formal testing is particularly impaired on tests that make demands on abstraction, planning, organizational and strategic functioning and mental flexibility, tasks that have traditionally been considered sensitive to frontal-lobe dysfunction.

The duration of illness is variable and may be prolonged, apparently relating to late development of striatal signs of akinesia and rigidity. Strikingly, physical health is characteristically preserved, although blood pressure may be low and labile. Early neurological signs in the majority of patients are confined to the emergence of primitive reflexes such as grasping, pouting, sucking and extensor plantar responses. Striatal signs of akinesia, rigidity and tremor typically become evident only in the late stages. Myoclonus is not seen and corticospinal weakness is not evident. Muscular wasting occurs only in that subgroup of patients who develop motor neurone disease. Ataxia does not occur.

Clinical subtypes of FTD

FTD is not clinically homogeneous, though all patients share the major features of gross change in personality and social conduct and exhibit a picture suggestive of 'frontal lobe' disorder on neuropsychological testing. Three major subsyndromes can be identified:

- a profile of disinhibition, inattention and overactivity;
- a profile of retardation, apathy and withdrawal; and
- a profile of stereotypic and ritualistic behaviours.

Disinhibited type

Some patients present with features reminiscent of hypomania. They are overactive, restless, inattentive and distractible, rushing unproductively from one activity to another with marked lack of application and persistence. Their demeanour is fatuous, inappropriately jocular, disinhibited and socially inappropriate. Patients may perform surprisingly well on cognitive tasks, at least in the early stages of disease.

Apathetic type

Some patients exhibit an opposite pattern of behaviour to that described above, and present in an apathetic, amotivational and pseudodepressed state. Their behaviour is characterized by loss of volition and inertia, so that, if left to their own devices, they would spend their day in bed or sitting unoccupied. All behaviours are economical, with minimal expenditure of mental effort. Response latencies to questions are often excessively prolonged, although once initiated, rate of execution of verbal or motor responses is unremarkable. With disease progression, patients becomes increasingly unresponsive, so that virtually no verbal or motor behaviour can be elicited. It is in these patients that perseverative behaviour, both verbal and motor, is the most pronounced and that marked loss of speech prosody is liable to occur.

Stereotypic type

In some patients, the dominant characteristic is of repetitive, ritualistic and idiosyncratic behaviours. Patients adhere to a rigid routine and become agitated if their daily schedule is altered. They adopt personal rituals that have a compulsive quality, although they lack the accompanying feelings of anxiety and release from anxiety that are characteristic of obsessive–compulsive states. Such patients exhibit extrapyramidal signs at a relatively early stage of the illness.

Neuropathological basis of the clinical subtypes

The distinct subtypes are based on the particular distribution of pathology within frontotemporal structures, with the apathetic type reflecting a dorsolateral frontal atrophy and the disinhibited type corresponding to an orbitobasal frontal degeneration. The stereotypic type is strongly related to severe striatal disease with lesser involvement of frontal or temporal neocortex.

Clinical investigations

Routine electroencephalography is normal, even in the context of severe dementia, a feature that helps to distinguish FTD from AD, in which there is a slowing of waveforms. Structural imaging (computed tomography) usually reveals a non-specific cerebral atrophy, although a pronounced widening of the interhemispheric and sylvian fissures sometimes suggests anterior frontotemporal atrophy. Emphasis of pathology in the frontal lobes is more readily demonstrated on magnetic resonance imaging.

Single photon emission computed tomography (SPECT) reveals reduced tracer activity (corresponding to blood flow) in the anterior frontal and temporal lobes. Abnormalities are typically bilateral but they may be symmetrical or asymmetrical. This pattern of anterior hemisphere dysfunction contrasts with the prototypical pattern of posterior hemisphere dysfunction of AD.[12] As might be anticipated from the topographic distribution of the pathology, SPECT reveals a relatively circumscribed deficit involving the orbitofrontal and anterior temporal lobes in the disinhibited type of patient, whereas in the apathetic type there is widespread anterior hemisphere abnormalities, with particular involvement of the dorsolateral convexity. In those patients with marked stereotypic behaviour, SPECT imaging reveals a widespread disorder of the frontal and temporal lobes

Neuropathological changes in FTD

Gross pathological changes

In prototypical cases[1,14,16] the brain shows an overall decline in weight. Most cases have brain weights of 1000–1250 g, although instances of brain weights that are well below 1000 g are not uncommon. Loss of brain weight is due to cerebral atrophy, principally within the cerebral hemispheres. It involves mostly the frontal, anterior parietal, cingulate, insular and temporal regions, and it results, in extreme cases, in 'knife-edge' atrophy. Even in severely affected cases, the motor, sensorimotor and posterior cerebral cortical regions are largely unaffected and the cerebellum and brainstem both appear externally normal.

On coronal section, the distinction between grey and white matter in atrophic areas is usually well maintained, although in severe cases there is great loss of axons and myelin and the white matter becomes brownish in colour and soft and 'rubbery' in texture. Atrophy in other cerebral cortical regions is less apparent, especially in the posterior third of the temporal lobe, where the superior temporal gyrus is conspicuously spared. The hippocampal formation, particularly the entorhinal cortex, and the amygdala are frequently atrophic,[16,51] as is the caudate nucleus, although the putamen, globus pallidus and thalamus are less affected. The corpus callosum is usually thinned, particularly anteriorly. The lateral ventricles are much enlarged, although the temporal horns are little changed, except in severe cases. In some cases the substantia nigra and locus caeruleus are noticeably underpigmented, but in others these regions appear normal. The cerebellum usually appears normal on section.

In FTD, atrophy of the prefrontal and anterior temporal lobes generally appears symmetrical or display a slightly greater involvement of the left cerebral hemisphere. The basal ganglia are also involved.[1] When the pathology affects the temporal lobes bilaterally and selectively, it produces the syndrome of semantic dementia.[1,52] If the left perisylvian frontotemporal regions are affected preferentially, progressive aphasia occurs.[1,53] When the parietal and motor regions are involved, progressive apraxia develops.[1] In another syndrome the histopathology of FTD combines with, or overlaps, that of classical motor neurone disease to produce motor neurone disease dementia.[54–61] It is the distribution, rather than the specific nature, of the pathological changes within the frontal and temporal lobes of the brain that determines these clinical syndromes

Histopathological changes

The histological changes of FTD have in the past been referred to as 'non-distinctive' or 'non-specific',[28] in the sense that 'specific' pathologies, such as plaques and tangles, Pick bodies or Lewy bodies, are not seen.[1,14–19,24,36,62]

Some cases display a microvacuolar change in the outer cortical laminae, mainly layer II and upper layer III, owing to shrinkage of nerve cell bodies and their processes. There is severe loss of the smaller pyramidal cells of layer II and the larger ones in layer III; nerve cells in the deeper laminae are shrunken rather than lost. Swollen, chromatolytic neurones are occasionally seen, especially in layers V and VI; these are strongly immunoreactive for β-crystallin[64] but less so for tau or ubiquitin protein.[17] Neuropil spheroids that are strongly immunoreactive for neurofilament (heavy chain) protein and suggestive of degeneration of presynaptic terminals have been reported to be widespread.[65] Astroglial reaction is slight and is usually confined to subpial regions or the border between grey and white matter. Loss of myelin and axons is often inconspicuous except in severely atrophic areas, and white matter gliosis is mild.[66] Microglial cell reaction is confined to white matter.[66,67]

Because distinctive inclusion bodies are not seen,[17] this type of cortical microvacuolar pathology has been designated as 'frontal lobe degeneration' (FLD).[14,15]

In other cases, there is severe pyramidal cell loss from the cerebral cortex and hippocampus, accompanied by transcortical tissue cavitation and florid astrocytosis. Intraneuronal inclusions, characterized by the presence of tau and ubiquitin and known as Pick bodies, are widespread in neurones in affected areas of the cortex and hippocampus, in conjunction with numerous β-crystallin-positive ballooned neurones.[14,15,17,68] These latter changes have been termed Pick type histology, and they form the basis for the modern definition of Pick's disease.[68]

The hippocampus in FLD is usually normal, although a severe loss of nerve cells from area CA1 sometimes occurs; on other occasions neurofibrillary tangles are present, especially among the stellate cells of layer II of the entorhinal cortex. In some cases there is pronounced cell loss from the substantia nigra, with residual pigment lying free within the neuropil or in macrophages; neurofibrillary tangles or Lewy bodies are absent.[17] Grumose bodies occur when neuronal cell loss is heavy. The locus caeruleus can also be affected, although is usually spared, sometimes even when nigral involvement is severe.[69]

In many cases, especially those with linkage to chromosome 17, neurofibrillary tangles that share the same immunohistochemical profile as those of AD are sparsely (or, more rarely, widely) present in subcortical structures such as the nucleus basalis of Meynert, the dorsal raphe nucleus, the pontine nuclei, the dentate nucleus and the reticular substance. Tau-positive glial cells can be seen in the internal capsule and globus pallidus.[36] In other cases there is no tau pathology whatsoever, either within cerebral cortex or elsewhere.

Although the basal ganglia and amygdala are often greatly atrophied,[16] no specific histopathological changes are evident except for a variable degree of astrocytosis.[36,70] This can be more severe and neuronal loss can be heavy, particularly in those cases in which stereotypic behaviours are prominent.[17]

Senile (neuritic) plaques are not generally seen, and any diffuse deposits of β-amyloid protein (mostly within the undamaged posterior cerebral cortex) are not beyond that expected for age.

Neurochemistry of FTD

The neurochemical changes of FTD contrast with those of AD[71] in that there is no cholinergic deficit. Serotonin receptors are lost from the frontal and temporal cortex whereas in AD they are lost from the temporal and parietal cortex. In FTD, there is no loss of kainate receptors, but there is loss of AMPA receptors from both temporal and frontal lobes; the pattern of this loss distinguishes patients with Pick-type histology from those with FLD.

Familial forms of FTD linked to chromosome 17

The clinical and pathological changes described above, which are mostly based on the observations made by the authors and other workers on cases of sporadic FTD, are typically seen in certain British families (Pickering-Brown, unpublished work), Dutch families[24] and Swedish families (in Karolinska)[37,63] with FTDP-17. However, an identical phenotype can be seen in many other patients from these countries in which there is no apparent family history, or in which the previous family history is not so well documented.[1,14,15,17] A very similar phenotype has also been reported in an Australian pedigree[34,72] and in a US pedigree (Duke 1684),[32,73] both of which show the same tau mutation as the British family. Other FTDP-17 cases in other parts of the world share the salient clinical and pathological features of FTD, but they may present significant additional features.

Hereditary frontotemporal dementia

Three Dutch families with HFTD linked to chromosome 17 have been described.[24] All basically conform to the clinical and pathological profile described above for FTD, based on observations of sporadic and familial cases (including FTDP-17 cases). Interestingly, Pick body-like structures were seen in the cortex of one patient from one of the families. These three families have been coded HFTD1, HFTD2 and HFTD3, although subsequent studies[40] have shown these to be genetically heterogeneous, with HFTD2 family relating to a different mutational event.

Similar clinical and pathological changes to those seen in these Dutch families have recently been described[39] in a further chromosome 17-linked family (family MN) of French–Canadian origin, which shares the same tau mutation as the HFTD1 and HFTD2 families. One family of US origin[74] and two others, again of French–Canadian ancestry,[75] have been described; none had previously been linked to chromosome 17 but all have the same mutation as the HFTD1 and MN families. Neurofibrillary tangles in neurones and tangles in glial cells were numerous in all these families; in some cases Pick-like inclusion bodies were seen in neurones.[39,75] Astrocytic plaques were described in some cases[74] and the substantia nigra was usually severely degenerated.

Dementia disinhibition parkinsonism amyotrophy complex

A family of Irish origin with DDPAC was first reported by Lynch *et al*.[23] Family members show personality changes and behavioural disorders that involve disinhibition, withdrawal, hyperphagia and alcoholism as early features, followed by memory loss, reduced speech, rigidity, bradykinesia and postural instability. Pathologically, there is microvacuolation of the superficial temporal, occipital and prefrontal lobes, with subpial gliosis and neuronal loss that is most severe in layers II, III and VI.[23,62] Occasional ballooned cells are seen but intraneuronal inclusions (Pick bodies) are not. The amygdala is severely affected, although hippocampal involvement is slight. Loss of cells from the substantia nigra is severe. Neurofibrillary tangle-like structures are widespread throughout the subcortical regions, but they are only sparse in cerebral cortex. Oligodendroglial tangles are widely present in the long white matter tracts and the corpus callosum. Some patients show muscle wasting and fasciculations, with anterior horn cell loss.

Hereditary dysphasic disinhibition dementia

HDDD is an inherited degenerative disorder originating in a German family who emigrated to USA in 1852. HDDD shares clinical and pathological features of FTD (Pick's disease) and AD. It was first described[25] in 1984 under the title of hereditary dysphasic dementia. Clinically, there is deterioration in language and cognitive abilities, behavioral change with hyperphagia, and variable parkinsonism. This family was coded HDDD1. Similar changes were observed in a second kindred, known as HDDD2, although it was only in this second family that linkage analysis was possible.[26]

The cortical pathology in both families is of the microvacuolar type of degeneration, and the amygdala and hippocampus are usually severely affected. Degeneration of the substantia nigra is variably present. Neurofibrillary tangles are sparsely present in the cortex, hippocampus and basal ganglia; glial tangles are likewise infrequent. Plaques are also sometimes present in HDDD2, but not in sufficient numbers with tangles to warrant a diagnosis of AD.[26] In HDDD1, however, neuritic plaques occur widely, mostly in the posterior hemisphere where the microvacuolar pathology is minimal.[25]

Rapidly progressive autosomal-dominant parkinsonism and dementia with pallidopontonigral degeneration

More than 39 individuals have been affected with PPND out of a kindred of over 310 dating back nine generations to a female 'founder' who was born in 1854 in the USA.[21,22] The age at onset ranges from 32 to 58 years, and the initial clinical signs include rapidly progressing parkinsonism and dystonia. Dementia, personality changes, ocular movement disorder, amyotrophy and frontal release signs occur later. At autopsy, there is severe neuronal loss and gliosis within the substantia nigra, pontine tegmentum and globus pallidus, with lesser involvement of the caudate nucleus and putamen.[22] The cerebral cortex shows only mild gliosis and neuronal loss, which is diffusely spread through frontal, temporal, occipital and parietal regions, although ballooned neurones are common. Neurofibrillary tangles are widely present[76] and glial fibrillary tangles are also seen, particularly in oligodendrocytes.[76,77]

Familial presenile dementia with psychosis

In a family designated as Seattle family A, cortical microvacuolation is absent and there are no ballooned cells; nor is there involvement of the substantia nigra or basal ganglia.[78] Neurofibrillary tangles, neuronal loss and gliosis are widely present in the neocortex, entorhinal cortex, parahippocampal gyrus and amygdala.[77–79] Such tangles appear morphologically identical, both in tissue sections and under the electron microscope, to those of AD; glial cell tangles are not present.[77–79]

Familial multiple system tauopathy with presenile dementia

In MSTD, the gross brain atrophy follows the pattern that is characteristic of FTD; the histopathological changes are those of microvacuolar degeneration.[27,42,77] There are abundant tau protein deposits, seen as neurofibrillary tangles and punctate staining, in neurones of the cerebral cortex, subcortex, brainstem and spinal cord. Tau deposits are also widely seen in glial cells (chiefly in oligodendrocytes) as coiled bodies.[27,42,77]

Duke family 1684

This family consists of five generations with 57 members, of whom 14 have been affected over three generations. The clinical picture is typical of FTD.[73] At autopsy, a microvacuolar type of cortical degeneration is seen, and tau deposits are widely present both in neurones and in glial cells, mostly oligodendroglia.[73,77] In two cases examined at autopsy there was severe degeneration of the substantia nigra.

Iowa family

This small family was described[80] as having 'autosomal-dominant dementia with widespread neurofibrillary tangles'. Although linkage analysis never formally established a causative locus on chromosome 17, subsequent studies have shown a mutation to be present in this family,[40] and in a second, Dutch family (HFTD4).[81] As the name implies, neurofibrillary tangles within neurones in the absence of senile plaques are widespread throughout cortical and subcortical brain regions in a distribution reminiscent of progressive supranuclear palsy. Ultrastructurally, however, the tangles are composed of paired helical filaments (see below) in a pattern that is characteristic of AD and not of the straight filaments of progressive supranuclear palsy. Tangles in glial cells are not seen.[80]

Familial progressive subcortical gliosis

This term familial progressive subcortical gliosis (FPSG) was introduced in 1967 by Neumann and Cohn[82] to describe a dementing disorder characterized by behavioural changes, speech reduction and psychiatric signs but with little motor impairment even in late stages of the illness. Although the disorder mostly appears to be sporadic, familial cases have been described.[29] In these cases, the pathological changes involve cerebral atrophy, predominantly of the white matter of the frontal and temporal cortex, with severe astroglial reaction; this occurs in subpial regions and at the junction between grey and white matter regions. Only a mild neuronal loss is seen,[29,82] although microvacuolation of the superficial laminae is sometimes present. The substantia nigra is affected with neuronal loss and astrocytic reaction. Tau deposits are extensively seen in both neurones and glial cells (in astrocytes these deposits are manifested as 'tufted' astrocytes and in oligodendrocytes they are manifested as coiled bodies) in many cortical and subcortical regions.[36,83] The neuronal tau deposits sometimes resemble neurofibrillary tangles but they are usually more punctate in appearance; Pick bodies are absent.

Summary of familial forms

As can be seen from the descriptions above, the range of clinical and pathological phenotypes associated with FTDP-17 is wide and it is not possible to identify definitively such cases from the general body of FTD cases on these criteria alone. Genetic analyses[84] of the frequency of tau mutations in unselected cases of non-Alzheimer degenerative dementia indicate that the frequency is extremely low (<0.2%) which confirms that cases of FTD caused by mutations on chromosome 17 are rare. Without prior knowledge of the presence of one of the disease causing mutations in other family members, it is unlikely that FTDP-17 will be predictable by clinical assessment or by autopsy examination of the brain after death.

How far the FTD phenotype extends is still not clear. Descriptions of families bearing a non-Alzheimer dementia phenotype often with movement disorder, have been published.[85–88] These descriptions show, to some degree, the same 'non-specific' features of FTD, such as neuronal loss and gliosis, often with neurofibrillary changes in the absence of neuritic plaques, and striatal and substantia nigral involvement. Whether these also need to be considered under FTD is uncertain – molecular genetic advances may define their nosology.

Molecular genetics and tau biochemistry of FTD

Linkage and mutations

As noted earlier, a previous history of a similar disorder has been claimed to occur in about 50% of patients with FTD families, with autosomal dominance being the likely mode of inheritance.[1] Genetic linkage studies[24,26,27,30–39] indicated a causative gene on the long arm of chromosome 17 (17q21–22). Affected families include FTD variants such as HFTD, HDDD, DDPAC, PPND MSTD and FPSG, as well as the more prototypical familial FTD cases (Table 2.1).

In most of these chromosome 17-linked families, researchers have now identified missense (exonic) mutations within coding regions of the tau gene or splice-site (intronic) mutations within regulatory regions of the gene (see Table 2.1).[40–42,89,90] Sequencing of the tau gene in other patients with FTD and in members of families with the FTD phenotype who have not been previously linked to chromosome 17 has revealed further instances of these particular disease-causing mutations,[39,74,75,91–94] as well as identifying other novel mutations (see Table 2.1).[95–98] Although these inherited forms of FTD associated with mutations in tau have a broadly microvacuolar type of histology, cases with the Pick-type of histology have also been shown to relate to (different) mutations in the tau gene (see Table 2.1).[98]

It is of great interest that the same mutation can occur in geographically different populations and in families who present with widely varying clinical phenotypes (see Table 2.1). Hence, the +16 splice site mutation occurs in several (probably related) British pedigrees[40,84,92] (Pickering-Brown, unpublished work), in an Australian pedigree,[34,40,72] in two US families (Duke 1684[32,73] and FTD002)[40] and in FPSG.[83] Likewise, the P301L mutation occurs in two Dutch families,[24,40,81] six French families,[92] four other French families[39,89] and two US families.[40,74] The N279K mutation, initially associated with PPND,[89] has also been found in a French family[91] and a Japanese family.[94] The R406W mutation occurs in one Dutch family[81] and one US family.[40] Other mutations, however, appear to be 'genetically private' and occur only in single pedigrees (e.g. G272T;[24,40,81]

Table 2.1 Mutations in tau gene associated with FTDP-17, together with their family origins. Brief details of the tau biochemistry in such mutations and the tissue pathology that such changes in tau induce are also given.

Family origins	Reference	Mutation	Tau pathology	Tissue pathology
Single case/British	98	K257T EX9	? 3R-tau ? 4R-tau	Pick bodies in neurones
HFTD2/Dutch	24, 40, 81	G272V EX9	? 3R-tau ? 4R-tau	Pick-like bodies in neurones
PPND/American French Japanese	89 91 94	N279K EX10	4R-tau	Flat wide twisted ribbons in neurones and glia
Single case/Dutch	24, 81	ΔK280 EX10	3R-tau	Not known
French Canadian	96	L284L EX10	4R-tau	Not known
HFTDI/Dutch Seattle DE/Oregon FTD003/American Montreal French/Canadian French American	24, 40, 81 41,89 40 39 92 74	P301L EX10	4R-tau Minor 3R-tau	Flat wide ribbons in neurones and glia
American	95	P301S EX10	4R-tau Minor 3R-tau	Flat ribbons in neurones and glia
Japanese	97	S305N EX10	4R-tau	Flat wide ribbons in neurones and glia

Seattle A/American	41,42	V337m Ex9	3R-tau 4R-tau	Paired helical and straight filaments in neurones
MSTD/American	42	+3 EX10	4R-tau	Flat wide ribbons in neurones and glia
Japanese	Unpublished	+12 EX10	Not known	?Flat wide ribbons in neurones and glia
Man 19/British	40	+13 EX10	4R-tau	?Flat wide ribbons in neurones and glia
DDPAC/Irish	23,40	+14 EX10	4R-tau	Flat twisted wide ribbons in neurones and glia
Man 6,23,49,125/British AUS1/Australian FTD002/American Duke 1684/American PSG/American	40,84,92,93 32,40,73 40 34,72 83	+16 EX10	4R-tau	Flat twisted wide ribbons in neurones and glia
Single case/British	98	G389R EX10	3R-tau 4R-tau	Pick bodies in neurones
FTD004/American FTD4/Dutch	40 91	R406W EX13	3R-tau 4R-tau	Paired helical filaments in neurones

P301S;[95] S305N;[96] L284L;[97] V337M;[41,42] +3 splice;[42] +13, +14 splice;[40] Δ280[81]) (see Table 2.1). Although in many instances the geographical distribution may be attributed to patterns of migration of founder family members, the possibility that certain mutations have arisen independently cannot be excluded. It is notable that in at least two families with linkage to chromosome 17 (the Karolinska family[37,63] and the HDDD2 family[28]), no mutations in the tau gene have as yet been determined; in the Karolinska family there is no tau pathology either.[63]

Pathogenetic considerations

The way in which tau mutations operate to produce neurodegeneration is not clear, but it seems to be brought about by several mechanisms, which may explain the phenotypy associated with the disorder.

The tau gene consists of 15 exons,[99] of which 11 encode the six major isoforms (ranging from 352 to 441 amino acids) that are normally produced by nerve cells from six messenger RNA (mRNA) transcripts. These differ according to the (alternatively spliced) inclusion of particular N-terminal domains (none, one or two 29 amino acid inserts) and three or four (imperfect) repeat domains of 31 or 32 amino acids within the C-terminal region of the molecule.[100] These latter domains, along with some adjoining sections of the molecule, are encoded by exons 9–12 and act as the microtubule-binding region, producing tau molecules known as 3- or 4-repeat tau (when exon 10 is excluded or included, respectively). Slightly more than half of the tau molecules that are normally produced are of the 3-repeat type; slightly less than half are therefore of the 4-repeat type.[100] Regulation of the exon 10 splice site is complex and is governed by several complementary and competing mechanisms. Firstly, there is a stem loop structure at the 3' end of exon 10 that regulates U1snRNP binding and the overall utilization of the splice donor site at that region.[40,42,101,102] Secondly, there is a splice-enhancing domain that occupies codons 276–281, which likewise increases the splicing in of exon 10.[96] Thirdly, there is a splice silencing element around codon 284 that reduces the inclusion of exon 10.[96]

All six isoforms of tau, however, play a particular role in the maintenance of microtubular structure. If one or more of the various forms fails to function, or if there is a stoichiometric imbalance in the different variants, microtubule formation becomes more difficult or the stability of microtubules so formed is compromised. Tau is thus critical to the maintenance of axonal transport and the stabilization of the neuronal cytoskeleton.[103] Any excess of unused tau (of any isoform composition) can be bundled into indigestible residue – tangles – that chokes the cell and impairs its function, possibly through a toxic action of the filaments.[104]

The mis-sense mutations in exons 9 (G272V), 10 (ΔK280, P301L, P301S), 12 (V337M) and 13 (R406W) produce tau proteins with conformational changes in the molecule, either within or close to the micro-tubule-binding region. These particular mutations affect all six isoforms of tau. All these former missense mutations, along with P301L and P301S mutations, result in an impaired efficiency to interact with α- and β-tubulin molecules, giving partial loss of microtubular function.[74,75,81,90,105] On the other hand, the effect of the intronic mutations is to destabilize the stem loop structure and increase U1snRNP binding and the inclusion of exon 10[40,42,101,102] (but see also D'Souza *et al*.[96]). This results in an increase in the proportion of tau mRNA transcripts that contain exon 10, thereby pro-ducing an imbalance in the relative formation of tau isoforms in favour of those containing 4-repeat tau (see Table 2.1). Mutations N279K and S305N do not alter the ability of tau to interact with microtubules but enhance the splicing in of exon 10,[89,90,96,106] also producing a relative excess of 4-repeat tau (see Table 2.1). The silent L284L mutation dramatically increases the proportion of 4-repeat tau (see Table 2.1) (no transcripts without exon 10 are produced in vitro), presumably by destroying the splice-silencing ele-ment at that codon.[96] The Δ280K mutation may destroy the function of the splice-enhancing domain, since in vitro this mutation results in a complete abolition of transcripts that contain exon 10.[96] Enigmatically, it also reduces the efficiency of microtubule binding.[96]

Because all six isoforms of tau are affected by the G272V, V337M and R406W mutations outside exon 10, the tangles so formed are made up of paired helical and straight filaments composed of a mixture of 3- and 4-repeat tau (see Table 2.1).[40–42,81,90,107] These structures, which appear only in neurones, are identical to the paired helical filaments of AD,[77] which themselves are similarly composed of equal amounts of 3- and 4-repeat tau. In the N279K, L284L, P301L, P301S and S305N mutations, and in the intronic (splice site) mutations that affect exon 10, the tangles are largely 4-repeat tau (with some 3-repeat tau) (see Table 2.1).[40,42,89,90,106,107] They appear as flat ribbons rather than as paired helical filaments, and they produce a pathology within neuronal and glial cells. The reason why cer-tain tau mutations produce a neuronal pathology and others neuronal and glial is not clear. It may reflect differing patterns of cellular expres-sion of tau, with neurones expressing all six isoforms but glial cells expressing only (or predominantly) 4-repeat tau. When pathological 3-repeat tau is in excess, the process favours assembly into paired helical filaments; when 4-repeat tau is in excess, flat, ribbon-like structures are formed.

Not only do the missense mutations impair the ability of tau to interact with microtubules, but the conformational changes they induce may, in some instances, favour the self-assembly of the mutant tau molecules into filamentous structures[108–110] or destabilize the cytoskeleton.[103] Hence, cellular tau pathology may represent a combination of predisposing changes in cell biology that include imbalances in stoichiometry of tau isoforms, impaired ability of tau to bind microtubules and enhanced propensity of mutant tau molecules to form fibrils. Additional effects, such as influences over the phosphorylation state of tau, remain to be determined. Even though none of the mutations that are known so far (except P301S) directly creates a novel phosphorylation site in tau, they could induce conformation changes that result in abnormal phosphorylation. The abnormal tau that accumulates in neurones is hyperphosphorylated, as it is in AD.[103] Although such changes may be well downstream from the primary pathogenetic events, they could nevertheless compound the functional disturbance – hyperphosphorylated tau is less effective at binding microtubules than normal tau – and hasten cellular demise. Obviously, the prevailing climate of biochemical changes may vary much with mutation type, but all will favour a net effect of producing redundant tau molecules that can eventually be assimilated into pathological structures.

Tau gene changes in Pick's disease

Two other mutations in tau, K257T and G389R, are associated with a Pick-type histology (see Table 2.1).[98] Again, both these mutations should affect all six isoforms of tau, but the mutant protein, instead of being assembled into paired helical filaments in the form of tangles, accumulates as intracytoplasmic Pick bodies. The K257T mutation lies in the microtubule-binding region of exon 9, and the G389R mutation, which is in exon 13, does not lie in any of the microtubule-binding regions of the protein but occurs in a region that is close to a microtubule domain. Again, the K257T and G389R mutations may confer upon tau a reduced ability to bind microtubules, and it may promote microtubule assembly, as has been shown for the other tau missense mutations. Biochemical investigations show that the abnormal tau in sporadic Pick's disease is composed of the 3-repeat isoform, with only trace amounts, if any, of the 4-repeat isoform.[112] However, the abnormal tau from the G389R case consists of 3- and 4-repeat tau, with proportionately more 4-repeat tau[97] than has been associated with sporadic Pick's disease cases. Moreover, it is quite distinct from that observed in AD and other tau gene mutations that lie outside exon 10 (see Table 2.1).[111]

It is of interest that in histopathological terms this particular case was atypical; in addition to the usual Pick inclusion bodies within nerve cells, an abundance of white matter changes in the form of 'coiled bodies' was also present.[98] Similar white matter alterations have also been seen in cases of FTD that are associated with the intronic mutations that favour the production of 4-repeat tau. Interestingly, the G272V mutation in tau is also characterized by the presence of Pick-like bodies, but the tau isoform composition of these, as with those of the K257T mutation, is not known.[91,107] Both these latter mutations in exon 9 affect all six tau isoforms, and so it might be anticipated that the Pick body-like structures are composed of some mixture of 3- and 4-repeat tau.

Other genetic factors

There have been claims that FTD, like AD,[113] is associated with an increased frequency of the ε4 allelic variant of the apolipoprotein gene.[49,114,115] However, other workers have not been able to confirm this, either in FTD overall[116–120] or specifically in cases of FTDP-17.[75,119,120] Moreover, and again in contrast to AD,[113,121,122] neither age at onset of disease nor duration of illness is modulated by the possession of ε4 allele in FTD generally[120] or in those families with FTDP-17.[75,119,120] It is unlikely, therefore, that possession of the ε4 allele has any impact on the likelihood of developing FTD or that it influences the age at onset or progression of the disorder in either familial or non-familial cases. Despite the superficial resemblance of the tissue cavitation in FTD to that in the human spongiform encephalopathies, no mutations in the prion gene have been associated with FTD, and deposits of the abnormal prion protein are not seen.[123,124]

Final considerations

The identification of mutations in tau gene associated with Pick's disease is of particular importance, since it ties both FLD- and Pick-type histologies into the same disease entity and settles controversial areas of nosology. The fact that such distinctive histological and clinical profiles can be generated in FTD by different tau mutations is not surprising – in the human spongiform encephalopathies, different prion gene mutations are associated with particular phenotypes. The varying pathology that characterize each disorder under the FTD umbrella is related to conformational or compositional changes in tau, directed by the mutational events.

How much of the FTD spectrum relates to tau pathology is still not clear. Are cases of 'sporadic' FTD caused by post-translational changes in tau or are they related to deleterious imbalances in regulatory elements of the tau gene, yet to be determined? Moreover, how do disorders such as motor neurone disease dementia, PA and semantic dementia, each of which share many of the clinical and histopathological features of FTD, relate genetically? To date, no mutations in the tau gene have been found in any patients with these particular disease phenotypes.

If mutations in tau occurred in these latter disorders, it would be necessary to explain the anterior preference for pathology in FTD and the temporal versus frontal involvement in semantic dementia and the lateral asymmetry in PA. Furthermore, does the tauopathy of FTD extend to include other non-Alzheimer forms of dementia such as progressive supranuclear palsy and corticobasal degeneration, in which tangles or a Pick type of histology are also present.[125] Cases of these disorders frequently show overlap in clinical presentation[126] and histopathological change[127] with FTD; indeed, some members of the FTDP-17 families have been reported as having symptomatologies consistent with either PSP[91,128] or CBD.[95] Investigations of the tau gene, in progressive supranuclear palsy at least, have repeatedly shown an increased frequency of a dinucleotide repeat in the intron between exons 9 and 10.[129–134] The tangles of progressive supranuclear palsy and corticobasal degeneration, as in FTDP-17, appear as ribbons of 4-repeat tau[135,136] and affect both nerve cells and glial cells. It is possible, therefore, that this particular dinucleotide repeat also facilitates the expression of exon 10 and the overproduction of 4-repeat tau; however, it is more likely that this genetic marker is in linkage disequilibrium with a function change closer to exon 10.[134] Even though the clinical phenotype attached to R406W mutation shares certain aspects with progressive supranuclear palsy, this particular mutation has not been found in 'typical' cases of sporadic PSP or CBD.[128] This lack of association might have been anticipated given the observations that the tangles in the FTDP-17 family with this mutation are a mix of 3- and 4-repeat tau and that they exist as paired helical filaments and not as the flat ribbons of 4-repeat tau (as in progressive supranuclear palsy). Further studies on the molecular genetics and biochemistry of tau may eventually reconcile many of these issues.

Finally, other families with a clinical FTD phenotype[137,138] have been linked to an as yet undetermined locus (or loci) on chromosome 3.[138–140] In one of these families there is evidence of anticipation,[141] which is suggestive of a possible trinucleotide gene expansion of the type seen in Huntington's disease,[142] although RED analysis failed to detect any trinucleotide expansions and immunohistochemistry did not visualize the characteristic intranuclear inclusion bodies.[141] Changes within the gene that are associated with this linkage might therefore explain other cases of both familial and sporadic FTD in which alterations in the tau gene and tau pathological changes seem not to be present

Molecular genetic advances have already distinguished mutations that are responsible for FTD in some familial cases and it is likely that further advances will clarify nosological issues that relate the status of the different histopathologies that underlie FTD to its relationship with other clinical syndromes that share those same histopathologies. Genetic advancement also holds the prospect of future treatment for this devastating form of dementia.

References

1. Snowden JS, Neary D, Mann DMA. Fronto-temporal lobar degeneration: Fronto-temporal dementia, progressive aphasia, semantic dementia. Edinburgh: Churchill Livingstone; 1996.

2. Pick A. Über die Bejiehungen des senilen Hirnatrophie zur Aphasie. Prager Med Wochenschr 1892;17:165–167.

3. Pick A. Über einen weiteren Symptomenkomplex in Rahmen der Dementia senilis, bedingt durch umschriebene starkere Hirnatrophie (gemischte Apraxie). Monatsschr Psychiatr Neurol 1906;19:97–108.

4. Schneider C. Über Picksche Krankheit. Monatsschr Psychiatr Neurol 1927;65:230–275.

5. Lowenberg K. Pick's disease. Arch Neurol Psychiatry 1935;36:768–789.

6. Ferrano A, Jervis GA. Pick's disease. Arch Neurol Psychiatry 1936;36:739–767.

7. Neumann MA. Pick's disease. J Neuropathol Exp Neurol 1949;8:255–282.

8. Gustafson L. Frontal lobe degeneration of non-Alzheimer type. II. Clinical picture and differential diagnosis. Arch Gerontol Geriatr 1987;6:209–223.

9. Gustafson L. Clinical picture of frontal lobe degeneration of non-Alzheimer type. Dementia 1993;4:143–148.

10. Gustafson L, Risberg J. Regional cerebral blood flow related to psychiatric symptoms in dementia with onset in the presenile period. Acta Psychiatr Scand 1974;50:516–538.

11. Neary D, Snowden JS, Bowen DM, et al. Neuropsychological syndromes in presenile dementia due to cerebral atrophy. J Neurol Neurosurg Psychiatry 1986;49:163–174.

12. Neary D, Snowden JS, Shields, RA, et al. Single photon emission tomography using 99mTc-HM-PAO in the investigation of dementia. J Neurol Neurosurg Psychiatry 1987;50:1101–1109.

13. Neary D, Snowden JS, Northen B, Goulding PJ. Dementia of frontal lobe type. J Neurol Neurosurg Psychiatry 1988;51:353–361.

14. Brun A. Frontal lobe degeneration of non-Alzheimer type. I. Neuropathology. Arch Gerontol Geriatr 1987;6:193–207.

15. Brun A, Englund E, Gustafson L. Frontal lobe degeneration of non-Alzheimer type revisited. Dementia 1993;4:126–131.

16. Mann DMA, South PW. The topographic distribution of brain atrophy in frontal lobe dementia. Acta Neuropathol 1993;85:335–340.

17. Mann DMA, South PW, Snowden JS, Neary D. Dementia of frontal lobe type: neuropathology and immunohistochemistry. J Neurol Neurosurg Psychiatry 1993;56:605–614.

18. Neary D, Snowden JS, Mann DMA. The clinical pathological correlates of lobar atrophy. A review. Dementia 1993;4:154–159.

19. Brun A, Englund E, Gustafson L. Clinical, neuropsychological and neuropathological criteria for fronto-temporal dementia. J Neurol Neurosurg Psychiatry 1994;57:416–418.

20. Neary D, Snowden JS, Gustafson L, et al. Frontotemporal lobar degeneration. A consensus on clinical diagnostic criteria. Neurology 1998;51:1546–1554.

21. Cordes M, Wszolek WK, Calne DB, *et al*. Magnetic resonance imaging studies in rapidly progressive autosomal dominant Parkinsonism and dementia with pallido-ponto-nigral degeneration. Neurodegeneration 1992;1: 217–224.

22. Wszolek ZK, Pfeiffer RF, Bhatt MH, *et al*. Rapidly progressive autosomal dominant Parkinsonism and dementia with pallido-ponto-nigral degeneration. Ann Neurol 1992;32:312–320.

23. Lynch T, Sano M, Marder KS, *et al*. Clinical characteristics of a family with chromosome 17-linked disinhibition–dementia–parkinsonism–amyotrophy complex. Neurology 1994;44:187–194.

24. Heutink P, Stevens M, Rizzu P, *et al*. Hereditary frontotemporal dementia is linked to chromosome 17q21–q22. A genetic and clinicopathological study of three Dutch families. Ann Neurol 1997;41:150–159.

25. Morris JC, Cole M, Banker BQ, Wright D. Hereditary dysphasic dementia and the Pick–Alzheimer spectrum. Ann Neurol 1984;16:455–466.

26. Lendon CL, Lynch T, Norton J, *et al*. Hereditary dysphasic disinhibition dementia: a frontotemporal dementia linked to 17q21–22. Neurology 1998;50: 1546–1555.

27. Spillantini MG, Crowther RA, Goedert M. Familial multiple system tauopathy: a new degenerative disease of the brain with tau neurofibrillary pathology. Proc Natl Acad Sci U S A 1997; 94:4113–4118.

28. Knopman DS, Mastri AR, Frey WH, *et al*. Dementia lacking distinctive histologic features: a common non-Alzheimer degenerative dementia. Neurology 1990;40:251–256.

29. Lanska DJ, Currier RD, Cohen M, *et al*. Familial progressive subcortical gliosis. Neurology 1994;44:1633–1643.

30. Wilhelmsen KC, Lynch T, Pavlov E, *et al*. Localization of disinhibition–dementia–parkinsonism–amyotrophy complex to 17q21–22. Am J Hum Genet 1994;55: 1159–1165.

31. Petersen RB, Tabaton, M, Chen SG, *et al*. Familial progressive subcortical gliosis: presence of prions and linkage to chromosome 17. Neurology 1995;45: 1062–1067.

32. Yamaoka LH, Welsh-Bohmer KA, Hulette CM, *et al*. Linkage of frontotemporal dementia to chromosome 17: clinical and neuropathological characterisation of phenotype. Am J Hum Genet 1996;59:1306–1312.

33. Wijker M, Wszolek ZK, Wolters ECM, *et al*. Localization of the gene for rapidly progressive autosomal dominant Parkinsonism and dementia with pallido-ponto-nigral degeneration to chromosome 17q21. Hum Mol Genet 1995;5:151–154.

34. Baker M, Kwok JBJ, Kucela S, *et al*. Localization of frontotemporal dementia with Parkinsonism in an Australian kindred to chromosome 17q21–22. Ann Neurol 1997;42:794–798.

35. Bird TD, Wijsman EM, Nochlin D, *et al*. Chromosome 17 and hereditary dementia: linkage studies in three non-Alzheimer families and kindreds with late onset FAD. Neurology 1997;48: 949–954.

36. Foster NL, Wilhelmsen K, Sima AAF, *et al*. Frontotemporal dementia and Parkinsonism linked to chromosome 17: a consensus conference. Ann Neurol 1997;41:706–715.

37. Froelich S, Basun H, Forsel C, *et*

al. Mapping of a disease locus for familial rapidly progressive frontotemporal dementia to chromosome 17q 20–21. Am J Med Genet 1997;74:380–385.

38. Murrell J, Koller D, Foroud T, *et al.* Familial multiple system tauopathy with presenile dementia localized to chromosome 17. Am J Hum Genet 1997;61: 1131–1138.

39. Nasreddine Z, Loginov M, Clark LN, *et al.* From genotype to phenotype: a clinical, pathological, and biochemical investigation of frontotemporal dementia and parkinsonism (FTDP-17) caused by the P301L mutation. Ann Neurol 1999;45:704–715.

40. Hutton M, Lendon CL, Rizzu P, *et al.* Association of missense and 5-splice-site mutations in tau with the inherited dementia FTDP-17. Nature 1998;393: 702–705.

41. Poorkaj P, Bird T, Wijsman E, *et al.* Tau is a candidate gene for chromosome 17 frontotemporal dementia. Ann Neurol 1998; 43:815–825.

42. Spillantini MG, Murrell JR, Goedert M, *et al.* Mutation in the tau gene in familial multiple system tauopathy with presenile dementia. Proc Natl Acad Sci U S A 1998;95:7737–7741.

43. Jagust WJ, Reed BR, Seab JP, Kramer JH, Budinger TF. Clinical–physiologic correlates of Alzheimer's disease and frontal lobe dementia. Am J Physiol Imaging 1989;4:89–96.

44. Miller BL, Cummings JL, Villanueva-Meyer J, *et al.* Frontal lobe degeneration: clinical, neuropsychological and SPECT characteristics. Neurology 1991; 41:1374–1382.

45. Miller BL, Chang L, Mena I, Boone K, Lesser IM. Progressive right frontotemporal degenera-tion: clinical, neuropsychological and SPECT characteristics. Dementia 1993;4:204–213.

46. Filley CM, Kleinschmidt-De Masters BK, Gross KF. Non Alzheimer frontotemporal degenerative dementia. A neurobehavioural and pathologic study. Clin Neuropathol 1994; 13:109–116.

47. Starkstein SE, Migliorelli R, Teson A, *et al.* Specificity of changes in cerebral blood flow in patients with frontal lobe dementia. J Neurol Neurosurg Psychiatry 1994;57:790–796.

48. Frisoni GB, Pizzolato G, Geroldi C, *et al.* Dementia of the frontal lobe type: neuropsychological and 99Tc-HM-PAO SPET features. J Geriatr Psychiatry Neurol 1995;8:42–48.

49. Stevens M, Van Duijn CM, Kamphorst W, *et al.* Familial aggregation in frontotemporal dementia. Neurology 1998;50:1541–1545.

50. Chow TW, Miller BL, Hayashi VN, Geschwind DH. Inheritance of frontotemporal dementia. Arch Neurol 1999;56:817–822.

51. Frisoni GB, Laakso MP, Beltramello A, *et al.* Hippocampal and entorhinal cortex atrophy in frontotemporal dementia and Alzheimer's disease. Neurology 1999;52:91–100.

52. Snowden JS, Griffiths H, Neary D. Semantic dementia: autobiographical contribution to preservation of meaning. Cognitive Neuropsychol 1994;11:256–288.

53. Snowden JS, Neary D, Mann DMA, *et al.* Progressive language disorder due to lobar atrophy. Ann Neurol 1992;31: 174–183.

54. Mitsuyama Y, Takamiya S. Presenile dementia with motor neuron disease in Japan. A new entity? Arch Neurol 1979;36: 592–593.

55. Hudson AJ. Amyotrophic lateral sclerosis and its association with dementia, Parkinsonism and other neurological disorders: a review. Brain 1981;104:217–247.

56. Salazar AM, Masters CL, Gajdusek DC, Gibbs CJ. Syndromes of amyotrophic lateral sclerosis and dementia: relation to transmissible Creutzfeldt–Jakob disease. Ann Neurol 1983;14:17–26.

57. Clark AW, White CL, Manz HJ, *et al.* Primary dementia without degenerative Alzheimer pathology. Can J Neurol Sci 1986; 13:462–470.

58. Morita K, Kaiya H, Ikeda T, Namba M. Presenile dementia combined with amyotrophy: a review of 34 Japanese cases. Arch Gerontol Geriatr 1987;6: 263–277.

59. Neary D, Snowden JS, Mann DMA, *et al.* Frontal lobe dementia and motor neurone disease. J Neurol Neurosurg Psychiatry 1990;53:23–32.

60. Okamoto, K, Murakami N, Kusaka H, *et al.* Ubiquitin-positive intraneuronal inclusions in the extramotor cortices of presenile dementia patients with motor neuron disease. J Neurol 1992;239:426–430.

61. Jackson M, Lennox G, Lowe J. Motor neurone disease-inclusion dementia. Neurodegeneration 1996;5:339–350.

62. Sima AAF, Defendini R, Keohane C, *et al.* The neuropathology of chromosome 17-linked dementia. Ann Neurol 1996; 39:734–743.

63. Basun H, Almkvist O, Axelman K, *et al.* Clinical characteristics of a chromosome 17-linked rapidly progressive familial frontotemporal dementia. Arch Neurol 1997;54:539–544.

64. Cooper PN, Jackson M, Lennox G, *et al.* Tau, ubiquitin and alpha β crystallin immunohistochemistry define the principal causes of degenerative fronto-temporal dementia. Arch Neurol 1995; 52:1011–1015.

65. Zhou L, Miller BL, McDaniel CH, Kelly L, Kim OJ, Miller CA. Frontotemporal dementia: neuropil spheroids and presynaptic terminal degeneration. Ann Neurol 1998;44:99–109.

66. Cooper PN, Siddons CA, Mann DMA. Patterns of glial cell activity in fronto-temporal dementia (lobar atrophy). Neuropathol Appl Neurobiol 1996;22:17–22.

67. Tolnay M, Probst A. Frontal lobe degeneration: novel ubiquitin-immunoreactive neurites within frontotemporal cortex. Neuropathol Appl Neurobiol 1995; 21:492–497.

68. Dickson DW. Pick's disease, a modern definition. Brain Pathol 1998;8:339–354.

69. Manaye KF, Woodward K, McIntyre DD, *et al.* Locus caeruleus cell loss in lobar atrophy. Neurodegeneration 1994;3:205–210.

70. Graff-Radford NR, Damasio AR, Hyman BT, *et al.* Progressive aphasia in a patient with Pick's disease: a neuropsychological, radiologic and anatomic study. Neurology 1990;40:620–626.

71. Procter AW, Qume M, Francis PT. Neurochemical features of frontotemporal dementia, Dementia Geriatr Cognitive Disord 1999;10(suppl 1):80–84.

72. Dark F. A family with autosomal dominant, non-Alzheimer's presenile dementia. Aust N Z J Psychiatry 1997;31:139–144.

73. Hulette CM, Pericak-Vance MA, Roses AD, *et al.* Neuropathological features of frontotemporal dementia and parkinsonism linked to chromosome 17q21–22 (FTDP-17): Duke family 1684. J

Neuropathol Exp Neurol 1999;58:859–866.

74. Mirra SS, Murrell JR, Gearing M, *et al*. Tau pathology in a family with dementia and a P301L mutation in tau. J Neuropathol Exp Neurol 1999;58:335–345.

75. Bird TD, Nochlin D, Poorkaj P, *et al*. A clinical pathological comparison of three families with frontotemporal dementia and identical mutations in the tau gene (P301L). Brain 1999; 122:741–756.

76. Reed LA, Schmidt ML, Wszolek ZK, *et al*. The neuropathology of a chromosome 17-linked autosomal dominant parkinsonism and dementia ('pallido-ponto-nigral-degeneration'). J Neuropathol Exp Neurol 1998;57: 588–601.

77. Spillantini MG, Bird TD, Ghetti B. Frontotemporal dementia and Parkinsonism linked to chromosome 17: a new group of tauopathies. Brain Pathol 1998; 8:387–402.

78. Spillantini MG, Crowther RA, Goedert M. Comparison of the neurofibrillary pathology in Alzheimer's disease and familial presenile dementia with tangles. Acta Neuropathol 1996;92: 42–48.

79. Sumi SM, Bird TD, Nochlin D, Raskind MA. Familial presenile dementia with psychosis associated with cortical neurofibrillary tangles and degeneration of the amygdala. Neurology 1992;42: 120–127.

80. Reed LA, Grabowski TJ, Schmidt ML, *et al*. Autosomal dominant dementia with widespread neurofibrillary tangles. Ann Neurol 1997;42:564–572.

81. Rizzu P, Van Swieten JC, Joosse M, *et al*. High prevalence of mutations in the microtubule-associated protein tau in a pop-ulation study of frontotemporal dementia in the Netherlands. Am J Hum Genet 1999;64: 414–421.

82. Neumann MA, Cohn R. Progressive subcortical gliosis, a rare form of pre-senile dementia. Brain 1967;90:405–427.

83. Goedert M, Spillantini MG, Crowther R, *et al*. Tau gene mutation in familial progressive subcortical gliosis. Nature Med 1999;5:454–457.

84. Houlden H, Baker M, Adamson J, *et al*. Frequency of tau mutations in three series of non-Alzheimer's degenerative dementia. Ann Neurol 1999; 46:243–248.

85. Mata MM, Dorovini-Zis K, Wilson M, Young AB. New form of familial Parkinson–dementia syndrome: clinical and pathologic findings. Neurology 1983;33: 1439–1443.

86. Rosenberg RN, Green JB, White CL III, *et al*. Dominantly inherited dementia and Parkinsonism with non-Alzheimer amyloid plaques: a new neurodegenerative disorder. Ann Neurol 1989;25: 152–158.

87. Golbe LI, Iorio G, Bonavita V, *et al*. A large kindred with autosomal dominant Parkinson disease. Ann Neurol 1990;27: 276–278.

88. Chapman SB, Rosenberg RN, Shobe A, Weiner MF. Autosomal dominant progressive syndrome of motor-speech loss without dementia. Neurology 1997; 49:1298–1306.

89. Clark LN, Poorkaj P, Wszolek Z, *et al*. Pathogenic implications of mutations in the tau gene in pallido-ponto-nigral degeneration and related neurodegenerative disorders linked to chromosome 17. Proc Natl Acad Sci U S A 1998;95:13103–13107.

90. Hong M, Zhukareva V, Vogelsberg-Ragaglia V, *et al.* Mutation-specific functional impairments in distinct tau isoforms of hereditary FTDP-17. Science 1998; 282:1914–1917.

91. Delisle MB, Murrell JR, Richardson R, *et al.* A mutation at codon 279 (N279K) in exon 10 of the tau gene causes a tauopathy with dementia and supranuclear palsy. Acta Neuropathol 1999;98:62–77.

92. Dumanchin C, Camuzat A, Campion D, *et al.* Segregation of a missense mutation in the microtubule-associated protein tau gene with familial frontotemporal dementia and parkinsonism. Hum Mol Genet 1998;7: 1825–1829.

93. Morris HR, Perez-Tur J, Janssen JC, *et al.* Mutation in the tau exon 10 splice site region in familial frontotemporal dementia. Ann Neurol 1999;45:270–271.

94. Yasuda M, Kawamata T, Komure O, *et al.* A mutation in the microtubule associated protein tau in pallido-nigro-luysian degeneration. Neurology 1999;53:864–868.

95. Bugiani O, Murrell JR, Giaccone G, *et al.* Frontotemporal dementia and corticobasal degeneration in a family with a P301S mutation in tau. J Neuropathol Exp Neurol 1999;58:667–677.

96. D'Souza I, Poorkaj P, Hong M, *et al.* Missense and silent tau gene mutations cause frontotemporal dementia with parkinsonism-chromosome 17 type, by affecting multiple alternative splicing regulatory elements. Proc Natl Acad Sci U S A 1999;96; 5598–5603.

97. Iijima M, Tabira T, Poorkaj P, *et al.* A distinct familial presenile dementia with a novel missense mutation in the tau gene. Neuro-Report 1999;10:497–501.

98. Pickering-Brown SM, Baker M, Yen SH, *et al.* Pick's disease is associated with mutations in the tau gene. 1999 (submitted for publication).

99. Andreadis A, Brown WM, Kosik KS. Structure and novel exons of the human tau gene. Biochemistry 1992;31:10626–10633.

100. Goedert M, Spillantini MG, Jakes R, *et al.* Multiple isoforms of human microtubule-associated protein tau: sequence and localization in neurofibrillary tangles of Alzheimer's disease. Neuron 1989;3:519–526.

101. Grover A, Houlden H, Baker M, *et al.* 5' Splice site mutations in tau associated with the inherited dementia FTDP-17 affect a stem-loop structure that regulates alternative splicing of exon 10. J Biol Chem 1999;274: 15134–15143.

102. Varani L, Hasegawa M, Spillantini MG, *et al.* Structure of tau exon 10 splicing regulatory element RNA and destabilization by mutations of frontotemporal dementia and parkinsonism linked to chromosome 17. Proc Natl Acad Sci U S A 1999; 96: 8229–8334.

103. Arawaka S, Usami M, Sahara N, *et al.* The tau mutation (val337met) disrupts cytoskeletal networks of microtubules. NeuroReport 1999;10:993–997.

104. Goedert M, Spillantini MG, Davies SW. Filamentous nerve cell inclusions in neurodegenerative diseases. Curr Opin Neurobiol 1998;8:619–632.

105. Hasegawa M, Smith MJ, Goedert M. Tau proteins with FTDP-17 mutations have a reduced ability to promote microtubule assembly. FEBS Lett 1998;437: 207–210.

106. Hasegawa M, Smith MJ, Iijima

M, *et al.* FTDP-17 mutations N279K and S305N in tau produce increased splicing of exon 10. FEBS Lett 1999;443:93–96.

107. Spillantini MG, Crowther RA, Kamphorst W, *et al.* Tau pathology in two Dutch families with mutations in the microtubule-binding region of tau. Am J Pathol 1998;153:1359–1363.

108. Goedert M, Jakes R, Crowther RA. Effects of frontotemporal dementia FTDP-17 mutations on heparin-induced assembly of tau filaments. FEBS Lett 1999;450:306–311.

109. Jicha GA, Rockwood JM, Berenfeld B, Hutton M, Davies P. Altered conformation of recombinant frontotemporal dementia-17 mutant tau proteins. Neurosci Lett 1999;260:153–156.

110. Nacharaju P, Lewis J, Easson C, *et al.* Accelerated filament formation from tau protein with specific FTDP-17 missense mutations. FEBS Lett 1999;447:195–199.

111. Arrasate M, Perez M, Armas-Portela R, Avila J. Polymerization of tau peptides into fibrillar structures. The effect of FTDP-17 mutations. FEBS Lett 1999;446:199–202.

112. Delacourte A, Sergeant N, Wattez, A, *et al.* Vulnerable neuronalsubsets in Alzheimer's and Pick's diseases are distinguished by their tau isoform distribution and phosphorylation. Ann Neurol 1998;43:193–204.

113. Corder EH, Saunders AM, Strittmatter WJ, *et al.* Gene dose of apolipoprotein E type 4 allele and the risk of Alzheimer's disease in late onset families. Science 1993;261:921–923.

114. Czech C, Forstl H, Monning U, *et al.* ApoE4 in clinically diagnosed Alzheimer's disease, frontal lobe degeneration and

non-demented controls. Neurobiol Aging 1994;15(suppl 1): S132.

115. Govoni S, Frisoni GB, Calabresi L, *et al.* Apolipoprotein E ϵ4 allele frequency in non-Alzheimer dementias. Neurobiol Aging 1994;15(suppl 1):S44.

116. Pickering-Brown SM, Roberts D, Owen F, Neary D. Apolipoprotein ϵ4 alleles and non-Alzheimer's disease forms of dementia. Neurodegeneration 1994;3:95–96.

117. Pickering-Brown SM, Siddons M, Mann DMA, Owen F, Neary D, Snowden JS. Apolipoprotein E allelic frequencies in patients with lobar atrophy. Neurosci Lett 1995;188:205–207.

118. Minthon L, Hesse C, Sjogren M, Englund E, Gustafson L, Blennow K. The apolipoprotein E ϵ4 allele frequency is normal in fronto-temporal dementia, but correlates with age at onset of disease. Neurosci Lett 1997; 226:65–67.

119. Houlden H, Rizzu P, Stevens M, *et al.* Apoliporotein E genotype does not affect age at onset of dementia in families with defined tau mutations. Neurosci Lett 1999;260:193–195.

120. Pickering-Brown SM, Owen F, Snowden JS, *et al.* Apolipoprotein E ϵ4 allele has no effect on age at onset or duration of disease in cases of frontotemporal dementia with Pick- or microvacuolar-type histology. Exp Neurol (in press).

121. Hardy J, Houlden H, Collinge J, *et al.* Apolipoprotein E genotype and Alzheimer's disease. Lancet 1993;342:737–738.

122. Nachmias B, Latorraca S, Piersanti P, *et al.* ApoE genotype and familial Alzheimer's disease: a possible influence on age at onset in APP717 Val $\rightarrow$ Ile

mutated families. Neurosci Lett 1995;183:1–3.

123. Clinton J, Mann DMA, Roberts GW. Frontal lobe dementia is not a variant of prion disease. Neurosci Lett 1993;164:1–4.

124. Owen F, Cooper PN, Pickering-Brown S, McAndrew C, Mann DMA, Neary D. The lobar atrophies are not prion encephalopathies. Neurodegeneration 1993;2:195–199.

125. Feany MB, Dickson DW. Neurodegenerative disorders with extensive tau pathology: a comparative study and review. Ann Neurol 1996;40:139–148.

126. Neary D, Kertesz A, Hachinski V. Frontotemporal dementia, Pick disease, and corticobasal degeneration. One entity or three? Arch Neurol 1997; 54: 1425–1429.

127. Jendroska K, Rossor M, Mathias CJ, Daniel SE. Morphological overlap between corticobasal degeneration and Pick's disease: a clinicopathologic report. Mov Disord 1995;10:111–114.

128. Higgins JJ, Litvan I, Nee LE, Loveless JM. A lack of the R406W tau mutation in progressive supranuclear palsy and corticobasal degeneration. Neurology 1999;52:404–406.

129. Conrad C, Andreadis A, Trojanowski JQ, et al. Genetic evidence for the involvement of τ in progressive supranuclear palsy. Ann Neurol 1997;41:277–281.

130. Higgins JJ, Litvan I, Pho LT, et al. Progressive supranuclear palsy is in linkage disequilibrium with the τ and not the α-synuclein gene. Neurology 1998;50: 270–273.

131. Oliva R, Tolosa E, Ezquerra E, et al. Significant changes in the tau A0 and A3 alleles in progressive supranuclear palsy and improved genotyping by silver detection. Arch Neurol 1998; 55:1122–1124.

132. Bennett P, Bonifati V, Bonuccelli U, et al. Direct genetic evidence for involvement of tau in progressive supranuclear paksy. European Study Group on Atypical Parkinsonism Consortium. Neurology 1998;51:982–985.

133. Morris HR, Janssen JC, Bandmann O, et al. The tau gene A0 polymorphism in progressive supranuclear palsy and related neurodegenerative diseases. J Neurol Neurosurg Psychiatry 1999;66:665–667.

134. Baker M, Litvan L, Houlden H, et al. Association of an extended haplotypein the tau gene with progressive supranuclear palsy. Hum Mol Genet 1999;8: 711–715.

135. Delacourte A, Buee L. Normal and pathological tau proteins as factors for microtubule assembly. Int Rev Cytol 1997;171: 167–224.

136. Sergeant N, Wattez A, Delacourte A. Neurofibrillary degeneration in progressive supranuclear palsy and corticobasal degeneration: tau pathologies with exclusively 'exon 10' isoforms. J Neurochem 1999;72:1243–1249.

137. Gydesen S, Hagen S, Klinken L, et al. Neuropsychiatric studies in a family with presenile dementia different from Alzheimer and Pick disease. Acta Psychiatr Scand 1987;76:276–284.

138. Podulso SE, Yin X, Hargis J, Brumback RA, Mastrianni JA, Schwankhaus J. A familial case of Alzheimer's disease without tau pathology may be linked with chromosome 3 markers. Hum Genet 1999;105:32–37.

139. Brown J. Chromosome 3-linked frontotemporal dementia. Cell Mol Life Sci 1998;54:925–927.

140. Brown J, Ashworth A, Gydesen S, *et al.* Familial non-specific dementia maps to chromosome 3. Hum Mol Genet 1995;4: 1625–1628.

141. Ashworth A, Lloyd S, Brown J, *et al.* Molecular genetic characterisation of frontotemporal dementia on chromosome 3. Dementia Geriatr Cognitive Disord 1999; 10(suppl 1):93–101.

142. Huntington's Disease Collaborative Research Group. A novel gene containing a trinucleotide repeat that is expanded and unstable on HD chromosome. Cell 1993;72:971–983.

3
Dementia with Lewy bodies

Ian McKeith

Introduction

Dementia in old age has traditionally been viewed as being due to Alzheimer's disease (AD), vascular dementia (VaD) or a mixture of these pathologies. Within the past decade however, advances in immunocytochemical techniques for examining post mortem brain[1] have identified an additional, common cause of dementia, which has been designated dementia with Lewy bodies (DLB).[2] Lewy bodies are neurofilament inclusion bodies that are indicative of neuronal dysfunction and loss. They were originally described in the nigrostriatal system of Parkinson's disease (PD) patients, but they are now recognized to occur more diffusely throughout the central and autonomic nervous system.[3,4] DLB accounted for 15–20% of cases of late-onset dementia in several hospital[5,6] and community-based[7] autopsy series, making it the second most common neurodegenerative cause of dementia after AD, with an estimated 100,000 DLB sufferers in the UK alone.

DLB patients typically exhibit a delirium-like presentation that consists of fluctuating confusion, attention deficits and psychiatric symptoms, particularly visual hallucinations.[8,9] Rigid–akinetic parkinsonism (often mild), intermittent loss of consciousness and falls are other common features.[10,11] This complex and distressing array of symptoms brings patients to psychiatric, geriatric medicine and neurology services[12–14] and requires expert management that is informed by knowledge of the underlying pathological and neurochemical deficits.[15]

Clinical features

Historical perspective – early reports

The first case reports that specifically described patients with DLB appeared in 1961, when Okazaki *et al.* published two cases,[16] both in elderly men who presented with cognitive decline and who subsequently developed severe dementia. Over the next 20 years, 34 similar autopsy confirmed cases were reported. Summarizing these, Kosaka *et al.* noted a 3:1 male predominance, with memory disturbance as the presenting feature in 67% of the cases, psychotic states [*sic*] in 17% and dizziness caused by orthostatic hypotension in 17%.[2] Progressive dementia with muscular rigidity eventually occurred in 80% of the cases, with only 25% of cases initially being diagnosed as parkinsonian.

In 1988, Burkhardt *et al.* listed 34 cases, including four from the USA, and carried out a simple meta-analysis.[17] Men were affected more than twice as often as women, the age of onset being, with few exceptions, between 50 and 80 years. The most common presentation was a 'neuro-behavioural syndrome'; memory impairment and other cognitive deficits were typical, and all but one of the 34 patients eventually became demented. Psychotic features such as depression, hallucinations and paranoia were seen in 10 patients (29%), and two patients were psychotic for many years before they developed other symptoms. Parkinsonian features, the most common of which was rigidity, were usually overshadowed by dementia; in only five cases (15%) were no extrapyramidal features present. The duration of illness was very variable (1–20 years) with an end-state of severe dementia, rigidity, akinetic mutism, quadriparesis in flexion and emaciation. The most common reported cause of death was aspiration pneumonia. Based on these observations, Burkhardt *et al.* were the first to attempt a general description of the clinical syndrome associated with diffuse Lewy body disease (DLBD – their preferred term), distinguishing it as separate from PD with dementia.[17] They concluded that, 'DLBD should be suspected in any elderly patient who presents with a rapidly progressive dementia, followed in short order by rigidity and other parkinsonian features. Myoclonus may be present'.

Crystal *et al.*, in 1990, criticized this approach on the grounds that 'extrapyramidal features occur in many patients with severe AD and since dementia occurs in many subjects with PD, the clinical criteria for the diagnosis of DLBD remain unclear'.[18] They proposed alternative criteria of 'progressive dementia with gait disorder, psychiatric symptoms and a burst pattern on EEG at the time of moderate dementia'. Agitation, hallucinations and delusions were the psychiatric features noted and these features were often present early. No particular characteristics of the pattern of cognitive impairment were noted. Although these early clinical definitions were important in drawing attention to the existence of DLB and in describing some of its salient characteristics, neither could be regarded as satisfactory for clinical diagnostic purposes, since they lacked detail and were not operationalized in a way that would allow acceptable inter-rater reliability.[19]

The Nottingham, Newcastle and San Diego cases

In the early 1990s, clinical reports about autopsy-confirmed DLB cases suddenly increased. The Nottingham group described the clinical characteristics of 15 new UK cases in considerable detail, making this the largest individual series published at that time.[9] Seven of the 15 cases were men, the mean age at onset was 72 years and the mean duration of illness was 5.5 years. Forty per cent presented with symptoms and signs of idiopathic Parkinson's disease, with cognitive impairment occurring 1–4 years later. A further 20% had parkinsonism and mild cognitive impairment at presentation, and the remaining 40% showed motor features later in their illnesses, gait disturbance and postural abnormalities being the most common. These latter cases had initially presented with neuropsychiatric features only – cognitive impairment, paranoid delusions and visual or auditory hallucinations. Fourteen of the 15 were demented before death, the exception presented with classical Parkinson's disease and later became depressed, irritable and mildly forgetful with frequent falls. Fluctuating cognition with episodic confusion for which no adequate underlying cause could be found was observed in 80% of the Nottingham cases, and the frequent occurrence of depression (20%) and psychosis (33%) was noted.

At about the same time, the Newcastle group also published details of two consecutive series of DLB cases ($n = 41$) and contrasted the clinical features with AD ($n = 57$) and VaD ($n = 9$) patients.[20,21] The DLB cases (designated in Newcastle at that time as 'senile dementia of Lewy body type') had generally been regarded as 'clinically atypical, causing much diagnostic perplexity'. Acute onset, fluctuating course, more rapid deterioration, early and prominent hallucinatory and behavioural disturbances and associated mild parkinsonian features were more often present in these patients, who were predominantly male (male to female ratio, 1.6:1). Other features noted were episodes of transient loss of consciousness and syncope and repeated, unexplained falls, each being present in about 25–40% of cases. A severe and often irreversible adverse reaction to antipsychotic medication (neuroleptic sensitivity) was described for the first time as a particular characteristic of DLB and accounted in part for the 50% reduction in mean survival time that was observed compared with AD.

In San Diego, detailed neuropsychological assessments of nine DLB cases (designated by researchers there as the LB variant of AD) revealed greater deficits in attention, fluency and visuospatial processing compared with AD patients who had been matched for age and degree of dementia.[6] Similar comparison of neurological examinations showed a significant increase in masked facies, essential tremor, bradykinesia, mild neck rigidity and slowing of rapid alternating movements. Extremity rigidity, flexed posture or other classic parkinsonian features were not, however, characteristic of the DLB group.

Review of recent reports

During the second half of the 1990s, sufficient clinical case reports about DLB patients have been published to allow the general characteristics of the disorder to be more clearly described.[3,22] Patients are almost twice as likely to be male, with a mean age of 70 years at onset (range of means 62–74 years) and a mean duration of illness of 6 years (range of means 2–10 years). Although mean age of onset and survival are similar to those of AD cases contained in the same case reports, some DLB patients do have a very rapidly progressive illness, with reports of death within 1 year of onset for some patients.[23] Some but not all of this reduced survival may be attributable to neuroleptic sensitivity reactions.[21]

Cognitive impairment is usually, but not always, the presenting feature of DLB. A relatively sudden onset of delirium is typical. Up to 20% of patients do not initially have significant cognitive impairment but present with a primary movement disorder, with mood disorders or psychosis, with dizziness and falls or with transient disturbances of consciousness and syncope.

All patients, by definition, develop a dementia syndrome with time. This has a characteristic profile, with prominent attention deficits and disproportionate frontal–subcortical and visuospatial dysfunction. In contrast to AD, recent memory and orientation may be well preserved in DLB, especially in the earlier stages. The rate of cognitive decline in DLB and AD appears to be similar.

Fluctuation occurs in half to three quarters of patients, but the range reported is very variable, probably because this is a difficult symptom to define. Fluctuating cognition and performance appear to originate from an unstable, underlying platform of attention and alertness, the basis of which is a dysregulation of the central cholinergic mechanisms that control level of consciousness. These variations may be subtle and transient, the patient simply appearing glazed or distant for brief periods. At the other extreme, there may be complete loss of consciousness that lasts for up to several hours, followed by spontaneous recovery.

Daytime somnolence is another manifestation of attentional fluctuation, and an associated feature is rapid eye movement (REM) sleep disorder, in which loss of normal REM sleep muscle atonia leads to jerking or complex vigorous movements of the limbs or body with associated dream recall.[24]

Patients often recall these experiences on waking and they can be difficult to distinguish from reports of visual hallucinations, which occur in up to 80% of DLB patients. These are typically colourful, three-dimensional images of animals and people, experienced and described in detail, usually occurring most days of the week. Insight into the unreal nature of these hallucinations is usually absent while they occur but is gained after the event. Auditory hallucinations also occurs in 20% of DLB subjects, but they are seldom present in AD.

Table 3.1 Clinical characteristics of DLB and AD cases as reported in autopsy-confirmed case series.

	DLB	AD
Dementia	+ + + +	+ + + +
Relatively sudden onset	+ +	−
Intermittent delirium	+ + +	+
Memory impairment as an early feature	+	+ + +
Disproportionate visuospatial impairment	+ + +	+
Impaired attention	+ + +	+
Fluctuating performance	+ + +	+
Persistent visual hallucinations	+ + +	−
Parkinsonism	+ + +	+
Recurrent falls	+ +	+
Systematized delusions	+ +	+ +
Depressed mood	+ + +	+
REM sleep behaviour disorder	+ +	−
Hippocampal atrophy on CT or MRI	+	+ + +
Reduced SPECT-HMPAO uptake	+ + +	+ + +
Early slowing of EEG	+ + +	+ +
Severe adverse reactions to neuroleptics	+ + +	+
Good response to cholinesterase inhibitors	+ +	+

A 38% prevalence of depressive symptoms in DLB is significantly greater than in AD and similar to rates reported in PD.[25,26]

Rates for motor features of parkinsonism vary considerably between different studies, being up to 100% for DLB patients identified via neurological departments that primarily receive movement disorder referrals. Taken overall, less than 50% of DLB cases have parkinsonism at presentation and 25% continue to have no evidence of parkinsonism at any point in their illness.[25] The inter-rater reliability and validity of assessment of mild extrapyramidal features in elderly demented subjects is difficult – bradykinesia, gait problems, tremor and reduced alternating movements can be normal findings in this age group, and their presence in isolation should not be overinterpreted.[27]

Finally, postural instability and recurrent falls occur in up to one-third of DLB cases, significantly more than in AD.[8,10] Neuroleptic sensitivity is also more common in DLB than in AD; it is detected in 60% of all DLB patients who receive neuroleptic agents but in only 15% of those with AD.[9,28] The key clinical features of DLB and AD are compared in Table 3.1.

Pathological features

Lewy bodies are spherical, intracytoplasmic, eosinophilic, neuronal inclusions. They have a dense hyaline core and a halo of radiating filaments that is composed of abnormally truncated and phosphorylated intermediate neurofilament proteins, which also contain ubiquitin and associated enzymes.[4] They were first described by the German neuropathologist Friedreich Lewy in brain stem nuclei of Parkinson's disease patients when he was working in Alzheimer's laboratory in Munich between 1910 and 1912.[29] Subcortical Lewy bodies are easily seen using conventional haematoxylin and eosin staining, but cortical Lewy bodies lack the characteristic core and halo appearance of their brainstem counterparts and were seldom detected until the development of antiubiquitin immunocytochemical staining methods allowed their true prevalence to be appreciated.[1] It is unlikely that DLB is a newly occurring disease; it is probably simply one that has only recently been recognized after this advance in neuropathological methods. Even more recently, α-synuclein antibodies have been shown to label purified Lewy bodies and give strong staining of Lewy bodies and Lewy neurites in post-mortem tissue.[30] α-Synuclein immunocytochemistry is now the most sensitive method of detecting DLB at autopsy, and it reveals an extensive neuritic involvement that was not previously appreciated.[31]

Current thinking about Lewy body disorders suggests that there is spectrum of disease, with the clinical presentation varying according to the site of Lewy body formation and neuronal loss:[4]

- nigrostriatal pathology produces an extrapyramidal movement disorder;
- cortical involvement generates neuropsychiatric features; and
- autonomic nervous system disease is associated with postural hypotension, dizziness and falls.

Although pure presentations are seen in clinical practice, heterogeneous combinations of parkinsonism, dementia and autonomic failure are most frequent in elderly patients.

Recommendations have recently been made as to which brain regions should be examined for Lewy bodies at autopsy, and a simple semiquantitative scoring system has been devised in which a score of 1 is given if any Lewy bodies are seen in a given area and a score of 2 is given if there are more than five Lewy bodies per field.[3] These scores are added to generate three pathological categories of DLB:

- brainstem predominant (0–2);
- limbic or transitional (3–6); and
- neocortical (7–10).

It has not yet been established to what extent these different patterns of pathological distribution correlate with different clinical profiles. Extensive neocortical pathology is certainly not essential for the development of dementia or other psychiatric symptoms, any of which may occur in the presence of limbic disease alone. It has been suggested that these consensus guidelines[3] are too inclusive for routine use, and a modification has been proposed that eliminates parietal and frontal association cortex from the analysis and cortical layers I and II from the sampling and that excludes cases without brainstem LB.[32]

A heated debate has surrounded the interpretation of the Alzheimer-type changes that are also seen in most DLB patients, some authorities describing DLB cases as the LB 'variant' of AD.[6] High senile plaque counts are found in the majority of cases, and these are morphologically indistinguishable from those found in pure AD.[33] They are, however, seldom tau-immunoreactive, and indeed in 80–90% of DLB cases there is no evidence of significant tau pathology, paired helical filaments or neocortical neurofibrillary tangles.[34] Therefore, whether or not DLB is considered to be a variant of AD depends on the pathological definition of AD that is used. Thus, 77% of LB pathology cases with dementia had 'plaque-only' AD, a concept derived from definitions of AD that are heavily dependent on plaque density.[35] By contrast, 80–90% of DLB cases fail to fulfil definitions of AD that require suprathreshold numbers of neocortical neurofibrillary tangles.[36] The new NIA–Regan Foundation criteria for Alzheimer's disease appear to be making a significant shift in this direction, with a proposed requirement for frequent neurofibrillary tangles equivalent to Braak stages 5 and 6.[37] DLB and pure AD will, according to such criteria, be pathologically distinct in the majority of cases.

A recent study of pathological burden versus clinical severity[38] examined correlations between two simple measures of cognitive ability and a range of lesion counts and neurochemical measures in the mid-frontal cortex of DLB cases. Dementia severity was significantly correlated with Lewy body density, plaque density and severity of cholinergic deficit but not with neurofibrillary tangle density or synaptophysin levels. In contrast, in AD cases it was tangle density and synaptophysin levels that were most highly correlated with clinical severity. This suggests that the dementias of DLB and AD may have different pathological substrates but similar neurochemical substrates. Another important correlate of the extensive cholinergic deficit of DLB is with the presence of hallucinations, which are a common clinical manifestation. Patients with hallucinations have significantly lower levels of choline acetyl transferase than non-hallucinators.[39]

Clinical diagnostic criteria for DLB

Early, accurate diagnosis of DLB is important since the condition is common and has a different clinical profile and treatment response from other dementia types. Several sets of criteria for the clinical diagnosis of DLB have been proposed,[9,20,40] and their potential to predict autopsy findings accurately has been provisionally assessed.[41–43] A recent consensus statement recommended that 'probable DLB' should be diagnosed in the presence of a dementia syndrome that has prominent attentional deficits, subcortical–frontal dysfunction and prominent visuospatial impairments and that is accompanied by any two of fluctuating cognition, persistent visual hallucinations and motor features of parkinsonism.[3] 'Possible DLB' is diagnosed when only one of these three features is present (Table 3.2).

Three retrospective chart reviews examining the validity of the consensus criteria have been published. Mega *et al.* reported on 24 cases with dementia or movement disorder, four of which had numerous cortical Lewy bodies at autopsy.[42] Three cases were correctly diagnosed clinically by the consensus criteria as probable DLB (sensitivity = 0.75), one case lacking evidence of any of the core features. The specificity (true negative) rate was 0.79. If an additional 11 cases with few (as opposed to no) cortical Lewy bodies were included, the specificity rose to 1.0 but the sensitivity fell to 0.40. Holmes *et al.* found that 12 out of 80 (15%) cases on a community based dementia case register in London had Lewy bodies at autopsy.[7] Nine were considered as primary DLB cases, and three others that were associated with infarcts were assigned to a 'mixed pathology' category. Chart review identified only two of these cases (sensitivity = 0.22), with no false-positive clinical diagnoses (specificity = 1.0). Most recently, Luis *et al.* compared consensus, CERAD and Newcastle criteria for DLB as applied to the case notes of 35 DLB and 21 AD cases. All were highly specific (range, 0.9–1.0) and although sensitivity was higher (range, 0.49–0.63) than in the study by Holmes *et al.*, a significant number of cases were not detected.[43]

Although retrospective validation studies give some indications about the performance of diagnostic criteria, they are usually confounded by items of clinical data that either were not recorded in the first instance or were recorded in insufficient detail. Lack of information reduces inter-rater reliability for specific items, and if these are required for diagnosis it will also reduce case detection rates, reflected in low sensitivity figures. For DLB diagnosis, the most problematic item to determine reliably from case notes is fluctuation. The necessary test is to apply diagnostic criteria actively to patients ante mortem and then to follow their progress to the time of death. One such study[44] has evaluated the first 50 cases to reach autopsy in a cohort to which consensus clinical diagnostic criteria for DLB, NINCDS-ADRDA criteria for AD and NINDS-AIREN criteria for VaD had been prospectively applied. Twenty-six clinical diagnoses of DLB 19 of AD and five of VaD were made. At autopsy, 29 cases of DLB, 15 of AD, five of VaD and one of progressive supranuclear palsy were identified. The sensitivity of a clinical diagnosis of probable DLB in this sample was 0.83; the specificity was 0.95. Of the five cases that received

Table 3.2 Three proposed clinical criteria for DLB.

Newcastle criteria[20]	CERAD criteria[40]	Consensus criteria[3]
A. Fluctuating cognitive impairment affecting both memory and higher cortical functions (such as language, visuospatial ability, praxis or reasoning skills). Fluctuation is marked, with the occurrence of both episodic confusion and lucid intervals, as in delirium, and is evident either on cognitive testing or by variable performance in activities of daily living	A. Clinical Dementia Rating Scale $\geqslant 0.5$	A. Progressive cognitive decline that interferes with social or occupational function
B. At least one of the following: 1. Visual and/or auditory hallucinations, which are accompanied by secondary paranoid delusions 2. Mild spontaneous extrapyramidal features or neuroleptic sensitivity syndrome 3. Repeated unexplained falls and/or transient clouding or loss of consciousness	B. Any two of the following: 1. Delusions or hallucinations 2. Extrapyramidal signs 3. Unexplained falls and/or changes in consciousness	B. Two of the following for probable DLB, one for possible DLB: 1. Fluctuating cognition with variations in attention and alertness 2. Well-formed, recurrent visual hallucinations 3. Spontaneous motor features of parkinsonism
C. Despite fluctuating pattern, clinical symptoms persist over a period of time and progress, often rapidly, to an end-stage of severe dementia.	C. One or more of the following: 1. Fluctuating course 2. Poor response to levodopa 3. Cognitive symptoms more severe than extrapyramidal signs 4. Cachexia, dysphagia, depression or dysthymia	C. Supportive features (not required): 1. Repeated falls 2. Syncope 3. Transient loss of consciousness 4. Neuroleptic sensitivity 5. Systematized delusions 6. Hallucinations in other modalities
D. Exclusion of other causes of delirium and vascular causes for decline	D. Exclusion of other causes of dementia	

a false-negative diagnosis of DLB, significant fluctuation was present in four but visual hallucinations and spontaneous motor features of parkinsonism were generally absent. Thirty-one per cent of the DLB cases had additional vascular pathology, and this contributed to a misdiagnosis of VaD in two cases. No correlations were found between the distribution of Lewy bodies and clinical features.

Differential diagnosis of DLB

There are four main categories of disorder that should be considered in the differential diagnosis of DLB. These are:

- other dementia syndromes;
- other causes of delirium;
- other neurological syndromes; and
- other psychiatric disorders.

Other dementia syndromes

Sixty-five per cent of autopsy-confirmed DLB cases meet the NINCDS-ADRDA clinical criteria for probable or possible AD, and this is the most frequent clinical misdiagnosis in DLB patients who present with a primary dementia syndrome.[41] This suggests that DLB should be routinely excluded when the diagnosis of AD is made. Up to one-third of DLB cases are additionally misclassified as VaD by the Hachinski Ischaemic Index by virtue of items such as fluctuating nature and course of illness. Pyramidal and focal neurological signs are, however, usually absent. The development of myoclonus in patients with a rapidly progressive form of DLB may lead the clinician to suspect Creutzfeldt–Jacob disease.[3]

Other causes of delirium

In patients with intermittent delirium, appropriate examination and laboratory tests should be performed during the acute phase to maximize the chances of detecting infective, metabolic, inflammatory or other aetiological factors. Pharmacological causes are particularly common in elderly patients. Although the presence of any of these features makes a diagnosis of DLB less likely, comorbidity is not unusual in elderly patients and the diagnosis should not be excluded simply on this basis.

Other neurological syndromes

In patients with a previous diagnosis of PD, the onset of visual hallucinations and fluctuating cognitive impairment may be attributed to side effects of antiparkinsonian medications, and this must be tested by dose reduction or withdrawal. Other atypical parkinsonian syndromes associated with poor levodopa response, cognitive impairment and postural instability include progressive supranuclear palsy and multisystem atrophy. Syncopal episodes in DLB are often incorrectly attributed to transient ischaemic attacks, despite an absence of focal neurological signs. Recurrent disturbances in consciousness accompanied by complex visual hallucinations may suggest complex partial seizures (temporal lobe epilepsy), and vivid dreaming with violent movements during sleep may meet criteria for REM sleep behaviour disorder. Both of these conditions have been reported as being uncommon presenting symptoms in autopsy-confirmed DLB.

Other psychiatric disorders

DLB should be considered if a patient spontaneously develops parkinsonian features or cognitive decline or shows excessive sensitivity to neuroleptic medication during the course of late-onset delusional disorder, depressive psychosis or mania.

Investigations

As with any patient who presents with cognitive impairment, a full history, mental state examination and physical examination are essential steps towards making a firm clinical diagnosis. As with suspected cases of Alzheimer's disease, the level and extent of laboratory investigations will vary according to the clinical picture, associated comorbidity and physical examination. However, the particular associations of DLB with fluctuations in attention and cognition and visual hallucinations, both of which are very commonly associated with a variety of other organic disorders, means that investigation of suspected cases of DLB requires very careful laboratory evaluation. This usually includes routine haematology and biochemistry, erythrocyte sedimentation rate or C-reactive protein, thyroid function tests, vitamin B12 and folate levels, syphilis serology and urinalysis. A chest X-ray should also be considered routine in view of the high incidence of lung carcinomas in the elderly, especially in smokers. As with the diagnosis of AD, neuroimaging investigations are often helpful both to exclude other intracranial disorders (including cerebrovascular disease) that may be responsible for the cognitive impairment and to provide supportive features for the diagnosis. Increasingly, some form of structural imaging is becoming essential to apply diagnostic criteria rigorously (e.g. the NINCDS/ADRDA criteria for AD, the NINCS-ADRDA criteria for VaD and the consensus criteria for DLB).

Structural imaging changes in DLB

Few studies have investigated computed tomography (CT) or magnetic resonance imaging (MRI) changes in DLB. In a longitudinal study of AD subjects who came to autopsy, Forstl et al.[45] reported more pronounced frontal lobe atrophy on CT in eight subjects who had Lewy body pathology at post mortem compared with pure AD cases. However, using MRI, Harvey et al.[46] found no differences in frontal lobe volumes between AD and DLB subjects, a finding replicated in a different and larger cohort by Barber et al.[47] While further studies are awaited, frontal lobe atrophy does not seem to be a particular feature of DLB. Similarly, DLB does not seem to differ from AD in terms of degree of ventricular enlargement or presence of white matter changes on MRI.[48]

The strong association between AD and atrophy of the medial temporal lobe, assessed either by a linear measurement of medial temporal lobe width on CT[49] or by visual or volumetric ratings of hippocampal atrophy on MRI,[50,51] led to an investigation of whether similar changes were associated with DLB. Jobst et al.[49] found medial temporal lobe atrophy of similar magnitude to AD in two of their four cases of DLB. However, subsequent case reports and controlled studies have shown DLB to be associated with preservation of temporal lobe structures relative to AD.[46,47,52,53] Barber et al.,[47] using visual ratings, found 38% of DLB subjects (compared with no AD subjects) had a normal rating of temporal lobe atrophy, which suggests that, at least in some cases, relative preservation of the hippocampus and medial temporal lobe may support a diagnosis of DLB. The reason for this variability in temporal lobe atrophy in DLB is unknown, although Harvey et al.,[46] using a very limited autopsy examination of four cases, suggested that temporal lobe atrophy on MRI may be a marker of concurrent AD pathology in DLB. However, although cross-sectional imaging may be helpful in some cases, it is clearly not a diagnostic marker. It remains to be determined whether accurate longitudinal assessment of regional volume change on MRI may improve accuracy of diagnosis, as may be the case for AD.[54]

In summary, the limited evidence available suggests that structural imaging in DLB reveals similar generalized atrophic changes to those seen in AD in most cases, although approximately 40% of DLB subjects show preservation of medial temporal lobe structures.

Functional imaging changes in DLB

Single photon emission computed tomography (SPECT) using blood flow markers such as technitium hexamethylpropylene amine oxime (Tc-HMPAO) has been extensively investigated in dementia. In AD the classical appearance is of posterior bilateral symmetrical temporoparietal hypoperfusion,[49,55] which contrasts with the frontal hypoperfusion that is characteristically seen in frontal lobe dementia.[56] VaD is associated with a mottled, uneven, patchy appearance that reflects the variable anatomical localization of vascular disease.[57] In PD, there is decreased blood flow in the basal ganglia; when PD is associated with dementia, biparietal changes similar to those seen in AD are reported.[58,59] Similarly, in the few SPECT studies of DLB, similar patterns of blood flow changes to AD have been found, though Donnemiller *et al.* also found a subtle difference in perfusion patterns, with a greater degree of occipital hypoperfusion in DLB than in AD.[60]

The more powerful, although still research-based, use of SPECT involves specific ligands for different neurochemical systems. Ligands have been developed for pre- and postsynaptic dopaminergic and cholinergic systems. Significant reductions in dopamine transporter activity in the nigrostriatal system have been demonstrated using a specific ligands (β- or FP-CIT) in DLB but not in AD.[60] This is what would be predicted from known neurochemical differences between the two disorders, and it may form the basis for an accurate and sensitive diagnostic marker.[61] Reduced dopamine-2 receptor density in basal ganglia using IBZM has also been reported in DLB. Using a marker of the choline transporter, significant differences between AD subjects and controls as well as between PD subjects with and without dementia have been found.[62] In summary, current evidence suggests that blood flow SPECT will show similar appearances in DLB to those seen in AD, although, as with AD, SPECT may still be useful in distinguishing DLB from frontal lobe dementia or VaD. However, new chemical imaging techniques, which are not yet clinically available, show great promise in differentiating DLB from other disorders and are an exciting area of current research.

Other investigations

A differentiated pattern of neuropsychological deficits may help to discriminate between DLB and AD patients who have been matched (as far as possible) for global severity. DLB patients perform better on tests of verbal memory but worse on visuospatial performance tasks (e.g. clock drawing and copying, block design and object assembly).[63–65] More refined computer-based tests demonstrate, in addition, the attention deficits of DLB, with poor performance on simple and choice reaction tasks and digit vigilance.[66–68]

Characteristic electroencephalographic (EEG) abnormalities have also been reported. Background posterior slowing and a frontally dominant burst pattern of slow waves were present in one series;[17] in another series, standard EEG recordings autopsy-confirmed cases of DLB showed slowing of dominant and non-dominant rhythms, with 50% of patients having temporal lobe slow wave transients (defined as episodes of θ- or δ-waves associated with sharply contoured monophasic components of less than 80 ms). These focal dysrhythmias were highly correlated with a history of episodes of loss of consciousness.[69] Similar records were seen in only 18% of an AD control group.

Treatment

Important management issues for DLB patients include:

- the issue of severe neuroleptic sensitivity reactions;
- the achievement of an optimal balance between antiparkinsonian treatment and potential exacerbation of psychiatric symptoms; and
- the possible preferential response to cholinesterase inhibitors.

Activity of the cholinergic enzyme choline acetyl transferase is lower in DLB than AD, particularly in temporal and parietal cortex.[70] Clouding of consciousness, confusion and visual hallucinations are recognized effects of anticholinergic drug toxicity, and the summative effects of subcortical and cortical cholinergic dysfunction probably play a major role in the spontaneous generation of similar fluctuating symptoms in DLB. Reductions in levels of choline acetyl transferase are correlated with severity of cognitive impairment,[71] and hallucinations may be related to hypocholinergic and (relatively) hypermonoaminergic neocortical neurotransmitter function.[70] Laevodopa responsiveness is less predictable in DLB than in Parkinson's disease.[23,69]

There have been several reports that patients who respond well to cholinesterase inhibitor treatments are more likely to be found to have DLB than AD at autopsy.[72,73] This is consistent with the neurochemical profile of DLB and the fact that postsynaptic cortical muscarinic receptors are functionally intact. Case reports suggest that cholinesterase inhibitors can reduce psychotic symptoms in DLB.[74,75] Although theoretically one might expect some worsening of parkinsonism with procholinergic therapy, this appears to be relatively mild and infrequent.[74] An early study using tacrine in severely impaired Parkinson's disease patients with dementia and psychosis found very significant motor improvements in addition to large improvements in hallucinations and Mini Mental State Examination scores.[76] The precise role of cholinergic drugs in the management of DLB needs to be properly established in extensive clinical trials and also further explored in the clinic.

The most important practical point in the management of a patient with DLB is caution in (or preferably avoidance of) the use of neuroleptic medications, which are the mainstay of antipsychotic treatment in other patient groups.[15,77] Severe neuroleptic sensitivity reactions can precipitate irreversible parkinsonism, further impair consciousness level and induce autonomic disturbances reminiscent of neuroleptic malignant syndrome. They occur in 40–50% of DLB patients who are treated with neuroleptic agents and are associated with a two- or three-fold increase in mortality.[21,28] Acute dopamine-2 receptor blockade is thought to mediate these effects, and despite some promising initial reports, atypical and novel antipsychotic agents such as risperidone[78] and olanzapine[79] seem to be about as likely to cause neuroleptic sensitivity reactions as older drugs. There are undeniably situations in which a trial of neuroleptic medication is unavoidable – to try and relieve distressing psychotic symptoms or to reduce agitation and aggression. Hospital admission during dose titration would seem a safe precaution in a patient who has previously been diagnosed with DLB. Regular records of motor, cognitive and neuropsychiatric state by experienced personnel should detect the earliest signs of neuroleptic sensitivity reactions, which should in turn prompt drug withdrawal.[77] Patients with prominent nocturnal hallucinations and behavioural disturbance may be experiencing REM sleep behaviour disorder and may respond to a small dose of clonazepam at bedtime.

Until safe and effective medications become available, there is no doubt that the mainstay of clinical management is to educate patients and caregivers about the nature of their symptoms and to suggest strategies to cope with them. For example, one patient with disturbing visual hallucinations of dogs in her house found that they disappeared when she went to pat them! Psychotic and confusional symptoms are both made worse by understimulation, reflecting a fundamental problem in spontaneously maintaining an adequate level of consciousness. This may be one of the reasons that fluctuation and hallucinations are seldom seen during the clinical interview (which, it is hoped, is a stimulating environment) even when they are reported to occur regularly at home. An active, reality orientation type of approach may be particularly productive in DLB, the aim being to use external stimulation and cueing to maintain the patient's level of alertness within an acceptable range. This suggestion remains to be tested in a formal study, and caregivers should equally be advised against excessive stimulation, which is likely to be counterproductive.

Conclusion

DLB now appears to be established as a common cause of dementia in old age. Comorbid Alzheimer-type and vascular pathological changes are frequently seen in these cases and their precise temporal and aetiological relationships remain to be established. The second DLB International Workshop[80] met in July 1998 to review developments since publication of consensus guidelines for the clinical and pathological diagnosis of DLB. It concluded that antiubiquitin immunocytochemistry is the method of choice for routine detection of Lewy bodies for diagnostic purposes in research and clinical practice. The use of α-synuclein antibodies to label Lewy bodies represents a major methodological advance, which is likely to be most useful in research laboratories, particularly for clinicopathological correlative studies. The consensus clinical diagnostic criteria should continue to be used in their current format, and they need to be further validated with research efforts focused on increasing sensitivity of case detection. There is now a pressing need to establish appropriately designed, randomized, controlled trials in DLB. Collaboration between dementia and movement disorder specialists will be essential for rapid progress in research and clinical protocols.

References

1. Lennox G, Lowe J, Landon M, Byrne EJ, Mayer RJ, Godwin-Austen RB. Diffuse Lewy body disease: correlative neuropathology using anti-ubiquitin immunocytochemistry. J Neurol Neurosurg Psychiatry 1989;52:1236–1247.

2. Kosaka K, Yoshimura M, Ikeda K, Budka H. Diffuse type of Lewy body disease: progressive dementia with abundant cortical Lewy bodies and senile changes of varying degree: a new disease? Clin Neuropathol 1984;3;185–192.

3. McKeith IG, Galasko D, Kosaka K, et al. Consensus guidelines for the clinical and pathologic diagnosis of dementia with Lewy bodies (DLB): report of the consortium on DLB international workshop. Neurology 1996;47:1113–1124.

4. Lowe JS, Mayer RJ, Landon M. Pathological significance of Lewy bodies in dementia. In: Perry R, McKeith I, Perry E, eds. Dementia with Lewy bodies. New York: Cambridge University Press; 1996:195–203.

5. Perry RH, Irving D, Blessed G, Fairbairn A, Perry EK. Senile dementia of Lewy body type. A clinically and neuropathologically distinct form of Lewy body dementia in the elderly. J Neurol Sci 1990;95:119–139.

6. Hansen L, Salmon D, Galasko D, et al. The Lewy body variant of Alzheimer's disease: a clinical and pathologic entity. Neurology 1990;40:1–8.

7. Holmes C, Cairns N, Lantos P, Mann A. Validity of current clinical criteria for Alzheimer's disease, vascular dementia and dementia with Lewy bodies. Br J Psychiatry 1999;174:45–51.

8. McShane R, Gedling K, Reading M, McDonald B, Esiri MM, Hope T. Prospective study of relations between cortical Lewy bodies, poor eyesight, and hallucinations in Alzheimer's disease. J Neurol Neurosurg Psychiatry 1995;59:185–188.

9. Byrne EJ, Lennox G, Godwin-Austen RB, et al. Dementia associated with cortical Lewy bodies. Proposed diagnostic criteria. Dementia 1991;2:283–284.

10. Kuzuhara S, Yoshimura M. Clinical and neuropathological aspects of diffuse Lewy body disease in the elderly. Adv Neurol 1993;60:464–469.

11. Louis ED, Klatka LA, Liu Y, Fahn S. Comparison of extrapyramidal

features in 31 pathologically confirmed cases of diffuse Lewy body disease and 34 pathologically confirmed cases of Parkinson's disease. Neurology 1997; 48:376–380.

12. McKeith IG, Galasko D, Wilcock GK, Byrne EJ. Lewy body dementia: diagnosis and treatment. Br J Psychiatry 1995;167:709–717.

13. Schultz DW, Lennox GG, Ironside JW, Warlow CP. Behavioural disturbance and visual hallucinations in a 78 year old man. J Neurol Neurosurg Psychiatry 1998;65: 933–938.

14. Scully RE, Mark EJ, McNeely WF, Ebeling SH, Philips LD. Case records of the Massachusetts General Hospital. N Engl J Med 1998;338:603–610.

15. Harrison RH, McKeith IG. Senile dementia of Lewy body type: a review of clinical and pathological features: implications for treatment. Int J Geriatr Psychiatry 1995;10:919–926.

16. Okazaki H, Lipton LS, Aronson SM. Diffuse intracytoplasmic ganglionic inclusions (Lewy type) associated with progressive dementia and quadrapesis in flexion. J Neurol Neurosurg Psychiatry 1961;20:237–244.

17. Burkhardt CR, Filley CM, Kleinschmidt-DeMasters BK, de la Monte S, Norenberg MD, Schneck SA. Diffuse Lewy body disease and progressive dementia. Neurology 1988;38:1520–1528.

18. Crystal HA, Dickson DW, Lizardi JE, Davies P, Wolfson LI. Antemortem diagnosis of diffuse Lewy body disease. Neurology 1990; 40:1523–1528.

19. Hansen LA, Galasko D. Lewy body disease. Curr Opin Neurol Neurosurg 1992;5:889–894.

20. McKeith IG, Perry RH, Fairbairn AF, Jabeen S, Perry EK. Operational criteria for senile dementia of Lewy body type (SDLT). Psychol Med 1992;22:911–922.

21. McKeith I, Fairbairn A, Perry R, Thompson P, Perry E. Neuroleptic sensitivity in patients with senile dementia of Lewy body type. BMJ 1992;305:673–678.

22. Papka M, Rubio A, Schiffer RB. A review of Lewy body disease, an emerging concept of cortical dementia. J Neuropsychiatry Clin Neurosci 1998;10:267–279.

23. Armstrong TP, Hansen LA, Salmon DP, et al. Rapidly progressive dementia in a patient with the Lewy body variant of Alzheimer's disease. Neurology 1991;41:1178–1180.

24. Boeve BF. REM sleep behaviour disorder and degenerative dementia: an association likely reflecting Lewy body disease. Neurology 1998;51:363–370.

25. McKeith IG. Dementia with Lewy bodies: clinical and pathological diagnosis. Alzheimer Rep 1998; 1:83–87.

26. Klatka LA, Louis ED, Schiffer RB. Psychiatric features in diffuse Lewy body disease: findings in 28 pathologically diagnosed cases. Neurology 1996;47:1148–1152.

27. Richards M, Stern Y, Mayeaux R. Subtle extrapyramidal signs can predict the development of dementia in elderly individuals. Neurology 1993;43:2184–2188.

28. Imamura T, Hirono N, Hashimoto M, et al. Clinical diagnosis of dementia with Lewy bodies in a Japanese dementia registry. Dementia 1999;10:210–216.

29. Lewy FH. Paralysis agitans. I. Pathologische anatomie. In: Lewandowsky M, ed. Handbuch der Neurologie, vol 3. Berlin: Springer; 1912:920–933.

30. Spillantini MG, Schmidt ML, Lee VMY, Trojanowski JQ, Jakes R, Goedert M. α-Synuclein in Lewy bodies. Nature 1997;388:839–840.

31. Trojanowski JQ. Dementia with Lewy bodies: histopathological aspects of differential diagnosis. Neurobiol Aging 1998;4S:S4.

32. Harding AJ, Halliday GM. Simplified neuropathological diagnosis of dementia with Lewy bodies. Neuropathol Appl Neurobiol 1998;24:195–201.

33. McKenzie JE, Edwards RJ, Gentleman SM, Ince PG, Royston MC, Roberts GW. A quantitative comparison of plaque types in Alzheimer's disease and senile dementia of Lewy body type. Acta Neuropathol 1996;91:526–529.

34. Harrington CR, Perry RH, Perry EK, *et al.* Senile dementia of Lewy body type and Alzheimer type are biochemically distinct in terms of paired helical filaments and hyperphosphorylated tau protein. Dementia 1994;5:215–228.

35. Hansen LA, Masliah E, Galasko D, Terry RD. Plaque-only Alzheimer disease is usually the Lewy body variant, and vice versa. J Neuropathol Exp Neurol 1993;52:648–654.

36. Perry RH, Irving D, Blessed G, Fairbairn A, Perry EK. Senile dementia of Lewy body type. A clinically and neuropathologically distinct form of Lewy body dementia in the elderly. J Neurol Sci 1990;95:119–139.

37. Ball M, Braak H, Coleman P, Dickson D, *et al.* Consensus recommendations for the postmortem diagnosis of Alzheimer's disease. Neurobiol Aging 1997;18(suppl 4): 51–52.

38. Samuel W, Alford M, Hofstetter CR, Hansen L. Dementia with Lewy bodies versus pure Alzheimer's disease: differences in cognition, neuropathology, cholinergic dysfunction, and synapse density. J Neuropathol Exp Neurol 1997;56:499–508.

39. Perry EK, Marshall E, Kerwin J, *et al.* Evidence of a monoaminergic-cholinergic imbalance related to visual hallucinations in Lewy body dementia. J Neurochem 1990; 55:1454–1456.

40. Hulette C, Mirra S, Wilkinson W, *et al.* The Consortium to Establish a Registry for Alzheimer's Disease (CERAD). Part IX. A prospective cliniconeuropathologic study of Parkinson's features in Alzheimer's disease. Neurology 1995;45:1991–1995.

41. McKeith IG, Fairbairn AF, Perry RH, Thompson P. The clinical diagnosis and misdiagnosis of senile dementia of Lewy body type (SDLT). Br J Psychiatry 1994;165:324–332.

42. Mega MS, Masterman DL, Benson F, *et al.* Dementia with Lewy bodies: reliability and validity of clinical and pathologic criteria. Neurology 1996;47:1403–1409.

43. Luis CA, Barker WW, Gajara K, *et al.* Sensitivity and specificity of three clinical criteria for dementia with Lewy bodies in an autopsy-verified sample. Int J Geriatr Psychiatry 1999;14:526–533.

44. McKeith IG, Ballard CG, Perry RH, *et al.* Prospective validation of concensus criteria for the diagnosis of dementia with Lewy bodies. Neurology 2000;54:1050–1058.

45. Forstl H, Burns A, Luthert P, *et al.* The Lewy body variant of Alzheimer's disease: clinical and pathological findings. Br J Psychiatry 1993;162:385–392.

46 Harvey GT, O'Brien JT, Hughes J, *et al.* Magnetic resonance imaging differences between dementia with Lewy bodies and Alzheimer's disease. Psychol Med 1999;29: 181–187.

47. Barber R, Gholkar A, Scheltens P, *et al.* Medial temporal lobe atrophy on MRI in dementia with Lewy bodies. Neurology 1999;52: 1153–1158.

48. Barber R, Gholkar A, Ballard C, *et al.* White matter lesions on MRI in dementia with Lewy bodies, Alzheimer's disease, Vascular dementia and normal ageing, J Neurol Neurosurg Psychiatry 1999;67:66–72.

49. Jobst KA, Barnetson LPD, Shepstone BJ. Accurate prediction of confirmed Alzheimer's disease and the differential diagnosis of dementia: the use of NINCDS-ADRDA and DSM IIIR criteria, SPET, X-ray CT and ApoE4 in medial temporal lobe dementias. Int Psychogeriatr 1998;10:271–302.

50. Jack CR Jr, Petersen RC, O'Brien PC, *et al.* MR-based hippocampal volumetry in the diagnosis of Alzheimer's disease. Neurology 1992;42:183–188.

51. O'Brien JT, Desmond P, Ames D, Schweitzer I, Chiu E, Tress B. Temporal lobe magnetic resonance imaging can differentiate Alzheimer's disease from normal ageing, depression, vascular dementia and other causes of cognitive impairment. Psychol Med 1997;27:1267–1275.

52. Robles A, Rodriguez RM, Aldrey JM, *et al.* Diagnostico clinico de la demencia asociada a cuerpos de Lewy corticales. Rev Neurol (Barc) 1995;23:62–66.

53. Hashimoto M, Kitagaki H, Imamura T, *et al.* Medical temporal and whole-brain atrophy in dementia with Lewy bodies: a volumetric MRI study. Neurology 1998;51:357–362.

54. Fox MC, Freeborough PA, Rossor MN. Visualisation and quantification of rates of atrophy in Alzheimer's disease. Lancet 1996;348:94–97.

55. O'Brien JT, Eagger S, Syed GS, Sahakian BJ, Levy R. A study of regional cerebral blood flow and cognitive performance in Alzheimer's disease. J Neurol Neurosurg Psychiatry 1992;55:1182–1187.

56. Neary D, Snowden JS, Shields RA, *et al.* Single photon emission tomography using 99mTc-HMPAO in the investigation of dementia. J Neurol Neurosurg Psychiatry 1987;50:101–109.

57. Read SL, Miller BL, Mena I, Kim R, Itabashi H, Darby A. SPECT in dementia: clinical and pathological correlation. J Am Geriatr Soc 1995;43:1243–1247.

58. Pizzolato G, Dam M, Borsato N, *et al.* [99mTc]-HM-PAO SPECT in Parkinson's disease. J Cerebr Blood Flow Metab 1988;8:S101–S108.

59. Habert MO, Spampinato U, Mas JL, *et al.* A comparative technetium 99m hexamethylpropylene amine oxime SPET study in different types of dementia. Eur J Nucl Med 1991;18:3–11.

60. Donnemiller E, Heilmann J, Wenning GK, *et al.* Brain perfusion scintigraphy with 99mTc-HMPAO or 99mTc-ECD and 123I-beta-CIT single-photon emission tomography in dementia of the Alzheimer-type and diffuse Lewy body disease. Eur J Nucl Med 1997;24:320–325.

61. Walker Z, Costa DC, Ince P, McKeith IG, Katona CLE. In vivo demonstration of dopaminergic degeneration in dementia with Lewy bodies. Lancet 1999; 354:646–647.

62. Walker Z, Costa DC, Janssen AG, Walker RW, Livingstone G, Katona CL. Dementia with Lewy bodies: a study of post-synaptic dopaminergic receptors with iodine-123 iodobenzamide single-photon emission tomography. Eur J Nucl Med 1997;24:609–614.

63. Salmon D, Galasko D. Neuropsychological aspects of Lewy body dementia. In: Perry R, McKeith I,

Perry E, eds, Dementia with Lewy bodies. New York: Cambridge University Press; 1996:99–114.

64. Gnanalingham KK, Byrne EJ, Thornton A, Sambrook MA, Bannister P. Motor and cognitive function in Lewy body dementia: comparison with Alzheimer's and Parkinson's diseases. J Neurol Neurosurg Psychiatry 1997;62: 243–252.

65. Shimomura T, Mori E, Yamashita H, *et al*. Cognitive loss in dementia with Lewy bodies and Alzheimer disease. Arch Neurol 1998;55:1547–1552.

66. Sahgal A, Galloway PH, McKeith IG, Edwardson JA, Lloyd S. A comparative study of attentional deficits in senile dementias of Alzheimer and Lewy body types. Dementia 1992;3:350–354.

67. Sahgal A, McKeith IG, Galloway PH, Tasker N, Steckler T. Do differences in visuospatial ability between senile dementias of the Alzheimer and Lewy body types reflect differences solely in mnemonic function. J Clin Exp Neuropsychol 1995;17:35–43.

68. Ayre GA, Sahgal A, McKeith IG, *et al*. Distinct profiles of cognitive impairment in dementia with Lewy bodies and Alzheimer's disease. Neurology 1999; in press.

69. Briel R. EEG findings in dementia with Lewy bodies and Alzheimer's disease. J Neurol Neurosurg Psychiatry 1999;66:401–403.

70. Perry EK, Marshall E, Kerwin J, *et al*. Evidence of a monoaminergic–cholinergic imbalance related to visual hallucinations in Lewy body dementia. J Neurochem 1990;55:1454–1456.

71. Samuel W, Alford M, Hofstetter CR, Hansen L. Dementia with Lewy bodies versus pure Alzheimer's disease: differences in cognition, neuropathology, cholinergic dysfunction, and synapse density. J Neuropathol Exp Neurol 1997;56:499–508.

72. Levy R, Eagger S, Griffiths M, *et al*. Lewy bodies and response to tacrine in Alzheimer's disease. Lancet 1994;343:176.

73. Wilcock GK, Scott MI. Tacrine for senile dementia of Alzheimer's or Lewy body type. Lancet 1994; 344:544.

74. Shea C, Macknight C, Rockwood R. Donepezil for treatment of dementia with Lewy bodies: a case series of nine patients. Int Psychogeriatr 1998;10:229–239.

75. Kaufer DI, Catt KE, Lopez EI, DeKosky ST. Dementia with Lewy bodies: response of delirium like features to donepezil. Neurology 1998;51:1512.

76. Hutchinson M, Fazzini E. Cholinesterase inhibitors in Parkinson's disease (letter). J Neurol Neurosurg Psychiatry 1996;61:324–325.

77. McKeith IG, Fairbairn AF, Harrison R. Management of the noncognitive symptoms of Lewy body dementia. In: Perry R, McKeith I, Perry E, eds. Dementia with Lewy bodies. New York: Cambridge University Press; 1996: 381–396.

78. McKeith IG, Ballard CG, Harrison RWS. Neuroleptic sensitivity to risperidone in Lewy body dementia. Lancet 1995;346:699.

79. Walker Z, Grace J, Overshot R, *et al*. Olanzapine in dementia with Lewy bodies: a clinical overview. Int J Geriatr Psychiatry 1999;14: 459–466.

80. McKeith IG, Perry EK, Perry RH for the Consortium on DLB. Report of the Second Dementia with Lewy Body International Workshop: Consortium on Dementia with Lewy Bodies. Neurology 1999;53:902–905.

4
Parkinsonism with dementia

Irene Litvan

Introduction

The study of parkinsonism with dementia is of increasing scientific interest because it helps to delineate the less well-known cognitive and behavioral roles of the basal ganglia. Disorders of the basal ganglia may interrupt, in addition to motor circuits, as many as three of the five fronto-subcortical circuits that unite regions of the frontal lobe with the striatum, globus pallidus and thalamus and that mediate cognition, motivation and behavior.[1-3] Involvement of the dorsolateral frontal circuit is manifest by:

- impaired execution of sequential actions;
- impaired shifting between tasks;
- concreteness in thinking;
- difficulty in retrieving information; and
- decreased verbal fluency.

Orbitofrontal circuitry dysfunction may be manifest as:

- depression; or
- behaviors that depend more on environmental stimuli than on the patient's own internal mental state.

Involvement of the mediofrontal circuit may be manifest as:

- apathy; or
- disturbances in attention.

Because the different basal ganglia disorders affect each of these circuits differently, it is not surprising that the cognitive and behavioral disturbances vary in different disorders and may precede or follow the development of parkinsonism. Moreover, whereas the diagnosis of parkinsonism (bradykinesia or hypokinesia associated with rigidity or tremor) is not influenced by the presence of dementia, the diagnosis of dementia in a patient with parkinsonism may, at times, be challenging. This is particularly true if one uses the definition of dementia outlined by the *Diagnostic and Statistical Manual of Mental Disorders* (DSM),[4] which requires a link between a patient's cognitive impairment and an inability to pursue social and work-related obligations, since it may be difficult to determine if such inability is related to motor disturbances, dementia or both. In addition, executive dysfunction – a critical disturbance observed in parkinsonism with dementia syndromes caused by disruption of dorsolateral frontal circuits – is not considered to be one of the multiple cognitive deficits required to define dementia in the DSM-IIIR criteria. Fortunately, this issue has been resolved in DSM-IV.[4]

Another methodologic issue to consider when diagnosing dementia in patients with parkinsonism is the tools that are used to assess cognition. Neuropsychological testing is usually more sensitive than bedside testing or clinical impressions in defining a patient's dementia, but the battery of such tests should be chosen carefully because patients with parkinsonism may be unduly penalized in timed tests. On the other hand, neurologists tend to minimize the motor problems of patients with dementia, which either delays the diagnosis of the various parkinsonism with dementia syndromes or means that they are not diagnosed appropriately.

In addition to problems in defining dementia in individual patients, different studies have used a variety of case ascertainment methods (prospective, retrospective, longitudinal, cross-sectional, hospital-based or community-based) to evaluate parkinsonism with dementia, which explains the difference in estimated figures.[5–9]

Nevertheless, an effort to make an early and accurate nosological diagnosis is necessary because complications, management and survival vary in the different parkinsonism with dementia disorders (Table 4.1).[10] It is particularly important to exclude treatable causes such as those induced by drugs, infections, vascular disorders, or tumors. A good history rules out drug-induced parkinsonism in patients with dementia (e.g. caused by neuroleptic agents) or drug-induced cognitive disturbances in those with parkinsonism (e.g. caused by anticholinergic agents). Similarly, ancillary tests (e.g. neuroradiological or cerebrospinal studies) help to diagnose infectious, vascular or tumoral causes when these are suspected from the history or physical examination.

Because there are at present no biological markers that can distinguish the different neurodegenerative dementia with parkinsonism disorders, the accurate diagnosis of these disorders may, at times, be a considerable task. Although there are no current treatments that can slow or stop the progression of these neurodegenerative disorders, an early and correct nosological diagnosis allows physicians to provide the appropriate care and to estimate their patients' survival. This chapter focuses on neurodegenerative parkinsonism with dementia disorders and reviews both clinicopathological and clinical studies while acknowledging that clinicopathological studies may include atypical cases and that cross-sectional clinical studies may include inaccurately diagnosed patients.

Table 4.1 Etiologies of parkinsonism with dementia syndromes.

Neurodegenerative disorders
Tauopathies (e.g. PSP, Pick's disease)
Synucleinopathies (e.g. PD, dementia with Lewy bodies)
Drug-induced
(e.g. combination of drugs, anticholinergics in patients with PD, dopamine
receptor blockers in patients with AD)
Infectious
(e.g. Whipple's disease, Creutzfeldt–Jakob disease, human immunodeficiency
virus infection)
Vascular
(e.g. multi-infarct, lacunar infarct)
Toxic
(e.g. Wilson's disease, manganese toxicity)
Tumor
(e.g. primary or secondary or chronic subdural hematomas)
Normopressure hydrocephalus
Post-traumatic
(e.g. dementia pugilistica)

The neurodegenerative disorders that include parkinsonism with
dementia can be broadly classified as tauopathies and synucleinopathies on the basis of the abnormal aggregation of proteins found in
the neuropathological lesions that characterize them (Table 4.2).[11]
Recent research has substantially advanced our understanding of the
tauopathies and synucleinopathies and provides the opportunity to
develop transgenic mouse models, which (it is hoped) will accelerate the
discovery of more effective therapies.[12]

Tauopathies

Tauopathies are disorders that exhibit an abnormal phosphorylated tau,
usually expressed as:

- neurofibrillary tangles (NFTs);
- neuropil threads; or
- abnormal tau filaments (e.g. Pick bodies).

These disorders can be grouped according to the pattern of tau bands
and their isoform composition. The normal brain has six tau isoforms,
generated by alternative mRNA splicing of the tau gene. These isoforms
differ by the presence or absence of one or two terminal inserts and by
the presence of three or four microtubule-binding repeats in the C-termi-
nal region.[13] The presence of three or four repeats depends on whether

Table 4.2 Tauopathies with parkinsonism and dementia

Disorder	Clinical and radiological presentation
Progressive supranuclear palsy	Progressive history of postural instability with falls, axial parkinsonism, pseudobulbar palsy, supranuclear gaze palsy, executive dysfunction (e.g. decreased fluency, difficulty in shifting concepts, planning or sequencing) or behavioral disturbances (e.g. apathy, less frequently disinhibition), bradyphrenia with or without mild memory or visuospatial dysfunction. Cognitive or behavioral disturbances may present at symptom onset. CT or MRI may show mid-brain atrophy and periaqueductal hyperintensities in the mid-brain. PET with fluorodeoxyglucose shows frontal hypometabolism
Corticobasal degeneration	Progressive lateralized cognitive disturbances (e.g. ideomotor apraxia, alien hand syndrome, aphasia, sensory or visual neglect) in a patient with progressive focal motor dysfunction (e.g. dystonia, parkinsonism, myoclonus). Cognitive or behavioral disturbances occur frequently at symptom onset. CT or MRI usually shows asymmetric frontal or parietal atrophy (wide sulci), focal hyperintensities in frontal, temporal, and/or parietal lobes and in corpus callosum. PET with fluorodeoxyglucose shows frontal, parietal or basal ganglia asymmetrical hypometabolism
Pick's disease	Progressive severe frontal lobe behavioral features (disinhibition, impulsivity, social misconduct, social unawareness, hyperphagia) and cognitive features (difficulty planning and sequencing, echolalia, aphasia). Parkinsonism usually develops at later stages. CT or MRI may show severe frontal or temporal atrophy. PET with fluorodeoxyglucose shows frontal hypometabolism
Alzheimer's disease	Progressive anterograde memory deficits, with eventual language, visual or praxis deficits in the absence of other disorders that could justify these features including delirium. Parkinsonism may occur at later stages. CT or MRI may show cortical or hippocampi atrophy. PET with fluorodeoxyglucose shows parietotemporal hypometabolism

CT, computerized tomography; MRI, magnetic resonance imaging; PET, positron emission tomography.

exon 10 is spliced out or in.[13] In Pick's disease there are three isoforms without exon 10, and in progressive supranuclear palsy (PSP) and corticobasal degeneration (CBD) there are four repeats with exon 10 isoforms. In Alzheimer's disease (AD), however, all six isoforms are present. Accordingly, the tau parkinsonism–dementia syndromes can be divided into three major groups according to the deposition of tau bands:

- those with the 64, 68 and 72 kDa tau bands include PSP, CBD and the familial multiple system tauopathy with presenile dementia, a form of frontotemporal dementia with parkinsonism that is associated with chromosome-17 (FTDP-17);
- those with tau bands of 60 and 64 kDa make up Pick's disease; and
- those in which the 60, 64 and 68 kDa tau bands and a minor band of 72 kDa tau band are observed include AD, Lytico–Bodig disease (previously called parkinsonism–dementia complex of Guam), Niemann–Pick disease type C and Gerstmann-Sträussler–Scheinker disease with tangles.

At an early stage some of these disorders manifest mainly as dementia (e.g. AD and Pick's disease), mainly as parkinsonism (e.g. Parkinson's disease (PD)) or as both (e.g. PSP, dementia with Lewy bodies or FTDP-17). However, at later stages, dementia and parkinsonism are usually apparent.

Progressive supranuclear palsy

Most PSP patients develop marked cognitive deficits and personality changes suggestive of frontal lobe dysfunction, leading to the concept of 'subcortical dementia.'[14] Although PSP patients develop early frontal lobe-type disturbances, in less than 10% of cases do these constitute the first symptoms.[15] These cognitive changes may be severe enough to warrant the diagnosis of dementia in 60% of cases 3 years after symptom onset.[16,17] Pillon et al.[17] found that cognitive deficits in PSP consistently progress and that executive functions are the most severely affected. Executive dysfunction and slowed information processing appear early, are relatively severe and help to differentiate PSP from other dementias.[18–24] Attention and memory, although also impaired, are less severely affected.[25,26]

PSP patients also exhibit severe behavioral symptoms.[27,28] A study of 34 PSP patients showed that the majority suffered from continuous apathy (mostly in the moderate to severe range) and that one-third exhibited moderate to severe disinhibition.[28] However, in contrast to what has been reported in PD, depression was infrequent (18%) and mostly mild.

From a neuropsychiatric point of view, PSP can be differentiated from dementia with Lewy bodies because hallucinations and delusions are very unusual (they have not been reported in any autopsy-confirmed PSP

Table 4.3 Clinical features of main parkinsonism with dementia disorders.

Characteristics	Tauopathies			Synucleinopathies	
	Progressive supranuclear palsy	Corticobasal degeneration	Alzheimer's disease	Parkinson disease	Dementia with Lewy bodies
Progession	Rapid	Rapid	Rapid	Slow	Rapid
Parkinsonism	Symmetric/Axial	Asymmetric/Distal	Late/Symmetric	Asymmetric/Distal	Symmetric/Distal
Levodopa response	Initial?⇒Absent	Absent	Absent	Moderate/Excellent	Minimal/Moderate
Cognitive disturbances*	Frontal (Severe)	Lateralized**	Cortical	Frontal⇒Cortical	Cortical
Psychiatric disturbances	Apathy	Depression	Depression, late psychotic features	Depression	Hallucinations
Myoclonus	Absent	Present	Late/Infrequent	Absent	Present
Dystonia	Axial (retrocollis)	Asymmetric/Limbs	Absent	Absent	Absent
Contracture*	Late	Present	Absent	Absent	Absent
Postural Instability	Initial	Present (late usually)	Absent	Absent	Present
Saccades latency	Normal	Impaired	Normal	Normal	Normal?
Saccades speed	Slow vert.⇒horiz.	Normal	Normal	Normal	Normal
Pyramidal signs	Late (Bilateral)	Unilateral⇒Bilateral	Absent	Absent	Late (Bilateral)
Cerebellar signs	Absent	Absent	Absent	Absent	Absent
Dysautonomia	Absent	Absent	Absent	Late	Present (Mild)
Gait	Ataxic	Apraxic/small-step	Late disturbances	Small-step	Small-step

*Not related to treatment

study). PSP can be differentiated from AD because language abnormalities, except for verbal adynamia (severely decreased active language initiation and search) have not been reported in any PSP autopsy-confirmed study (Table 4.3).[29] PSP can also be distinguished from CBD because PSP patients do not exhibit focal or lateralized cognitive features (e.g. visual or sensory neglect, alien limb syndrome, aphasia). PSP patients may exhibit use of body parts when ideomotor praxis is tested for, but moderate to severe ideomotor apraxia or other focal abnormalities are infrequent in autopsy-confirmed patients.[30,31] In addition to bedside testing and interviews, neuropsychological tests may provide additional quantitative information to support the diagnosis of PSP and to exclude these other disorders.

PSP patients usually present with early postural instability and falls, and they eventually develop a peculiar, wide-based, slow and unsteady gait.[32] The parkinsonism in PSP is characterized by the presence of axial involvement more than limb involvement, symmetrical limb involvement and a lack of response to levodopa therapy. Patients with PSP usually develop early dysarthria and dysphagia, but what defines and allows us to make the diagnosis of this disease is the presence of supranuclear vertical gaze palsy, which is later followed by horizontal gaze abnormalities. This disorder is a good example of impairment of the five frontal–subcortical circuits, although prefrontal, frontal, hippocampal and brainstem lesions contribute to the features.[33]

Corticobasal degeneration

CBD can present at onset with focal motor or cognitive problems or, rarely, with bilateral parkinsonism and global cognitive disturbances (see Table 4.2).[32,34,35] Eventually patients with CBD may develop multiple cognitive deficits and memory deficits and develop full-blown dementia with cortical features (e.g. aphasia, ideomotor or ideatory apraxia, sensory cortical deficits) as well as frontal deficits.[32] However, dementia is infrequent at symptom onset in CBD and, when dementia does occur, the disorder is rarely diagnosed as such.[35]

As a result of the involvement in CBD of the frontal and parietal cortical areas, these patients may present with ideomotor and ideatory apraxis, alien hand syndrome, aphasia, marked cortical sensory dysfunction or hemispatial deficits.[36–43] However, frontal deficits in CBD are not as severe as those found in PSP.[39] Since none of the neurodegenerative disorders, except for Pick's disease, usually present with lateralized cognitive features, a progressive lateralized cognitive dysfunction, particularly in a patient with asymmetrical onset of motor extrapyramidal disturbances, is highly suggestive of CBD (see Table 4.2) and helps to differentiate it from PD and PSP.[42] CBD is frequently misdiagnosed as PSP,[42] but diagnostic accuracy may improve if one considers that PSP patients do not develop focal cognitive disturbances and usually have bilateral and symmetrical motor involvement. However, PSP patients infrequently present asymmetrical motor findings and limb levitation, making it almost impossible to differentiate PSP from CBD.[35,44] In addition, the oculomotor disturbances usually differ (e.g. whereas CBD patients have difficulty initiating horizontal and vertical saccades, PSP patients develop slowed vertical saccades but normal saccade latency (see Table 4.3)).[45] In fact, a recent clinicopathological study that retrospectively examined the clinical features of 51 patients who had been pathologically diagnosed with PSP or CBD, identified two sets of predictors (models) for CBD patients using logistic regression analysis. One set consisted of asymmetric parkinsonism, cognitive disturbances at onset and instability and falls at first clinic visit; the other set consisted of asymmetric parkinsonism, cognitive disturbances at symptom onset and speech disturbances. In contrast, PSP patients often had severe postural instability at onset, symmetric parkinsonism, vertical supranuclear gaze palsy, speech disorders and frontal lobe-type features. CBD patients who presented with an alternate phenotype characterized by early severe frontal dementia and bilateral parkinsonism were generally misdiagnosed.[32]

When CBD patients present with a progressive aphasia they are difficult to differentiate from those with Pick's disease, although CBD patients do not usually exhibit the severe behavioral disturbances Pick's disease patients do.[46] Frontotemporal dementias associated with abnormalities in chromosome 17 may manifest clinically as CBD.[47,48] A P301S mutation in exon 10 of the tau gene may appear in affected patients as frontotemporal dementia or as CBD, demonstrating that the same primary gene defect in tau can lead to two distinct clinical phenotypes.[48] Although family history may help to differentiate these two disorders, it is a challenge to differentiate the frontoparietal focal form of AD from CBD.[49,50] Accurate diagnosis is difficult since the constellation of clinical features that is considered characteristic of CBD (e.g. asymmetric motor features, including parkinsonism, dystonia, myoclonus and asymmetric focal cognitive impairment such as aphasia and apraxia) may be associated with heterogeneous pathologies, which may present with asymmetric frontoparietal cortical degeneration.

Pick's disease

Classically, Pick's disease is characterized by the presence of early personality changes, deterioration of social skills, prominent language abnormalities with initial preservation of memory and praxis, and later presentation of parkinsonism (see Table 4.2).[51] Pick's disease is underdiagnosed[52] but diagnostic accuracy improves with the use of the Lund and Manchester diagnostic criteria, which have been found to be reliable and accurate.[53] It is more challenging to make the diagnosis of Pick's disease when patients present with early memory disturbances.[52,54,55] Memory disturbances in Pick's disease may be due to both frontal and hippocampal involvement. On the other hand, a diagnosis of Pick's disease should be seriously considered when patients present with striking personality changes at symptom onset such as disinhibition, euphoria, apathy, aberrant motor behavior or inappropriate social behavior.[56] However, the frontal dementia syndrome needed to diagnose Pick's disease is nonspecific, since many disorders (such as PSP, dementia with Lewy bodies and CBD) cause a frontal dementia syndrome. Nonetheless, the frontal dementia syndrome in most of these disorders is less severe at onset or presents at later stages of the disease. However, occasionally PSP patients also present with cognitive and behavioral disturbances, including florid frontal symptomatology, but PSP patients do not usually exhibit euphoria or aphasia, which are features usually associated with Pick's disease.[27,56]

Alzheimer's disease

AD may present not only cognitive but also extrapyramidal symptomatology (see Table 4.2). However, the extrapyramidal symptomatology characterized by parkinsonism usually develops at a later stage. There are difficulties in differentiating AD from dementia with Lewy bodies (see Table 4.3),[57,58] particularly because both disorders are frequently associated, but also because dementia with Lewy bodies may present without parkinsonism. When Lewy bodies are the main pathology, clinicopathological studies show that early hallucinations and delusions unrelated to medications are suggestive of dementia with Lewy bodies, features that usually develop at a later stage in AD. In addition, whereas the earliest cognitive feature in PD with dementia is a frontal dysfunction, in AD it is amnesia; thus, at early stages these disorders may be differentiated.[59] Such differentiation is important for care management as well as for prognosis.

A recent study[53] evaluated the inter-rater reliability and validity of clinical diagnostic criteria for AD, PSP and frontotemporal lobe dementia in a mixed sample of patients with cortical and subcortical neurodegenerative processes. Four experienced clinicians who reviewed first-visit clinical data abstracted form the records of 40 pathologically diagnosed demented subjects, applying the NINCDS-ADRDA criteria for AD and the Consensus Guidelines for the Clinical Diagnosis of Dementia with Lewy Bodies, found that the reliability to diagnose AD was substantial ($\kappa = 0.73$) while that for dementia with Lewy bodies was only fair ($\kappa = 0.37$). The reliability for the diagnosis of dementia with Lewy bodies was significantly worse than that achieved when diagnosing AD, PSP and frontotemporal dementia (κ pool test). Although the sensitivity for diagnosing AD was good (95%), for dementia with Lewy bodies it was 34%. The mean specificity for AD was 79% and for dementia with Lewy bodies it was 94%, suggesting that inter-rater reliability for diagnosing AD among clinicians is improved compared with earlier studies. However, clinicians overdiagnosed AD and misdiagnosed dementia with Lewy bodies as AD. The heterogeneity of the clinical presentation of dementia with Lewy bodies significantly affected inter-rater agreement and accuracy.[53]

Lytico–Bodig disease

Lytico–Bodig (also called Guam amyotyrophic lateral sclerosis or parkinsonism–dementia complex) is a neurodegenerative condition endemic to the native Chamorros of Guam. It usually occurs in the fifth to seventh decade. When it is clinically characterized by a parkinsonism–dementia syndrome it is called Bodig disease; when it presents with amyotrophic lateral sclerosis, it is called Lytico disease. In addition to the parkinsonism (mainly bradykinesia and rigidity, but also tremor that less frequently includes pill-rolling tremor), the Bodig form may also present with shuffling gait, pyramidal signs and supranuclear gaze palsy. Both variants of Lytico–Bodig may present with a retinal pigment epitheliopathy (56% of the subjects) which is also present in 16% of the Chamorros.[60] There are no studies that evaluate in detail the different cognitive and behavioral characteristics of the dementia in Lytico disease. Neuropathologically, Bodig is characterized by abundant NFT lesions similar to those of AD but without amyloid plaques.[61] However, the NFT distribution is similar to that in PSP.[62] Although several hypotheses have been proposed (e.g. neurotoxins such as β-*N*-methylamino-*l*-alanine from the *Cycas circinalis* seeds, viral genetic), the etiology of Lytico–Bodig is still unknown. A clinically similar atypical parkinsonian and frontal dementia neurodegenerative disorder was recently described in the West Indies.[63] At present there are no autopsies that link this disorder to other tauopathies. Interestingly, epidemiological studies found that this atypical parkinsonism from the West Indies is associated with the consumption of pawpaw fruit and herbal tea that contains a common neurotoxic alkaloid (benzyltetrahydroisoquinoline).[63]

Frontal lobe dementia with parkinsonism associated with chromosome 17

FTDP-17 is clinically characterized by frontal behavioral disturbances (disinhibition, withdrawal, hyperorality) and cognitive disturbances (executive dysfunction, nonfluent aphasia) and parkinsonism.[64,65] There is phenotypic and genetic heterogeneity in the different FTDP-17 kindreds.[66,67]

Neuropathological changes include frontotemporal atrophy, which is often associated with atrophy of the basal ganglia, substantia nigra and amygdala. The diagnostic lesions of FTDP-17 brains are characterized by tau-rich filaments in the cytoplasm of specific subpopulations of neurons and glial cells that have an increased ratio of 4-repeat to 3-repeat tau isoforms.[68,69] NFTs are seen in some families but not all. Inheritance is autosomal dominant and the gene has been regionally localized to chromosome 17q21–22.[65] Several exonic and intronic tau mis-sense and splice site mutations were identified in more than 20 FTDP-17 families.[70–72]

Some families with an abnormality in chromosome 17q21–22 manifest with frontal lobe dementia, parkinsonism and amyotrophy.[64,73,74] Frontal lobe behavioral disturbances usually present at onset but eventually develop in all affected subjects. Patients also develop non-levodopa-responsive parkinsonism and postural instability. At later stages, some develop amyotrophy.

FTDP-17 with a mutation at codon 301 of the tau gene may present in families with early-onset dementia and parkinsonism who exhibit either frontal dementia or a CBD phenotype as well as extensive tau pathology.[48,68,75] Neuronal and glial inclusions, neuropil threads and astrocytic plaques similar to those seen in CBD were described in some affected subjects. Sequencing of exon 10 revealed a C-to-T transition at codon 301, resulting in a Pro-to-Leu substitution.[68]

FTDP-17 families with a G-to-A transition in the intron following exon 10 of the tau gene (familial multiple system tauopathy) may manifest supranuclear gaze palsy in addition to frontal and parkinsonian disturbances and a 4-repeat tauopathy.[76] On the other hand, FTDP with a mis-sense mutation (Ser305Asn) in the tau gene may present with hereditary frontotemporal dementia characterized by personality changes followed by memory disturbances but minimal parkinsonism.[77] Brain examination at autopsy showed ring-shaped NFTs that partially surrounded the nucleus and were most prominent in the frontal, temporal, insular and postcentral cortices, as well as in dentate gyrus.

Pallido ponto nigral degeneration is also linked to chromosome 17q21–22. This is an autosomal-dominant, rapidly progressive disorder that is characterized by a parkinsonism–dementia syndrome, dystonia, pyramidal signs and ocular disturbances.[78–81] Morphologic and biochemical lesions in this disorder overlap with those seen in sporadic CBD and PSP. Average disease onset is at 43 years and average survival is 8.6 years. Patients present either with parkinsonism (asymmetric limb bradykinesia and rigidity) or with frontal lobe-type dementia. Later on, patients develop postural instability, axial rigidity, and occasionally mild tremor. They also develop dysarthria and dysphagia, eye movement abnormalities (vertical supranuclear gaze palsy), eyelid apraxia and, at end-stages, dystonia that is unrelated to treatment. Clinically, this condition resembles PSP, but the familiar nature, earlier age of presentation and axial and limb parkinsonism may assist in the differentiation. Two mis-sense mutations in exon 10 of the tau gene that segregate with the disease have been found.[79,82,83]

Occurrence of the FTDP-17 mutations in dementia is generally rare. A study evaluated their frequency in three patient series: a community-based dementia series, a clinicopathological tauopathy referral series (P301L mutations in 3.6% of cases but 9.4% of familial cases) and a pathologically confirmed familial frontotemporal dementia series (three splice-site mutations in 13.6% of cases). The data indicated variable but less than 15% of cases with FTDP-17, depending on the sample referral and criteria used.[84]

FTDP-17 should be differentiated from the rigid variant of Huntington's disease, which has an autosomal-dominant inheritance and presents at later stages with parkinsonism and frontal lobe-type dysfunction. The abnormalities in the short arm of chromosome 4 should be helpful for its diagnosis.

Synucleinopathies

Initially this group of disorders were called α-synucleinopathies. This was because α-synuclein gene mutations were found in rare familial PD kindreds and α-synuclein is a major component of Lewy bodies in sporadic PD and dementia with Lewy bodies. However, recent work by Galvin *et al.* broadened the concept of α-synucleinopathies to synucleinopathies since they found that, in addition to α-synuclein, β-synuclein and γ-synuclein are found in dystrophic neurites of PD and in dementia with Lewy bodies patients.[85] These findings suggest these three synucleins are involved in the process of abnormal protein aggregation and synaptic dysfunction leading to the onset or progression of PD and dementia with Lewy bodies.[85]

Parkinson's disease

At early stages, PD patients may experience frontal disturbances but do not exhibit dementia (see Table 4.3).[57,86] In fact, the presence of dementia or neuropsychiatric disturbances at early stages points towards an alternative diagnosis (Table 4.4).[87] When dementia occurs in PD it may be due to:

- an association between PD and AD;
- the presence of cortical Lewy bodies ('pure' DLB); or
- an association of PD, AD and cortical Lewy bodies.

Moreover, because it may be clinically challenging to differentiate the

Table 4.4 Synucleinopathies with parkinsonism and dementia.

Disorder	Clinical and radiological presentation
Parkinson's disease with dementia	Progressive memory disturbances and frontal lobe features with/without visuospatial disturbances in a patient with longstanding PD (unilateral onset of parkinsonism). PD patients without dementia may exhibit a progressive frontal lobe cognitive disturbances (e.g. decreased fluency, difficulty in shifting concepts, planning or sequencing) but no other disturbances
Dementia with Lewy bodies	Early memory disturbances, hallucinations or delusions that are unrelated to therapy, cortical or frontal dementia, neuroleptic sensitivity, marked fluctuations in alertness or cognitive abilities. Parkinsonism is usually bilateral and may have mild to moderate benefits from levodopa therapy, but it may be associated with gait disturbances and postural instability. Patients may present at onset with either or with both parkinsonism or cognitive and behavioral disturbances

various etiologies that lead to dementia in PD (e.g. patients with PD and AD, dementia with Lewy bodies, PD and vascular disease or drug-induced cognitive disturbances or other atypical parkinsonian disorders), studies without autopsy confirmation should be interpreted cautiously. Interestingly, the UK PD brain bank described demented PD cases without anatomopathological abnormalities that might explain the cognitive disturbances.[88] Synaptic abnormalities that contribute to AD dementia were not found in patients who had PD and dementia or in those who had dementia with Lewy bodies.[89] It is unclear whether impaired cognition may be drug-induced or related to neurochemical abnormalities.

In addition, because of different dementia definitions and varied PD populations included in the clinical studies (e.g. patients at different stages of parkinsonism, the absence of a standardized definition of PD), it is not surprising that the reported frequency of dementia in PD varies widely (range, 4–93%).[8,9,17,90–94] This is not a trivial issue since the presence of dementia significantly increases PD mortality.[6,95]

To overcome some of the limitations of the DSM-IIIR dementia definition, Pillon *et al.* used an operational definition of dementia that consisted of a global intellectual performance that was two standard deviations below the mean control values when they tested 44 patients with AD, 164 patients with PD and 45 patients with PSP.[17] They found that only 18% of the PD patients were demented whereas 93% of the AD patients were classified as demented. The fact that not all the AD patients were classified as demented suggests that the criteria used were quite strict. The estimated values are similar to those of other hospital and community-based studies.[5,9,90,93] Using the DSM-III or DSM-IIIR criteria, clinically demented PD patients tend to be older than non-demented subjects.[5,96] Similarly, dementia is three times more frequent when PD starts after age 70 years than when the disease begins earlier. In fact, Mayeux *et al.* found that the highest incidence of dementia in PD occurs between the ages of 65 and 75 years.[5] A prospective cohort study that determined the incidence of dementia in PD by evaluating the clinical features of 250 non-demented PD patients who were followed up for 5 years found that the risk of developing dementia was increased:[97]

- after the age of 70 years (odds ratio, 2.7; CI, 1.4–5.5);
- in patients with a PD rating scale score over 25 (odds ratio, 3.0; CI, 1.5–6.2);
- in depressed patients (odds ratio, 2.7; CI, 1.5–6.6);
- in patients who were confused or psychotic on levodopa (odds ratio, 3.3; CI, 1.3–8.7); and
- in patients who had facial masking as a presenting sign (odds ratio, 6.1; CI, 1.4–26.9).

Although demented PD patients are older at the onset of motor manifestations and have a more rapid motor disability progression than non-demented patients,[7] symptom duration, levodopa use and the presence of tremor or depression are similar in demented and non-demented PD patients. However, the fact that clinically demented PD patients progress rapidly and often respond poorly to levodopa suggests that they may not have idiopathic PD, because autopsy studies indicate that a fast progression of symptoms and poor levodopa response are not features of idiopathic PD. Because many of the clinical studies include postural instability in the criteria for PD (a symptom that occurs late in PD but early in most atypical parkinsonian disorders[57,87]), the presence of misdiagnosed patients in these studies may be frequent.

When selected aspects of memory, executive function and visuospatial function are compared in PD and AD patients with similar degrees of clinical dementia, the neurobehavioral differential patterns are relative rather than absolute.[59,86,98] However, since it is clinically difficult to exclude AD in PD patients with clinically diagnosed dementia relative differences may reflect some degree of misdiagnosis. Despite this, semantic and episodic memory are more impaired in AD than in PD, whereas demented PD patients are more compromised in performing executive tasks. In addition, since the neuropsychological pattern that characterizes the preclinical stage of dementia in PD (frontal lobe dysfunction) differs from that of preclinical AD (memory dysfunction) (see Table 4.2),[99-101] the dementia in PD is probably superimposed on previous cognitive changes. Thus, it appears that the dementing process in PD involves different systems and pathologies than those involved in non-demented PD. Although frontal lobe dysfunction (e.g. difficulty in shifting or planning) is the pattern of cognitive disturbance in non-demented PD, the dementia of PD is more difficult to differentiate from that of AD.

There is disagreement as to whether PD and dementia with Lewy bodies (including diffuse Lewy body disease and Lewy body variant of AD)[102] represent two distinct nosological entities or whether they are the ends of the spectrum of a single disorder (i.e. Lewy body disease).[57] Such debate is the logical consequence of considerable clinicopathological overlap. For example, extrapyramidal features occur in many patients with severe AD[103-105] and dementia occurs in many PD patients.[5,59,88,106] Despite the presence of Lewy bodies in both PD and dementia with Lewy bodies, the relationship between these disorders is debatable.[88,107-110] However, because of different prognosis of PD and DLP, most investigators have considered them to be different disorders.

Dementia with Lewy bodies

Dementia with Lewy bodies is underdiagnosed even when the diagnostic criteria proposed by the International Consortium are used.[102] These proposed criteria are specific but they have a low sensitivity and reliability.[53,57,111] However, although these criteria have hardly improved the differentiation of DLB from other disorders,[57] they are still the recommended criteria for its diagnosis.[112] It is difficult to select features that distinguish early-stage dementia with Lewy bodies from AD and PD or dementia with Lewy bodies with and without AD (see Tables 4.3 and 4.4).[113]

Autopsy-confirmed studies that have evaluated early clinical features suggest that the presence of early hallucinations and cortical dementia and the absence of gait or balance disturbances point towards dementia with Lewy bodies, whereas asymmetric parkinsonism, levodopa response, rest tremor and the absence of cognitive disturbances point towards PD.[57] However, findings differ in various studies. For example, Louis *et al.* found that rest tremor is more common in PD (85% of subjects) than in dementia with Lewy bodies (55%), whereas myoclonus is more common in dementia with Lewy bodies (18.5%) than in PD (0%); however, they found no other difference in extrapyramidal features.[114] They also found that myoclonus, absence of rest tremor, no response to levodopa or no perceived need to treat with levodopa were 10 times more frequent in dementia with Lewy bodies than in PD. Differences in findings may be partially explained by different stages of the disease examined, since they searched for ante mortem, between-group differences whereas Litvan *et al.*[57] looked for early disease predictors. Different stages of the disease may also explain why hallucinations – a good predictor of dementia with Lewy bodies in some studies[57,111] – is not as accurate in the same group of patients.[115]

Multiple system atrophy

Multiple system atrophy is also a synucleinopathy; however, although patients may have frontal dysfunction, they rarely exhibit dementia.[116,117] In fact, if dementia is associated with autonomic disturbances at onset, dementia with Lewy bodies rather than multiple system atrophy should be suspected. Currently, it is difficult to understand why patients with multiple system atrophy lack more severe cognitive disturbances when this disorder also affects the three frontosubcortical circuits.

Summary

In summary, recognizing the features that differentiate these different neurodegenerative disorders (see Table 4.3) requires a detailed clinical history as well as focused neurological, oculomotor, cognitive and psychiatric evaluations. It also requires that the less obvious disease presentations should be recognized and that an increased index of suspicion should be developed. Using validated criteria improves diagnostic accuracy, which in turn allows better patient care as well as the possibility of early enrollment of patients into research studies.

References

1. Alexander GE, DeLong MR, Strick PL. Parallel organization of functionally segregated circuits linking basal ganglia and cortex. Annu Rev Neurosci 1986; 9:357–381.

2. Alexander GE, Crutcher MD, DeLong MR. Basal ganglia–thalamocortical circuits: parallel substrates for motor, oculomotor, 'prefrontal' and 'limbic' functions. In: Uylungs HBM, Van Eden CG, De Bruin JPC, Corner MA, Feenstra MGP, eds. The profrontal cortex, its structure, function and pathology. Progress on Brain Research, Vol 85. New York: Elsevier Science Publishers; 1990:266–271.

3. Cummings JL. Anatomic and behavioral aspects of frontal–subcortical circuits. Ann N Y Acad Sci 1995;769:1–13.

4. American Psychiatric Association. Diagnostic and statistical manual of mental disorders. DSM-IV. Washington DC: American Psychiatric Association; 1994.

5. Mayeux R, Chen J, Mirabello E, *et al.* An estimate of the incidence of dementia in idiopathic

Parkinson's disease. Neurology 1990;40:1513–1517.

6. Marder K, Leung D, Tang M, *et al.* Are demented patients with Parkinson's disease accurately reflected in prevalence surveys? A survival analysis. Neurology 1991;41:1240–1243.

7. Mayeux R, Denaro J, Hemenegildo N, *et al.* A population-based investigation of Parkinson's disease with and without dementia. Relationship to age and gender. Arch Neurol 1992;49:492–497.

8. Tison F, Dartigues JF, Auriacombe S, Letenneur L, Boller F, Alperovitch A. Dementia in Parkinson's disease: a population-based study in ambulatory and institutionalized individuals. Neurology 1995;45:705–708.

9. Aarsland D, Tandberg E, Larsen JP, Cummings JL. Frequency of dementia in Parkinson disease. Arch Neurol 1996;53:538–542.

10. Litvan I. Parkinsonism–dementia syndromes. In: Jankovic J, Tolosa E, eds. Parkinson's disease and movement disorders, 3rd ed. New York: Williams and Wilkins; 1998:819–836.

11. Spillantini MG, Goedert M. Tau protein pathology in neurodegenerative diseases. Trends Neurosci 1998;21:428–433.

12. Trojanowski JQ, Lee VM. Transgenic models of tauopathies and synucleinopathies. Brain Pathol 1999;9:733–739.

13. Goedert M, Spillantini MG, Davies SW. Filamentous nerve cell inclusions in neurodegenerative diseases. Curr Opin Neurobiol 1998;8:619–632.

14. Albert ML, Feldman RG, Willis AL. The 'subcortical dementia' of progressive supranuclear palsy. J Neurol Neurosurg Psychiatry 1974;37:121–130.

15. Litvan I, Mangone CA, McKee A, *et al.* Natural history of progressive supranuclear palsy (Steele–Richardson–Olszewski syndrome) and clinical predictors of survival: a clinicopathological study. J Neurol Neurosurg Psychiatry 1996;60:615–620.

16. Maher ER, Smith EM, Lees AJ. Cognitive deficits in the Steele–Richardson–Olszewski syndrome (progressive supranuclear palsy). J Neurol Neurosurg Psychiatry 1985;48:1234–1249.

17. Pillon B, Dubois B, Ploska A, Agid Y. Severity and specificity of cognitive impairment in Alzheimer's, Huntington's, and Parkinson's diseases and progressive supranuclear palsy. Neurology 1991;41:634–643.

18. Pillon B, Dubois B, Lhermitte F, Agid Y. Heterogeneity of cognitive impairment in progressive supranuclear palsy, Parkinson's disease, and Alzheimer's disease. Neurology 1986;36:1179–1185.

19. Pierrot-Deseilligny C, Turell E, Penet C, *et al.* Increased wave P 300 latency in progressive supranuclear palsy. J Neurol Neurosurg Psychiatry 1989; 52:656–658.

20. Grafman J, Litvan I, Gomez C, Chase TN. Frontal lobe function in progressive supranuclear palsy. Arch Neurol 1990;47:553–558.

21. Johnson RJ, Litvan I, Grafman J. Progressive supranuclear palsy: altered sensory processing leads to degraded cognition. Neurology 1991;41:1257–1262.

22. Johnson RJ. Event-related brain potentials. In: Litvan I, Agid Y, eds. Progressive supranuclear palsy: clinical and research approaches. New York: Oxford University Press; 1992:122–154.

23. Dubois B, Pillon B, Legault F,

Agid Y, Lhermitte F. Slowing of cognitive processing in progressive supranuclear palsy. A comparison with Parkinson's disease. Arch Neurol 1988;45: 1194–1199.

24. Rosser AE, Hodges JR. The dementia rating scale in Alzheimer's disease, Huntington's disease and progressive supranuclear palsy. J Neurol 1994;241:531–536.

25. Litvan I, Grafman J, Gomez C, Chase T. Memory impairment in patients with progressive supranuclear palsy. Arch Neurol 1989;46:765–767.

26. Pillon B, Deweer B, Michon A, Malapani C, Agid Y, Dubois B. Are explicit memory disorders of progressive supranauclear palsy related to damage to striatofrontal circuits? Comparison with Alzheimer's, Parkinson's, and Huntington's diseases. Neurology 1994;44:1264–1270.

27. Litvan I, Mega MS, Cummings JL, Fairbanks L. Neuropsychiatric aspects of progressive supranuclear palsy. Neurology 1996;47:1184–1189.

28. Litvan I, Paulsen JS, Mega MS, Cummings J. Neuropsychiatric behavioral assessment of patients with hyperkinetic and hypokinetic movement disorders. Arch Neurol 1998;55: 1313–1319.

29. Esmonde T, Giles E, Xuereb J, Hodges J. Progressive supranuclear palsy presenting with dynamic aphasia. J Neurol Neurosurg Psychiatry 1996;60: 403–410.

30. Pharr V, Litvan I, Brad DG, Troncoso J, Reich SG, Stark M. Ideomotor apraxia in progressive supranuclear palsy: a case study. Mov Disord 1999;14: 162–166.

31. Leiguarda RC, Pramstaller PP, Merello M, Starkstein S, Lees AJ, Marsden CD. Apraxia in Parkinson's disease, progressive supranuclear palsy, multiple system atrophy and neuroleptic-induced parkinsonism. Brain 1997;120:75–90.

32. Litvan I, Grimes DA, Lang AE, et al. Clinical features differentiating patients with postmortem confirmed progressive supranuclear palsy and corticobasal degeneration. J Neurol 1999; 246:S1–S5.

33. Verny M, Duyckaerts C, Agid Y, Hauw JJ. The significance of cortical pathology in progressive supranuclear palsy. Clinicopathological data in 10 cases. Brain 1996;119:1123–1136.

34. Wenning GK, Litvan I, Jankovic J, et al. Natural history and survival of 14 patients with corticobasal degeneration confirmed at postmortem examination. J Neurol Neurosurg Psychiatry 1998;64:184–189.

35. Bergeron C, Davis A, Lang AE. Corticobasal ganglionic degeneration and progressive supranuclear palsy presenting with cognitive decline. Brain Pathol 1998;8:355–365.

36. Gimenez-Roldan S, Mateo D, Benito C, Grandas F, Perez-Gilabert Y. Progressive supranuclear palsy and corticobasal ganglionic degeneration: differentiation by clinical features and neuroimaging techniques. J Neural Transm Suppl 1994;42: 79–90.

37. Kertesz A, Hudson L, Mackenzie IR, Munoz DG. The pathology and nosology of primary progressive aphasia. Neurology 1994;44:2065–2072.

38. Leiguarda R, Lees AJ, Merello M, Starkstein S, Marsden CD. The nature of apraxia in corticobasal degeneration. J Neurol

Neurosurg Psychiatry 1994;57: 455–459.

39. Pillon B, Blin J, Vidailhet M, *et al.* The neuropsychological pattern of corticobasal degeneration: comparison with progressive supranuclear palsy and Alzheimer's disease. Neurology 1995;45:1477–1483.

40. Rey GJ, Tomer R, Levin BE, Sanchez-Ramos J, Bowen B, Bruce JH. Psychiatric symptoms, atypical dementia, and left visual field inattention in corticobasal ganglionic degeneration. Mov Disord 1995;10: 106–110.

41. Kertesz A. Pick complex and Pick's disease: the nosology of frontal lobe dementia, primary progressive aphasia, and corticobasal ganglionic degeneration. Eur J Neurol 1996;3: 280–282.

42. Litvan I, Agid Y, Goetz C, *et al.* Accuracy of the clinical diagnosis of corticobasal degeneration: a clinicopathological study. Neurology 1997;48:119–125.

43. Frattali CM, Grafman J, Patronas N, Maclhouf F, Litvan I. Language disturbances in corticobasal degeneration. Neurology 2000;54:990–992.

44. Barclay C, Bergeron C, Lang A. Arm levitation in progressive supranuclear palsy. Neurology 1999;52:879–882.

45. Vidailhet M, Rivaud S, Gouider-Khouja N, *et al.* Eye movements in Parkinsonian syndromes. Ann Neurol 1994;35:420–426.

46. Litvan I, Cummings JL, Mega M. Neuropsychiatric features of corticobasal degeneration. J Neurol Neurosurg Psychiatry 1998;65:717–721.

47. Brown J, Lantos P, Rossor M. Familial dementia lacking specific pathological features presenting with clinical features

of corticobasal degeneration. J Neurol Neurosurg Psychiatry 1998;65:600–603.

48. Bugiani O, Murrell J, Giaccone G, *et al.* Frontotemporal dementia and corticobasal degeneration in a family with a P301S mutation in tau. J Neuropathol Exp Neurol 1999;58:667–677.

49. Horoupian D. Alzheimer's disease pathology in motor cortex in dementia with Lewy bodies clinically mimicking corticobasal degeneration. Acta Neuropathol (Berl) 1999;98:317–322.

50. Boeve B. Pathologic heterogeneity in clinically diagnosed corticobasal degeneration. Neurology 1999;53:795–800.

51. The Lund and Manchester Groups. Clinical and neuropathological criteria for frontotemporal dementia. J Neurol Neurosurg Psychiatry 1994;57: 416–418.

52. Litvan I, Agid Y, Sastry N, *et al.* What are the obstacles for an accurate clinical diagnosis of Pick's disease? A clinicopathologic study. Neurology 1997; 49:62–69.

53. Lopez OL, Litvan I, Catt KE, *et al.* Accuracy of four clinical diagnostic criteria for the diagnosis of neurodegenerative dementias. Neurology 1999;53: 1292–1299.

54. Binetti G, Locascio JJ, Corkin S, Growdon JH. Pick's disease and Alzheimer's disease have different cognitive profiles (abstract). Soc Neurosci 1996;22.

55. Mendez M, Selwood A, Mastri A, Frey W. Pick's disease versus Alzheimer's disease: a comparison of clinical characteristics. Neurology 1993;43:289–292.

56. Levy ML, Miller BL, Cummings JL, Fairbanks LA, Craig A. Alzheimer disease and frontotemporal dementias. Behav-

ioral distinctions. Arch Neurol 1996;53:687–690.

57. Litvan I, MacIntyre A, Goetz CG, *et al.* Accuracy of the clinical diagnoses of Lewy body disease, Parkinson disease, and dementia with Lewy bodies: a clinicopathologic study. Arch Neurol 1998;55:969–978.

58. Litvan I, McKee A. Clinicopathologic case report. Dementia with Lewy bodies (DLB). J Neuropsychiatry Clin Neurosci 1999;11: 107–112.

59. Litvan I, Mohr E, Williams J, Gomez C, Chase TN. Differential memory and executive functions in demented patients with Parkinson's and Alzheimer's disease. J Neurol Neurosurg Psychiatry 1991;54:25–29.

60. Cox TA, McDarby JV, Lavine L, Steele JC, Calne DB. A retinopathy on Guam with high prevalence in Lytico–Bodig. Ophthalmology 1989;96:1731–1735.

61. Mawal-Dewan M, Schmidt ML, Balin B, Perl DP, Lee VMY, Trojanowski JQ. Identification of phosphorylation sites in PHF–Tau from patients with Guam amyotrophic lateral sclerosis/parkinsonism–dementia complex. J Neuropathol Exp Neurol 1996;55:1051–1059.

62. Geddes JF, Hughes AJ, Lees AJ, Daniel SE. Pathological overlap in cases of parkinsonism associated with neurofibrillary tangles. A study of recent cases of postencephalitic parkinsonism and comparison with progressive supranuclear palsy and Guamanian parkinsonism–dementia complex. Brain 1993;116:281–302.

63. Caparros-Lefebvre D, Elbaz A. Possible relation of atypical parkinsonism in the French West Indies with consumption of tropical plants: a case-control study.

Caribbean Parkinsonism Study Group. Lancet 1999;354: 281–286.

64. Wilhelmsen KC, Lynch T, Pavlou E, Higgins M, Nygaard TG. Localization of disinhibition–dementia–parkinsonism–amyotrophy complex to 17q21–22. Am J Hum Genet 1994; 55: 1159–1165.

65. Poorkaj P, Bird TD, Wijsman E, *et al.* Tau is a candidate gene for chromosome 17 frontotemporal dementia. Ann Neurol 1998;43:815–825.

66. D'Souza I, Poorkaj P, Hong M, *et al.* Missense and silent tau gene mutations cause frontotemporal dementia with parkinsonism–chromosome 17 type, by affecting multiple alternative RNA splicing regulatory elements. Proc Natl Acad Sci U S A 1999;96:5598–5603.

67. Spillantini MG, Crowther RA, Kamphorst W, Heutink P, van Swieten JC. Tau pathology in two Dutch families with mutations in the microtubule-binding region of tau. Am J Pathol 1998;153:1359–1363.

68. Mirra SS, Murrell JR, Gearing M, *et al.* Tau pathology in a family with dementia and a P301L mutation in tau. J Neuropathol Exp Neurol 1999;58:335–345.

69. Varani L, Hasegawa M, Spillantini MG, *et al.* Structure of tau exon 10 splicing regulatory element RNA and destabilization by mutations of frontotemporal dementia and parkinsonism linked to chromosome 17. Proc Natl Acad Sci U S A 1999;96: 8229–8234.

70. Grover A, Houlden H, Baker M, *et al.* 5' splice site mutations in tau associated with the inherited dementia FTDP-17 affect a stem-loop structure that regulates alternative splicing of exon

10. J Biol Chem 1999;274: 15134–15143.

71. Hong M, Zhukareva V, Vogelsberg-Ragaglia V, *et al.* Mutation-specific functional impairments in distinct tau isoforms of hereditary FTDP-17. Science 1998; 282:1914–1917.

72. Hutton M, Lendon CL, Rizzu P, *et al.* Association of missense and 5'-splice-site mutations in tau with the inherited dementia FTDP-17. Nature 1998;393: 702–705.

73. Lynch T, Sano M, Marder KS, *et al.* Clinical characteristics of a family with chromosome 17-linked disinhibition–dementia–parkinsonism–amyotrophy complex. Neurology 1994;44: 1878–1884.

74. Sima AA, Defendini R, Keohane C, *et al.* The neuropathology of chromosome 17-linked dementia. Ann Neurol 1996;39: 734–743.

75. Nasreddine ZS, Loginov M, Clark LN, *et al.* From genotype to phenotype: a clinical pathological, and biochemical investigation of frontotemporal dementia and parkinsonism (FTDP-17) caused by the P301L tau mutation. Ann Neurol 1999;45: 704–715.

76. Spillantini MG, Murrell JR, Goedert M, Farlow MR, Klug A, Ghetti B. Mutation in the tau gene in familial multiple system tauopathy with presenile dementia. Proc Natl Acad Sci U S A 1998; 95:7737–7741.

77. Iijima M, Tabira T, Poorkaj P, *et al.* A distinct familial presenile dementia with a novel missense mutation in the tau gene. NeuroReport 1999;10:497–501.

78. Wszolek ZK, Pfeiffer RF, Bhatt MH, *et al.* Rapidly progressive autosomal dominant parkinsonism and dementia with pallido-

ponto-nigral degeneration. Ann Neurol 1992;32:312–320.

79. Wijker M, Wszolek ZK, Wolters EC, *et al.* Localization of the gene for rapidly progressive autosomal dominant parkinsonism and dementia with pallido-ponto-nigral degeneration to chromosome 17q21. Hum Mol Genet 1996;5:151–154.

80. Yamaoka LH, Welsh-Bohmer KA, Hulette CM, *et al.* Linkage of frontotemporal dementia to chromosome 17: clinical and neuropathological characterization of phenotype. Am J Hum Genet 1996;59:1306–1312.

81. Wszolek ZK, Lagerlund TD, Steg RE, McManis PG. Clinical neurophysiologic findings in patients with rapidly progressive familial parkinsonism and dementia with pallido-ponto-nigral degeneration. Electroencephalogr Clin Neurophysiol 1998;107:213–222.

82. Clark LN, Poorkaj P, Wszolek Z, *et al.* Pathogenic implications of mutations in the tau gene in pallido-ponto-nigral degeneration and related neurodegenerative disorders linked to chromosome 17. Proc Natl Acad Sci U S A 1998;95:13103–13107.

83. Reed LA, Schmidt ML, Wszolek ZK, *et al.* The neuropathology of a chromosome 17-linked autosomal dominant parkinsonism and dementia ('pallido-ponto-nigral degeneration'). J Neuropathol Exp Neurol 1998;57: 588–601.

84. Houlden H, Baker M, Adamson J, *et al.* Frequency of tau mutations in three series of non-Alzheimer's degenerative dementia. Ann Neurol 1999;46: 243–248.

85. Galvin JE, Uryu K, Lee VM, Trojanowski JQ. Axon pathology in Parkinson's disease and Lewy body dementia hippocampus

contains alpha-, beta-, and gamma-synuclein. Proc Natl Acad Sci U S A 1999;96: 13450–13455.

86. Stern Y, Richards M, Sano M, Mayeux R. Comparison of cognitive changes in patients with Alzheimer's and Parkinson's disease. Arch Neurol 1993;50: 1040–1045.

87. Litvan I. Parkinsonian features: when are they Parkinson disease? JAMA 1998;280:1654–1655.

88. Hughes AJ, Daniel SE, Blankson S, Lees AJ. A clinicopathologic study of 100 cases of Parkinson's disease. Arch Neurol 1993;50:140–148.

89. Hansen LA, Daniel SE, Wilcock GK, Love S. Frontal cortical synaptophysin in Lewy body diseases: relation to Alzheimer's disease and dementia. J Neurol Neurosurg Psychiatry 1998;64: 653–656.

90. Brown RG, Marsden CD. How common is dementia in Parkinson's disease? Lancet 1984;1: 1262–1265.

91. Dubois B, Boller F, Pillon B, Agid Y. Cognitive deficits in Parkinson's disease. In: Boller F, Grafman J, eds. Handbook of neuropsychology. Amsterdam: Elsevier Science Publication; 1991.

92. Marder K, Tang MX, Cote L, Stern Y, Mayeux R. The frequency and associated risk factors for dementia in patients with Parkinson's disease. Arch Neurol 1995;52:695–701.

93. Mayeux R, Stern Y, Rosenstein R, *et al.* An estimate of the prevalence of dementia in idiopathic Parkinson's disease. Arch Neurol 1988;45:260–262.

94. Portin R, Rinne UK. Predictive factors for cognitive deterioration and dementia in Parkinson's disease. Adv Neurol 1986;45: 413–416.

95. Louis ED, Marder K, Cote L, Tang M, Mayeux R. Mortality from Parkinson disease. Arch Neurol 1997;54:260–264.

96. Biggins CA, Boyd JL, Harrop FM, *et al.* A controlled, longitudinal study of dementia in Parkinson's disease. J Neurol Neurosurg Psychiatry 1992;55: 566–571.

97. Stern Y, Marder K, Tang MX, Mayeux R. Antecedent clinical features associated with dementia in Parkinson's disease. Neurology 1993;43:1690–1692.

98. Mohr E, Litvan I, Williams J, Fedio P, Chase TN. Selective deficits in Alzheimer and parkinsonian dementia: visuospatial function. Can J Neurol Sci 1990;17:292–297.

99. Jacobs DM, Marder K, Cote LJ, Sano M, Stern Y, Mayeux R. Neuropsychological characteristics of preclinical dementia in Parkinson's disease. Neurology 1995;45:1691–1696.

100. Piccirilli M, D'Alessandro P, Finali G, Piccinin GL, Agostini L. Frontal lobe dysfunction in Parkinson's disease: prognostic value for dementia? Eur Neurol 1989;29:71–76.

101. Petersen RC, Smith GE, Waring SC, Ivnik RJ, Tangalos EG, Kokmen E. Mild cognitive impairment: clinical characterization and outcome. Arch Neurol 1999;56:303–308.

102. McKeith IG, Galasko D, Kosaka K, *et al.* Consensus guidelines for the clinical and pathological diagnosis of dementia with Lewy bodies (DLB): report of the Consortium on DLB International Workshop. Neurology 1996;47: 1113–1124.

103. Lopez OL, Wisnieski SR, Becker JT, Boller F, DeKosky ST. Extrapyramidal signs in patients with probable Alzheimer dis-

ease. Arch Neurol 1997;54: 969–975.

104. Morris JC, Drazner M, Fulling K, Grant EA, Goldring J. Clinical and pathological aspects of parkinsonism in Alzheimer's disease. Arch Neurol 1989;46: 651–657.

105. Mosla PK, Martila RJ, Rinne UK. Extrapyramidal signs in Alzheimer's disease. Neurology 1984;34:1114–1116.

106. Mindham RHS, Biggins CA, Boyd JL, *et al.* A controlled study of dementia in Parkinson's disease over 54 months. In: Narabayashi H, Nagatsu T, Yanagisawa N, Mizuno Y, eds. Advances in neurology. New York: Raven Press; 1993.

107. Calne D. Is 'Parkinson's disease' one disease? J Neurol Neurosurg Psychiatry 1989;52(suppl): 18–21.

108. Greenfield JG, Bosanquet FD. The brain-stem lesions in parkinsonism. J Neurol Neurosurg Psychiatry 1953;16: 213–226.

109. Perry EK, Perry RH, McKeith IG. Is dementia with Lewy bodies a distinct entity? Mov Disord 1996;11(suppl 1):19.

110. Smith MA, Perry G. Is a Lewy body always a Lewy body? In: Korczyn AD, ed. Dementia in Parkinson's disease. Bologna: Monduzzi Editore; 1995: 187–193.

111. Mega MS, Masterman DL, Benson F, *et al.* Dementia with Lewy bodies: reliability and validity of clinical and pathologic criteria.

Neurology 1996;47:1403–1409.

112. McKeith IG, Perry EK, Perry RH. Report of the Second Dementia with Lewy Body International Workshop: diagnosis and treatment. Consortium on Dementia with Lewy Bodies. Neurology 1999;53:902–905.

113. Gomez-Tortosa E, Newell K, Irizarry MC, Albert M, Growdon JH, Hyman BT. Clinical and quantitative pathologic correlates of dementia with Lewy bodies. Neurology 1999;53: 1284–1291.

114. Louis ED, Klatka LA, Liu Y, Fahn S. Comparison of extrapyramidal features in 31 pathologically confirmed cases of diffuse Lewy body disease and 34 pathologically confirmed cases of Parkinson's disease. Neurology 1997; 48:376–380.

115. Klatka LA, Louis ED, Schiffer RB. Psychiatric features in diffuse Lewy body disease: a clinicopathologic study using Alzheimer's disease and Parkinson's disease comparison groups. Neurology 1996;47: 1148–1152.

116. Pillon B, Gouider-Khouja N, Deweer B, *et al.* Neuropsychological pattern of striatonigral degeneration: comparison with Parkinson's disease and progressive supranuclear palsy. J Neurol Neurosurg Psychiatry 1995;58:174–179.

117. Robbins TW, James M, Lange KW, Owen AM, Quinn NP, Marsden CD. Cognitive performance in multiple system atrophy. Brain 1992;115:271–291.

5
Subcortical vascular dementia

Timo Erkinjuntti and Leonardo Pantoni

This chapter presents emerging information on subcortical vascular dementia. It is divided into two parts, a section that introduces general concepts about vascular dementia (VaD) and a section that focuses on subcortical VaD, its clinical picture, radiological and pathological aspects, its pathogenesis and some therapeutic perspectives.

Vascular dementia

Historical and conceptual background

As early as 1896 Emil Kraepelin, following the then-recent ideas of Alois Alzheimer and Otto Binswanger, separated 'arteriosclerotic dementia' (referring to a vascular form of dementia) from 'senile dementia' (referring to Alzheimer's disease (AD)).[1] Nevertheless, until the 1970s it was thought that cerebral atherosclerosis, by causing chronic strangulation of blood supply to the brain, was the most common cause of dementia, and AD was regarded as a rare cause that affected only younger patients. The seminal work of Tomlinson *et al.*[2] proposed AD as the most frequent cause of dementia. In 1974, Hachinski *et al.* used the term 'multi-infarct dementia' (MID) to underline the mechanism by which they considered cognitive impairment to be produced on a vascular basis.[3] As the pendulum swung in the direction of AD, vascular forms of dementia became relegated to a position of relative obscurity.[4] Until the 1990s the concept of VaD had been that it was a form of cognitive impairment caused by small or large brain infarcts, basically similar to MID.[3,5] VaD has come full circle with the resurgence of interest in the whole spectrum of vascular causes of dementia and cognitive impairment.[6]

VaD is the second most common cause of dementia. It accounts for 10–50% of cases of dementia depending on the geographical area, patient population and clinical methods used to define it.[7,8] The prevalence and incidence of VaD increase with age, and men seem to have a higher prevalence of VaD than women. In recent studies, the frequency of VaD has been found to be higher than was previously reported,[9] and it has become evident that cerebrovascular diseases are associated with a high risk of cognitive impairment and dementia.[10,11] Moreover, vascular factors such as coexisting stroke and white matter lesions (WMLs) also play a role in AD.[12,13] Thus, vascular causes may even be the leading basis of cognitive impairment world-wide.[14]

Because vascular causes of cognitive impairment are common, may be preventable and may benefit from therapy, early detection and accurate diagnosis of vascular cognitive impairment[15] and VaD are an important challenge.

Concept and causes

VaD as a clinical syndrome relates to various vascular mechanisms and changes in the brain, and it has various causes and clinical manifestations. VaD not only includes the traditional form of MID.[5,16] The pathophysiology of VaD incorporates interactions between vascular etiologies (cerebrovascular disorders and vascular risk factors), changes in the brain (infarcts, WMLs, atrophy), host factors (age, education) and cognition.[17-21]

Primary vascular mechanisms

Primary vascular mechanisms related to VaD include:[22-26]

- large artery disease (e.g. artery-to-artery embolism, occlusion of an extracranial or intracranial artery);
- cardiac embolic events;
- small vessel disease (ischemic WMLs, lacunar infarcts); and
- hemodynamic mechanisms.

However, individual roles that these factors may play in causing VaD have not yet been identified in detail.[4,16-18,20,26]

Secondary vascular factors

Secondary vascular factors related to VaD include risk factors for cerebrovascular diseases, stroke and WMLs, but also the causes of any cognitive decline and AD.[21]

Changes in the brain

Changes in the brain related to VaD include:[17,18,22,23]

- arterial territorial infarcts;

- distal field (watershed) infarcts;
- lacunar infarcts;
- ischemic WMLs; and
- incomplete ischemic injury, including laminar necrosis, focal gliosis, granular atrophy and incomplete white matter infarction.[27,28]

In addition, both focal functional ischemic changes (around the ischemic lesion) and remote functional ischemic changes (disconnection, diaschisis) relate to VaD.[29] An obstacle to research has been the limited technologies that are routinely available for detecting and verifying lesions that result from incomplete ischemic injury and functional ischemic changes.[30]

Cognition

The relationship between vascular factors and cognition is very important. Therefore, critical clinical issues include:

- whether the identified vascular factors cause or compound the VaD syndrome or only coexist with it;[11,31]
- whether they contribute to the risk and clinical picture of AD;[12,20] and
- which type, extent, side, site and tempo of vascular lesions in the brain relate to different types of VaD.[17–19,22]

Diagnostic criteria

Since the 1970s several clinical criteria for VaD have been used.[32–34] The most widely used criteria include criteria in the fourth edition of the *Diagnostic and Statistical Manual of Mental Disorders* (DSM-IV),[35] the *International Classification of Diseases*, 10th revision (ICD-10),[36] the State of California Alzheimer's Disease Diagnostic and Treatment Centers (ADDTC),[37] and the *National Institute of Neurological Disorders and Stroke, and l'Association Internationale pour la Recherche et l'Enseignement en Neurosciences* (NINDS-AIREN).[38]

The two cardinal elements implemented in the clinical criteria for VaD are:

- the definition of the cognitive syndrome of dementia;[39] and
- the definition of the vascular cause of dementia.[33,34,40]

Variations in defining these two critical elements cause different definitions to give different point prevalence estimates as well as identifying different groups of subjects and consequently also identifying different types and distribution of brain lesions.[9,34,39,41,42] This heterogeneity may have been a factor in the negative results in previous clinical trials in VaD.[43]

All the clinical criteria used are consensus criteria, which are neither derived from prospective community-based studies on vascular factors that affect cognition nor based on detailed natural histories.[32,33,37,38,44] All the criteria listed above are mainly based on the ischemic infarct concept and are designed to have high specificity, although they have been poorly implemented and validated.[32,44]

The DSM-IV definition for VaD requires focal neurological signs and symptoms or laboratory evidence of focal neurological damage that is clinically judged to be related to the disturbance.[35] The course is specified by sudden cognitive and functional losses. The DSM-IV criteria do not detail brain imaging requirements. The DSM-IV definition for VaD is reasonably broad and lacks detailed clinical and radiological guidelines.

The ICD-10 criteria[36] require unequal distribution of cognitive deficits, focal signs as evidence of focal brain damage, and significant cerebrovascular disease that is judged to be etiologically related to dementia. The criteria do not detail brain imaging requirements. The shortcomings of these criteria include lack of detailed guidelines (e.g. unequal cognitive deficits and neuroimaging), lack of etiological cues, and heterogeneity.[34,40]

The ADDTC criteria have been developed exclusively for ischemic VaD.[37] They require:

- evidence of two or more ischemic strokes by history, neurological signs or neuroimaging studies (computed tomography (CT) or T1-weighted magnetic resonance imaging (MRI)); or
- in a case of a single stroke, a clearly documented temporal relationship (not specified in detail);
- in all cases radiological evidence of at least one infarct outside the cerebellum.

The list of criteria includes features supporting the diagnosis as well as features that cast doubt on a diagnosis of probable ischemic VaD.

The NINDS-AIREN research criteria for VaD[38] include:

- dementia syndrome;
- cerebrovascular disease; and
- a relationship between the two.

Cerebrovascular disease is defined by the presence of focal neurological signs and detailed brain imaging evidence of ischemic changes in the brain. A relationship between dementia and cerebrovascular disorder is based on the onset of dementia within 3 months of a recognized stroke, on an abrupt deterioration in cognitive functions or on a fluctuating, stepwise progression of cognitive deficits. The criteria include a list of features that are consistent with the diagnosis, as well as a list of features that make the diagnosis uncertain or unlikely. Also, different levels of certainty of the clinical diagnosis (probable, possible, definite) are included. The NINDS-AIREN criteria recognize heterogeneity of the syndrome[33] and the variability of the clinical course in VaD, and they highlight detection of ischemic lesions and a relationship between lesion and cognition, as well as between stroke and dementia onset. The inter-rater reliability of the NINDS-AIREN criteria has been shown to be moderate to substantial ($\kappa = 0.46$–0.72).[45]

The DSM-IV[35] and the ICD-10[36] criteria for VaD do not specify any brain imaging requirements. The ADDTC criteria for ischemic VaD[37] require for the diagnosis of probable ischemic VaD 'evidence of two or more ischemic strokes by history, neurologic signs, and/or neuroimaging studies (CT or T1-weighted MRI), and evidence of at least one infarct outside the cerebellum by CT or T1-weighted MRI'. The diagnosis is further supported by 'evidence of multiple infarcts in brain regions known to affect cognition', but the sites are not detailed. Moreover, features that are thought to be associated with ischemic VaD but are awaiting further research include 'periventricular and deep white matter changes on T2-weighted MRI that are excessive for age'. In the category of possible ischemic VaD, the criteria include Binswanger's syndrome, with 'extensive white matter changes on neuroimaging', which are not otherwise specified. Ischemic white matter changes on CT or MRI do not qualify as brain imaging evidence of probable ischemic VaD, but they may support a diagnosis of possible ischemic VaD.

The NINDS-AIREN criteria for probable VaD[38] require 'evidence of relevant cerebrovascular disorder by brain imaging (CT or MRI) including multiple large-vessel stroke or a single strategically placed infarct (angular gyrus, thalamus, basal forebrain, posterior or anterior cerebral artery territories), as well as multiple basal ganglia and white matter lacunes or extensive periventricular white matter lesions, or combinations thereof'. The criteria state that 'white matter lesions on CT/MRI alone may be considered evidence for cerebrovascular disease; however, to be significant, these changes must be diffuse and extensive, and characterized by irregular periventricular hyperintensities on T1 and T2 MRI extending to the deep white matter but sparing the areas thought to be protected from perfusion insufficiency (e.g. subcortical U-fibers, external capsule, claustrum, and extreme capsule). Changes observed only on T2 MRI may be insignificant', and that 'it has been suggested that, in VaD, white matter changes involve at least one-fourth of the total white matter'. The criteria also list features that make the diagnosis of VaD uncertain or unlikely, including 'absence of cerebrovascular lesions on brain CT/MRI rules out probable VaD'. However, the class of 'possible VaD' may include patients who have 'focal neurologic signs but in the absence of brain imaging confirmation of definite cerebrovascular disorder'.

The current criteria for VaD are not interchangeable; they identify different figures and clusters of patients labeled as VaD.[39] The DSM-IV criteria are less restrictive compared to the ICD-10, the ADDTC and the NINDS-

AIREN criteria.[40,46] The ADDTC criteria seem to be more sensitive and the NINDS-AIREN criteria more specific.[47]

The NINDS-AIREN criteria are currently the most widely used in clinical drug trials in VaD, despite their limitations. In a pathological series, sensitivity of the NINDS-AIREN criteria was 58% and specificity was 80%.[47] The criteria successfully excluded AD in 91% of cases, and the proportion of combined cases misclassified as probable VaD was 29%.[47] Compared with the ADDTC criteria, the NINDS-AIREN criteria were more specific and better excluded combined cases (54% versus 29%).[47]

Subtypes of vascular dementia in current clinical criteria

Classification of VaD may be used on:

- the primary vascular etiological mechanism;
- the primary type of ischemic brain lesions;
- the primary location of brain lesions; or
- the primary clinical syndrome.

The currently proposed subtypes of VaD (Table 5.1) incorporate a variable combination of the given categories, which reflects the heterogeneity discussed above.

The subtypes of VaD included in current classifications (Table 5.2) are:[23,25,38,45–51]

- the cortical type of VaD or MID;
- subcortical VaD or small vessel dementia; and
- strategic infarct dementia.

Table 5.1 Subtypes of vascular dementia

Cortical vascular dementia
or
Multi-infarct dementia

Subcortical vascular dementia
or
Small vessel dementia

Strategic infarct dementia

Hypoperfusion dementia

Hemorrhagic dementia

Hereditary vascular dementia

Other vascular dementia

Alzheimer's disease with cerebrovascular disease (combined or mixed dementia)

Table 5.2 Vascular mechanisms and changes in the brain in main subtypes of vascular dementia

Vascular mechanisms	Changes in the brain
Cortical vascular dementia or multi-infarct dementia	
Large vessel disease	Arterial territorial infarction
Cardiac embolic events	Distal field (watershed) infarction
Hypoperfusion	
Subcortical vascular dementia or small vessel dementia	
Small vessel disease	Lacunar infarction
Hypoperfusion	Focal and diffuse white matter lesions
	Incomplete ischemic injury
Strategic infarct dementia	
Large vessel disease	Arterial territorial infarction
Cardiac embolic events	Distal field (watershed) infarction
Small vessel disease	Lacunar infarction
Hypoperfusion	Focal and diffuse white matter lesions

Many authors also include hypoperfusion dementia,[23,38,50,52] and further suggested subtypes include hemorrhagic dementia, hereditary VaD, and combined or mixed dementia (AD with cerebrovascular disease).

One question is whether these suggested subtypes are distinct disorders with specific pathological and clinical features and responses to therapy.[25] The goal is to identify homogeneous subtypes, which would improve comparability of independent studies and benefit multicenter collaboration.[37]

The current clinical criteria differ in their classification of VaD into subtypes. None of these sets contains detailed criteria for their subtypes. The DSM-IV criteria[35] do not specify subtypes. The ICD-10 criteria[36] include six subtypes with rather superficial clinical descriptions (acute onset, multi-infarct, subcortical, mixed cortical and subcortical, other, and unspecified). The ICD-10 criteria are selective in that only a subset of cases that fulfill the general criteria for VaD can be classified into defined subtypes.[34,40] The ADDTC criteria[37] do not specify detailed subtypes, but they highlight that classification of ischemic VaD for research purposes should specify features of the infarcts that may differentiate the disorder, such as location (cortical, white matter, periventricular, basal ganglia or thalamus), size (volume), distribution (large, small or microvascular), severity (chronic ischemia versus infarction) and etiology (embolism, atherosclerosis, arteriolosclerosis, cerebral amyloid angiopathy or hypoperfusion). The NINDS-AIREN criteria[38] include, without detailed description, cortical VaD, subcortical VaD, Binswanger's disease and thalamic dementia.

Clinical features of the main subtypes of vascular dementia

Cortical VaD

Cortical VaD relates to large vessel disease, cardiac embolic events and also, in some instances, hypoperfusion (see Table 5.2). From the pathological point of view, predominantly cortical and cortical–subcortical arterial territorial and distal field (watershed) infarcts are found. Typical clinical features are focal sensorimotor changes and abrupt onset of cognitive impairment and aphasia.[49] In addition, it has been suggested that some combinations of cortical neuropsychological syndromes are present in cortical VaD.[53] This group shows heterogeneity with regard to etiology, vascular mechanisms, changes in the brain and clinical manifestations.

Strategic infarct dementia

Focal, often small, ischemic lesions involving specific sites that are critical for higher cortical functions have been classified separately (see Table 5.2). The hippocampal formation and the angular gyrus are examples of the cortical sites. The subcortical sites include the thalamus, the gyrus cinguli, the fornix, the basal forebrain, the caudate, the globus pallidus, and the genu or anterior limb of the internal capsule.[5,17,22] This group shows the highest degree of heterogeneity.

Subcortical VaD

This type of VaD incorporates the old entities, 'lacunar state' and 'Binswanger's disease'. It relates to small vessel disease and hypoperfusion; from the pathological point of view, it is predominantly characterized by lacunar infarcts, focal and diffuse ischemic WMLs and incomplete ischemic injury.[49,53,54] Clinically, small vessel dementia is characterized by pure motor hemiparesis, bulbar signs and dysarthria, gait disorders, urinary disorders, depression and emotional lability, and in particular, deficits in executive functioning.[53–57] Subcortical VaD is a candidate for a more homogeneous subgroup (see below).

Challenging clinical criteria of vascular dementia

The heterogeneity of the patient populations that are derived by using current criteria for VaD has raised the need for an updated systematization. One suggestion has been that a more homogeneous group of patients could be identified by dividing VaD into subtypes.

The new criteria should be based on homogeneity in:

- etiology (primary vascular mechanism);
- changes in the brain (type and location of brain lesions); and
- clinical syndrome.

They should show predictable results in terms of:

- phenomenology and clinical picture;
- clinical course and natural history; and
- outcomes and treatment responses.

In addition, they should be reproducible (i.e. there should be intra- and inter-rater reliability) and practicable in various clinical settings. In this way, they should be able to identify homogeneous and representative patient samples. A proposal for a more homogeneous subtype with a more predictable outcome is subcortical VaD.

Subcortical vascular dementia

Concept

Subcortical VaD incorporates small vessel disease as the primary vascular etiology, lacunar infarcts and ischemic WMLs as the primary types of brain lesions, and subcortical location as the primary location of lesions (Table 5.3). The ischemic lesions in VaD affect especially the prefrontal–subcortical circuit, including the prefrontal cortex, caudate nucleus, globus pallidus, thalamus and the thalamocortical circuit (genu or anterior limb of the internal capsule, anterior centrum semiovale and anterior corona radiata).[58] Accordingly, the subcortical syndrome is the primary clinical manifestation.

Pathology

Thus far, no large and systematic study has been carried out to evaluate the pathological aspects of subtypes of VaD. Accordingly, knowledge must be extrapolated mainly from selected case series and from studies that have assessed the pathological–radiological correlates in patients with a clinical or radiological picture that is consistent with that of subcortical VaD (e.g. subjects with extensive WMLs but without large territorial infarcts). Large cortical lesions, by definition, exclude the diagnosis of subcortical VaD, but the possible role of microscopic alterations of the cortex in cases of subcortical VaD has never been systematically evaluated. However, cortical gliosis or granular atrophy that is related to incomplete ischemic injury in areas of selective vulnerability[59] may coexist with damage of subcortical structures and may go undetected in

Table 5.3 Etiology and brain changes in subcortical vascular dementia

Etiology

Primary vascular mechanisms
Small vessel disease
    Obliteration and occlusion
    Increased resistance
    Decreased autoregulation
    Cerebral blood flow fluctuations
    Endothelium changes
    Blood–brain barrier and carrier changes
    Perivascular changes

Primary risk factors
    Arterial hypertension
    Age

Secondary vascular mechanisms
    Hemodynamic changes of systemic vascular, cardiac or carotid origin

Secondary risk factors
    Hypotension
    Hypoxic–ischemic events
    Blood pressure fluctuations
    Diabetes mellitus
    Hyperlipidemia
    Low education level

Brain changes

Primary type
Ischemic white matter lesions
    Araiosis
    État criblé
    Demyelination
    Axonal loss
    Changes in oligodendrocytes and glial cells
    Incomplete infarcts
Lacunar infarcts
Incomplete ischemic injury
    Laminar necrosis
    Focal gliosis
    Granular atrophy
    Incomplete white matter infarcts

Primary location
    White matter lesions (extending periventricular and deep white matter lesions affecting especially the genu or anterior limb of the internal capsule, anterior corona radiata and anterior centrum semiovale)
    Lacunes (in the caudate, globus pallidus, thalamus, internal capsule, corona radiata and frontal white matter)

routine evaluations. Even so, there are some types of lesion that can be consistently recognized in subcortical VaD, particularly WMLs and lacunar infarcts.

WLMs can be diffuse or focal; the two types often coexist. The diffuse changes of white matter are characterized in brain sections prepared with staining for myelin by pallor sparing of the U fibers.[60-64] Sometimes these diffuse lesions are accompanied by the presence of an increased number of reactive astrocytes (astrogliosis).[60,65,66] The white matter rarefaction corresponds to spongiosis (vacuolization of white matter), *état criblé* (widening of perivascular spaces), loss of myelinated axons and decreased number of oligodendrocytes without clear aspects of necrosis.[61-63,67-69] In these areas, alterations of the small penetrating vessels are almost invariably found. These changes are typical of arteriolosclerosis and are characterized by thickening of the wall, replacement of the smooth muscle cells by fibrohyaline–lipid material and narrowing of the lumen.[60,61,63,65,70-73]

All of the changes noted above are mainly found in the deep hemispheric white matter (centrum semiovale, watershed areas), but in most cases of ischemic subcortical VaD alterations of the white matter are also evident in the periventricular regions. The less extensive periventricular white matter changes correlate with decreased myelin content,[64,65,71,72,74-77] loss of ependymal cell layer and reactive gliosis at the tip of the frontal horns,[64,65,74,76-78] as well as with increased content of extracellular fluid.[77] Because small lesions in the periventricular white matter can be found in all age groups,[75,77] the authors suggest that they should not be considered to be characteristic alterations of subcortical VaD.[79]

The focal, non-confluent, alterations of white matter can be regarded as being mainly lacunar infarcts and probably have the same significance. Lacunar infarcts are small areas of coagulative necrosis, by definition less than 15 mm in diameter, and they can be seen in different stages of pathological evolution.[80-82] In most cases of ischemic subcortical VaD, lacunar infarcts are seen in the chronic stage, i.e. they correspond to cavitated lesions seated in the regions of the small penetrating vessels, including the deep thalamic perforating and long medullary arteries, and in caudate, globus pallidus, thalamus, internal capsule, corona radiata and frontal white matter.[60,68,77,83,84] Lacunar infarcts must be distinguished from other types of focal cavitated changes, such as enlarged perivascular spaces.[64,76] Microscopically, enlarged perivascular spaces are characterized by lack of necrotic aspects (absence of macrophages and tissue debris) and by the presence of a small vessel within the lacuna. In addition to the traditional focal cavitated lacunes, a non-cavitated subtype has been identified as being related to incomplete ischemic injury.[85] According to an alternative hypothesis, such lesions may represent early stages of enlarged perivascular spaces.[86]

Brain imaging

The radiological hallmarks of subcortical VaD include:

- extending diffuse periventricular and deep ischemic focal WMLs that affect especially the genu or anterior limb of the internal capsule, the anterior corona radiata and centrum semiovale; and
- lacunar infarcts in the caudate nucleus, globus pallidus, thalamus, internal capsule, corona radiata and frontal white matter.

WMLs and lacunar infarcts can be detected by CT and MRI, but the two methods have different sensitivity and, possibly, different specificity.

WMLs are seen as bilateral, symmetric, areas of hypodensity on CT scans or as areas of hyperintensity on T2-weighted MRI. They are located in the periventricular or deep subcortical white matter. They can be distinguished from territorial infarcts because do not have well-defined margins, are not wedge-shaped, do not involve the cortex and are not associated with enlargement of the ipsilateral sulci or ventricle; moreover, they do not follow a specific vascular territory.[87]

WMLs detected by CT and MRI are not completely superimposable as to number, site and extension.[88-94] Moreover, many different rating scales exist for WMLs.[79,95] Most of these scales are based on the visual evaluation of the WMLs and are subject to high inter-rater variability. The simplest scales, especially those based on CT findings, classify WMLs into:

- periventricular WMLs, anterior or posterior WMLs; and
- deep subcortical WMLs, which are usually subclassified as either focal or diffuse.

Almost all the MRI visual rating scales for WMLs are more detailed than this. Periventricular lesions may be classified into:

- areas of hyperintensity that surround the tip of the frontal or occipital horns of the lateral ventricles (also called caps);
- tiny or more extensive areas of hyperintensity along the lateral wall of the cella media of the lateral ventricles (with a thin lining and smooth halo); alternatively, these lesions may extend from the periventricular areas towards the deeper white matter regions; and
- deep or centrum semiovale lesions; this type is usually distinguished as being focal, more or less confluent, or diffuse.

It has been shown that different scales attribute different significance to the same radiological picture.[79]

Rating of WMLs can be based on systematic identification of basic types of WMLs, as described below. WMLs can be rated in distinct white matter areas including periventricular, deep or centrum semiovale, watershed and subcortical areas (Table 5.4).[79,96] On MRI, periventricular WMLs (hyperintensities) are in contact with the ventricular wall whereas deep

Table 5.4 A proposal for classification of cerebral white matter lesions as detected by MRI

Periventricular hyperintensities around frontal and occipital horns

Small frontal or occipital caps (5 mm or less in diameter)
Large frontal/occipital caps (6–10 mm in diameter)
Extending frontal/occipital cap (> 10 mm in diameter as measured parallel to
   ventricle)

Periventricular hyperintensities along the lateral ventricles

Thin lining (≤ 5 mm in diameter)
Smooth halo (6–10 mm in diameter)
Irregular halo (> 10 mm wide, irregular margins, extending into deep white
   matter)

Hyperintensities in other white matter areas

Small focal lesions (5 mm in diameter, mostly rounded)
Large focal lesions (6–10 mm in diameter, mostly rounded)
Confluent hyperintensities (11–25 mm in diameter, irregular shape)
Diffusely confluent hyperintensities (> 25 mm in diameter, irregular shape)
Extensive white matter changes (diffuse hyperintensities without focal lesions)

hyperintensities are separated from the ventricular system by a strip of normal-looking white matter and are located outside watershed areas. The subcortical region is considered to represent the area less than 5 mm beneath the cortex.

Periventricular hyperintensities around the frontal and occipital horns are classified on the basis of their size and shape into small caps, large caps and extending caps. Small caps are hyperintensities that are 5 mm or less in diameter; they are rounded and have regular margins. Large caps are 6–10 mm in diameter, have mostly regular margins. Extending caps are more than 10 mm in diameter and have irregular margins. The size of the cap is measured in a direction parallel to the axis of the ventricular horn.

Periventricular hyperintensities along the bodies of lateral ventricles are classified on the basis of their thickness and shape into thin lining, smooth halo and irregular halo. Thin lining is a hyperintense lining that is 5 mm or less in diameter and has regular margins. A smooth halo is 6–10 mm in diameter, is smooth and has mostly regular margins. An irregular halo is more than 10 mm broad, has irregular margins and extends into the deep white matter.

Hyperintensities in other white matter areas are classified on the basis of their size (greatest diameter) and shape into small focal, large focal, focal confluent, diffusely confluent and extensive WMLs. Small focal lesions are punctate hyperintensities that are 5 mm or less in diameter;

they are mostly rounded. Large focal lesions are 6–10 mm in diameter and are mostly rounded. Focal confluent lesions are 11–25 mm in diameter, can have various shapes and may have irregular borders. Diffusely confluent lesions are over 25 mm and mostly have irregular borders. Extensive white matter changes implies diffuse hyperintensities without distinct focal lesions affecting the majority of the white matter area.

The reliability of these visual ratings was tested by having three raters review 60 MRI scans independently.[79] The weighted κ values for intraobserver agreement were 0.90 for periventricular caps, 0.93 for linings and halos and 0.95 for deep white matter hyperintensities. The corresponding κ values for interobserver agreement were 0.84, 0.82 and 0.84, and 0.82, 0.72 and 0.77 respectively. All values are over 0.61, indicating good intrarater and inter-rater agreement.

MRI has higher sensitivity than CT in detecting WMLs, but some of the WMLs detected on MRI are thought to represent normal radiological findings without pathological significance. WMLs detected by CT are commonly believed to be more indicative of disease than those detected by MRI.[97]

Lacunar infarcts are seen as more or less cavitated lesions according to different stages of evolution. They are round or oval in shape and have a diameter of less than 15 mm (this limit is arbitrary but seems reasonable). It should be kept in mind that the size of a radiologically detected lacunar infarct is slightly larger than that of the same lesion at autopsy. In the chronic stage, lacunar infarcts are hypodense on CT scans and hyperintense on T2-weighted MRI scans. On proton density-weighted images they can be isointense or hyperintense. According to some authors,[78,98] MRI can be used to distinguish lacunar infarcts from enlarged perivascular spaces, which are frequently found in the same brain regions, although the radiological criteria for such a distinction are debatable. Foci with smooth margins (as opposed to irregular margins) and with a putaminal location (as opposed to a thalamic location) are more likely to represent enlarged perivascular spaces than lacunar infarcts.[99] In addition, lesions that are smaller than 1×2 mm are more likely to be enlarged perivascular spaces than infarcts.

Pathophysiology

The causes of subcortical VaD have not been fully ascertained. However, information is accumulating about the risk factors and mechanisms of damage to the cerebral subcortical structures related to the pathogenesis of subcortical VaD. There is still a lack of studies that have a specific focus on subcortical forms, while studies including all the heterogeneous subtypes of VaD do not provide sufficient information.[5,100]

The two main types of lesion in subcortical VaD are WMLs and lacunar infarcts, and thus a way of understanding the pathogenesis of subcortical VaD is to refer to the mechanisms that underlie these two lesion types.

The pathogenesis of lacunar infarcts is considered to be reasonably well established[82,101] despite discordant opinions.[102] Conversely, the pathogenesis of white matter changes is less well established. Some clinical observations and instrumental and experimental data suggest that vascular mechanisms (more specifically ischemic mechanisms) are responsible for these alterations.[27]

In any case, alteration of deep small vessels is considered to play such a central role in subcortical VaD that the name 'small vessel dementia' has been proposed for this entity.[38] The small vessel pathology is related to aging, arterial hypertension and diabetes mellitus.[103–105] These changes may result in stenosis or occlusion of the vessels with consequent sudden or more chronic ischemia of the parenchyma. The effect of ischemia can be either:

- acute, severe and localized, leading to small areas of veritable necrosis (lacunar infarction); or
- chronic, less severe and diffuse, with histological alterations consistent with the definition of incomplete infarct.

In the white matter, incomplete infarction is considered to be characterized by rarefaction of the myelin sheaths, moderate loss of oligodendrocytes and reactive gliosis.[106] Moreover, the arteriolosclerotic changes cause the small arteries and arterioles of the deep white matter and basal ganglia to loose their physiologic capacity to autoregulate by dilating and constricting in response to variations in systemic blood pressure. Accordingly, the areas supplied by these vessels may suffer from fluctuations in cerebral blood flow (either a decrease or an increase) in response to changes in systemic blood pressure.[107] Both of these types of mechanisms may be particularly harmful to the brain parenchyma since the blood supply of the deep cerebral structures is of the terminal type with scarce, if any, anastomoses.[108–110] This vascular damage to the white matter is sufficient to provoke complete necrosis of the tissue (with the exception of some areas where true lacunar infarcts are recognizable) but it can cause selective damage to some histological components. Brun and Englund were among the first to propose that the diffuse changes of the white matter seen in demented patients should be considered to be a form of incomplete infarction.[106] Although this remains a hypothesis, there are now experimental data showing that white matter components are extremely vulnerable to ischemia and can be damaged in the absence of neuronal injury.[111,112]

Other hypotheses have been raised as alternatives to the possible ischemic origin of diffuse WMLs. In the authors' view, these mechanisms are not mutually exclusive and may occur together in the development of the final pathological picture. For example, the small vessel alterations could also lead to damage of the blood–brain barrier and to chronic leakage of fluid and macromolecules in the white matter. The increased interstitial fluid concentration in abnormal white matter may be also a consequence of arterial hypertension. The blood–brain barrier may be leaky, and the capillary permeability to proteins may be increased in patients with systemic hypertension.[113] Abnormalities in the blood–brain barrier, in the form of increased concentration of cerebrospinal fluid proteins, have been described in a group of patients with radiologically detected white matter changes[114] and in a pathological series of patients with subcortical vascular encephalopathy.[115] In addition to the effects of sustained hypertension, hypertensive bouts of short duration could cause fluid transudation and protein leakage.

Besides acquired vascular risk factors and conditions, other genetically determined factors could play an important role in the development of subcortical ischemic VaD, and there is at least one form of subcortical VaD with a clearly determined genetic origin. Cerebral autosomal-dominant arteriopathy with subcortical infarcts and leukoencephalopathy (CADASIL) is clinically characterized by recurrent strokes and progressive neurological deterioration in middle-aged subjects; it eventually results in pseudobulbar palsy and dementia.[116,117] Radiologically, CADASIL patients present with diffuse cerebral white matter alterations associated with small focal lesions of the lacunar type.[118] Histological studies have shown a degeneration of small vessel smooth muscle cells with deposition of granular osmiophilic material in the vessel wall.[119,120] Genetic linkage analysis has allowed the location of the altered gene to be defined as being on chromosome 19p13.1.[121]

Presently, the epidemiological relevance of these hereditary forms appears limited; however, other unknown forms of hereditary subcortical VaD that are linked to as yet undiscovered gene alterations may exist and may be unrecognized because of different patterns of transmission or penetrance. It is also possible that some genetic factors contribute, by interaction with conventional risk factors, to the development of white matter injury in non-familial cases. For example, polymorphism of angiotensin converting enzyme has been found to increase the risk of lacunar infarcts[122] and, more recently, of diffuse white matter changes.[122] Other factors such as apoE ϵ4 allele[124] have been found to be associated with damage to cerebral subcortical structures. Although their possible specific role in the origin of WMLs is yet to be explored, the influence of these genetic aspects could explain why not all patients with vascular risk factors (e.g. hypertension) develop white matter alterations at follow-up.

Clinical features

The cognitive syndrome of subcortical VaD is characterized by:

- dysexecutive syndrome, including slowed information processing;
- memory deficit that may be mild; and
- behavioral and psychological symptoms.

The dysexecutive syndromin subcortical VaD includes impairment in goal formulation, initiation, planning, organizing, sequencing, executing, set-shifting and set-maintenance, as well as in abstracting.[50,53,125] The memory deficit in subcortical VaD may be milder than, for example, in AD, and it is specified by impaired recall, relative intact recognition, less severe forgetfulness and better benefits from cues.[125] Behavioral and psychological symptoms in subcortical VaD include, in particular, depression, personality change, emotional lability and incontinence, as well as inertia, emotional bluntness and psychomotor retardation.[38,50,53]

Neurological findings, particularly early in the course of subcortical VaD, include episodes of mild upper motor neuron signs (drift, reflex asymmetry, incordination), gait disorder (apractic–atactic or small-stepped), imbalance and falls, urinary frequency and incontinence, dysarthria, dysphagia and extrapyramidal signs (hypokinesia, rigidity).[38,49,54–56] However, these focal neurological signs are often subtle.[126,127] VaD has been traditionally thought to be characterized by a relative abrupt onset (days to weeks), a stepwise deterioration (with some recovery after worsening) and a fluctuating course (e.g. a day-to-day difference in severity) of cognitive functions. This is seen in patients with multiple lesions affecting cortical and cortical–subcortical brain structures. In patients with subcortical VaD, however, the onset of cognitive symptoms is relatively insidious and the course is more slowly progressive.[37,38,54,88,126,127]

The mean duration of VaD is around 5 years,[7] and patient survival is shorter than that of the general population or AD patients.[9,128] Detailed studies on the natural history of subcortical VaD are lacking, and little is known or can be predicted about the rate and pattern of cognitive decline or the prognosis in subcortical VaD.[129]

Diagnostic criteria

Selection of patients with subcortical VaD for clinical studies and trials could be mainly based on brain imaging features, as these seem to be the most consistent findings and can be easily adapted for multicenter use. The brain imaging criteria should reflect the essential changes (construct validity) and all the main aspects of the changes (content validity). In subcortical VaD the essential changes, as well as the main aspects of the lesions, include:

- extensive ischemic WMLs; and
- lacunar infarcts in the deep gray and white matter structures.

A protocol for brain imaging requirements for subcortical VaD is given in Table 5.5.[79,96,130–132] The brain imaging criteria should cover cases with predominantly WMLs (the old 'Binswanger type') and cases with predominantly lacunar infarcts (the old 'lacunar state type').

Clinical criteria for subcortical VaD may be based on a modification of the NINDS-AIREN criteria[38] (Table 5.6). The main modifications include a definition of the cognitive syndrome and evidence of relevant cerebrovascular disease by brain imaging.

The cognitive syndrome includes both the executive syndrome and some degrees of memory deficit. This memory deficit has to interfere at

Table 5.5 Brain imaging criteria for subcortical VaD

CT

Extending periventricular and deep white matter lesions: patchy or diffuse symmetrical areas of low attenuation (intermediate density between that of normal white matter and that of intraventricular cerebrospinal fluid) with ill-defined margins extending to the centrum semiovale, *and* at least one lacunar infarct

and

no cortical or cortical–subcortical non-lacunar territorial infarcts and watershed infarcts, presence of hemorrhages, signs of normal pressure hydrocephalus, and specific causes of white matter lesions (e.g. multiple sclerosis, sarcoidosis, brain irradiation)

MRI

1. To include predominantly 'white matter cases': extending periventricular and deep white matter lesions; extending caps (> 10 mm as measured parallel to ventricle) or irregular halo (> 10 mm wide, irregular margins and extending into deep white matter) *and* diffusely confluent hyperintensities (> 25 mm, irregular shape) or extensive white matter changes (diffuse hyperintensity without focal lesions), *and* lacune(s) in the deep gray matter.

or

2. To include predominantly 'lacunar cases': multiple lacunes (e.g. more than five) in the deep gray matter *and* at least moderate white matter lesions; extending caps or irregular halo or diffusely confluent hyperintensities or extensive white matter change.

and

no cortical or cortical–subcortical non-lacunar territorial infarcts and watershed infarcts, presence of hemorrhages, signs of normal pressure hydrocephalus, and specific causes of white matter lesions (e.g. multiple sclerosis, sarcoidosis, brain irradiation)

Table 5.6 Proposal for clinical criteria of subcortical VaD

I. The criteria for the clinical diagnosis of subcortical VaD include all of the following:

A. Cognitive syndrome, including both:

Dysexecutive syndrome (impairment in goal formulation, initiation, planning, organizing, sequencing, executing, set-shifting and set-maintenance, abstracting) *and*

Memory deficit (may be mild) (impaired recall, relative intact recognition, less severe forgetting, benefit from cues)

These must indicate deterioration from a higher level of functioning, and are interfering with complex (executive) occupational and social activities not caused by physical effects of cerebrovascular disease alone

B. Cerebrovascular disease, including both:

Evidence of relevant cerebrovascular disease by brain imaging and

Presence or a history of neurologic signs (as evidence for cerebrovascular disease such as hemiparesis, lower facial weakness, Babinski sign, sensory deficit, dysarthria, gait disorder and extrapyramidal signs consistent with subcortical brain lesions)

II. Clinical features that support the diagnosis of subcortical vascular dementia include the following:

- Episodes of mild upper motor neuron involvement (e.g. drift, reflex asymmetry, incordination)
- Early presence of a gait disturbance (small-step gait or march à petits pas magnetic, apraxic–ataxic or parkinsonian gait)
- History of unsteadiness and frequent, unprovoked falls
- Early urinary frequency, urgency, and other urinary symptoms not explained by urologic disease
- Dysarthria, dysphagia, extrapyramidal signs (e.g. hypokinesia, rigidity)
- Behavioral and psychological symptoms (e.g. depression, personality change, emotional incontinence, psychomotor retardation)

III. Features that make the diagnosis of subcortical vascular dementia uncertain or unlikely include:

- Early onset of memory deficit and progressive worsening of memory and other cognitive functions such as language (transcortical sensory aphasia), motor skills (apraxia) and perception (agnosia), in the absence of corresponding focal lesions on brain imaging
- Absence of relevant cerebrovascular disease lesions on brain CT or MRI

least with the more complex executive social activities. Cerebrovascular disease is defined by evidence of relevant findings on brain imaging (see Table 5.4) and the presence of focal neurological signs consistent with cerebrovascular disease. Since these two elements include the assumption of causality, no further requirement is included. The criteria include clinical features that support the diagnosis of subcortical VaD, as well as those that make the diagnosis unlikely.

Prevention and treatment

At present, no drug has been definitely accepted as effective in VaD. A recent review has examined trials that aimed to test drug efficacy in VaD and commented on possible reasons for the partially disappointing results so far achieved.[43]

Prevention

A number of risk factors have been identified as having a possible relationship with vascular damage of subcortical cerebral structures and cognitive impairment of vascular origin. By controlling these risk factors it should be possible, theoretically, to avoid, slow or delay the onset of subcortical VaD. Arterial hypertension, which is probably the main risk factor for subcortical VaD, diabetes mellitus, smoking and hyperlipidemia can all be effectively controlled, but there are no preliminary data to confirm that subcortical VaD can be prevented by so doing, although it is reasonable to suppose this. In a small study, Meyer *et al.* showed that control of vascular risk factors, such as arterial hypertension and smoking, was able to stabilize or improve the cognitive status of patients diagnosed with MID.[133] The same authors observed that a too marked reduction in systolic blood pressure levels was associated with progression of mental deterioration.[133] The Syst-Eur trial, a randomized, double-blind, placebo-controlled trial for treating systolic hypertension, has provided the first clear-cut evidence that controlling hypertension reduces the incidence of dementia.[134] Lowering systolic blood pressure by at least 20 mmHg to a value of less than 150 mmHg by the administration of a calcium channel blocker, with the possible addition of an angiotensin converting enzyme inhibitor or a diuretic, reduced the incidence of dementia by 50%. This clinical trial provided no data about the mechanism by which control of hypertension reduced the risk of dementia (AD, mixed dementia or VaD). The authors suggest that calcium channel blockers used in this study may have a direct neuroprotective effect or may alter production of β-amyloid or neurotransmission. In contrast, another large therapeutic trial, the Systolic Hypertension in the Elderly Program (SHEP) trial,[135] using a thiazide diuretic and a β-blocker as antihypertensive treatment, failed to demonstrate a protective effect against cognitive impairment, which suggests that dementia cannot be prevented simply by lowering blood pressure.

The role of antiplatelet or anticoagulant agents in preventing VaD has also not been conclusively proved. A survey about the use of antithrombotic treatments that was carried out in Canada among neurologists and geriatricians showed that the most commonly employed treatment in subcortical VaD was aspirin, although the majority of the specialists pointed out the need of a randomized clinical trial to assess the efficacy of aspirin in VaD.[136]

Although oral anticoagulants are definitely effective in preventing cerebral infarcts of cardioembolic origin and, therefore, presumably may prevent or ameliorate MID, one recent trial comparing the safety and efficacy of oral anticoagulants and aspirin in the secondary prevention of stroke disclosed that oral anticoagulants are associated with an increased risk of cerebral hemorrhage in patients with WMLs on CT scan that are consistent with small vessel subcortical disease and chronic ischemia.[137,138] This result may indicate that drugs that are potentially beneficial in some subtypes of VaD may be harmful in other subtypes.

Treatment

A number of drugs have been tested in patients diagnosed with VaD. This topic has been summarized in recent reviews.[43,139] Objects of targeted treatment of VaD include:

- symptomatic improvement of core symptoms (e.g. cognitive or behavioral symptoms);
- slowing progression of the disorder; and
- treatment of secondary factors that affect cognition (e.g. depression, anxiety or agitation).

Classes of drugs include:

- antithrombotic drugs (e.g. aspirin);[140,141]
- ergot alkaloids (e.g. hydergine, nicergoline);[142,143]
- xantine derivatives (e.g. pentoxifylline, propentofylline);[144–148]
- calcium antagonists (e.g. nimodipine)
- posatirelin (a TRH analog);[149]
- EGb761 (a particular extract of Ginkgo biloba);[150]
- memantine (a low-affinity, voltage-dependent, non-competitive NMDA receptor antagonist).[151–153]

Studies on symptomatic improvement in VaD have mostly involved small numbers of patients, short treatment periods and variations in diagnostic criteria and tools, and they have often included mixed populations and had variations in the application of clinical end-points. In some of the above-mentioned trials, the target population was patients with dementia or cognitive impairment and data on VaD patients was derived from subgroup analysis. Of those trials that specifically referred to VaD, it is to be noted that none took into account a specific subtype of VaD, since all of them used the global definition of VaD or MID.

Recently, nimodipine, memantine and propentofylline have all raised expectations about the symptomatic treatment of VaD. Memantine, a low-affinity, voltage-dependent, non-competitive NMDA receptor antagonist, has raised expectations about both symptomatic and neuroprotective treatment of dementia.[151] In a first double-blind, placebo-controlled trial in severe dementia of mixed etiology, memantine (20 mg, given once) was well tolerated, and patients treated with the drug showed functional improvement and reduction of care dependency compared with placebo patients.[152,153] Currently, two pivotal trials in mild to moderate VaD are ongoing in Europe (Moebius HJ, personal communication).

Propentofylline is a neuroprotective glial cell modulator. The molecular effects include selective adenosine reuptake inhibition and selective phosphodiesterase inhibition, and the cellular effects include reduced microglial activation and improved astrocyte function.[147] Activation of glial cells, increased production of cytokines, free radicals and glutamate and dedifferentiation of astrocytes have been related to VaD.[147] Thus, propentofylline has been regarded as a candidate for symptomatic and neuroprotective treatment of VaD. Early phase III trials of propentofylline have shown an effect on both cognition and global impression of change, and also on progression of VaD.[146,147,154,155]

Preliminary results of an European–Canadian, double-blind, placebo-controlled, randomized, parallel-group trial on efficacy and safety of long-term treatment with propentofylline (300 mg, three doses) in patients with mild-to-moderate VaD according to NINDS-AIREN criteria have been presented.[156] The study involved two segments, a 24-week, traditional parallel-group design and a 24-week, combined randomized delayed-start–withdrawal design. The primary efficacy variables were the Alzheimer's Disease Assessment Scale – cognitive subscale (ADAS-Cog) and the Clinician's Interview Based Impression of Chance (CIBIC-Plus). The study showed significant symptomatic improvement and long-term efficacy in ADAS-Cog and CIBIC-Plus up to 48 weeks. In addition, sustained treatment effects could be shown for at least 12 weeks after withdrawal, indicating an effect on disease progression. Propentofylline was well tolerated, with no negative effects after withdrawal (B Kittner, personal communication).

An international study group has compared the efficacy of pentoxifylline (400 mg three times daily) with that of placebo over a period of 9 months.[148] The intention-to-treat analysis for those patients who completed the study ($n = 239$) showed a statistically significant difference of 3.5 points on the Gottfries–Bråne–Steen scale in favor of active treatment.[148]

As mentioned above, very few attempts have so far been made to test drugs in specific subtypes of VaD. One example is the use of nimodipine, a dihydropyridine calcium channel blocker, in subcortical VaD. Nimodipine exerts a vasoactive effect without a steal effect, reduces influx of calcium ions into depolarized neurons, and may have a neuroprotective effect that is not strictly related to improvement in cerebral blood flow.[157] Moreover, the drug has a specific effect on small vessels.[158,159]

One open-label study was designed to test the efficacy and safety of nimodipine in patients with a clinical–radiological syndrome consistent

with that of subcortical VaD.[130] Some encouraging results in this preliminary trial led to a subgroup analysis of the larger double-blind, placebo-
controlled, Scandinavian Multi-Infarct Dementia trial. Patients were
divided in MID and subcortical VaD groups according to blindly
assessed CT findings. The results indicate that nimodipine has a beneficial effect on attention and psychomotor performances in the subcortical
group, whereas no clear advantage is shown in the general sample.[160,161]
(Pantoni *et al.*, submitted). These preliminary results are currently being
tested in an international, multicenter, randomized, double-blind trial that
is enrolling patients with subcortical VaD defined on clinical–radiological
basis.

Future perspectives in the treatment of VaD include actions on delayed
neuronal death and on neurotransmission (e.g. cholinergic transmission),
and AD type strategies such as actions to decrease β-protein expression
and amyloid accumulation.

Conclusion

Subcortical VaD may offer a solution to enable a more homogeneous and
representative group of patients to be identified, which would improve
the comparability of independent studies and benefit multicenter collaboration.

Further empirical research and international debate is especially
needed to:

- define the cognitive syndrome and the stages of vascular cognitive
  impairment, including the most severe one of VaD;
- refine the selection, definitions and measures of domains related to the
  construct, including cognitive functions (e.g. memory, executive functions, aphasia, apraxia, agnosia), behavioral and psychological symptoms (e.g. depression, anxiety, psychotic symptoms, apathy, emotional
  control, personality) and social functions (e.g. work, executive activity
  of daily living (ADL), instrumental ADL and basic ADL);
- validate further the proposed brain imaging criteria for subcortical
  VaD;[162]
- characterize in large community samples the natural history and outcomes of the syndrome;
- identify the outcome measures for clinical trials (cognition, behavioral
  and psychological symptoms, functional and social activities) and the
  length of follow-up; and
- investigate biochemical correlates of WMLs in blood and cerebrospinal
  fluid.

References

1. Berchtold NC, Cotman CW. Evolution in the conceptualization of dementia and Alzheimer's disease: Greco–Roman period to the 1960s. Neurobiol Aging 1998;19:173–189.

2. Tomlinson BE, Blessed G, Roth M. Observations on the brains of demented old people. J Neurol Sci 1970;11:205–242.

3. Hachinski VC, Lassen NA, Marshall J. Multi-infarct dementia. A cause of mental deterioration in the elderly. *Lancet* 1974;ii: 207–210.

4. Brust JC. Vascular dementia is overdiagnosed. Arch Neurol 1998;45:799–801.

5. Erkinjuntti T, Hachinski VC. Rethinking vascular dementia. Cerebrovasc Dis 1993;3: 3–23.

6. Hachinski VC. The decline and resurgence of vascular dementia. Can Med Assoc J 1990; 142:107–111.

7. Hebert R, Brayne C. Epidemiology of vascular dementia. Neuroepidemiology 1995;14:250–257.

8. Rocca WA, Hofman A, Brayne C, *et al.* The prevalence of vascular dementia in Europe: facts and fragments from 1980–1990 studies. EURODEM-Prevalence Research Group. Ann Neurol 1991;30:817–824.

9. Skoog I, Nilsson L, Palmertz B, Andreasson LA, Svanborg A. A population-based study on dementia in 85-year-olds. N Engl J Med 1993;328:153–158.

10. Tatemichi TK, Desmond DW, Mayeux R. Dementia after stroke: baseline frequency, risks, and clinical features in a hospitalized cohort. Neurology 1992;42:1185–1193.

11. Tatemichi TK, Paik M, Bagiella E, *et al.* Risk of dementia after stroke in a hospitalized cohort: results of a longitudinal study. Neurology 1994;44:1885–1891.

12. Snowdon DA, Greiner LH, Mortimer JA, Riley KP, Greiner PA, Markesbery WR. Brain infarction and the clinical expression of Alzheimer disease. The Nun Study. JAMA 1997;277:813–817.

13. Stewart R. Cardiovascular factors in Alzheimer's disease. J Neurol Neurosurg Psychiatry 1998;65:143–147.

14. Hachinski V. Preventable senility: a call for action against the vascular dementias. Lancet 1992;340:645–648.

15. Bowler JV, Hachinski V. Vascular cognitive impairment: a new approach to vascular dementia. Baillieres Clin Neurol 1995;4: 357–376.

16. Chui HC. Rethinking vascular dementia: moving from myth to mechanism. In: Growdon JH, Rossor MN, eds. The dementias. Boston: Butterworth–Heinemann; 1998:377–401.

17. Tatemichi TK. How acute brain failure becomes chronic. A view of the mechanisms and syndromes of dementia related to stroke. Neurology 1990;40: 1652–1659.

18. Chui HC. Dementia: a review emphasizing clinicopathologic correlation and brain–behavior relationships. Arch Neurol 1989; 46:806–814.

19. Desmond DW. Vascular dementia: a construct in evolution. Cerebrovasc Brain Metab Rev 1996;8:296–325.

20. Pasquier F, Leys D. Why are stroke patients prone to develop dementia? J Neurol 1997;244: 135–142.

21. Skoog I. Status of risk factors for

vascular dementia. Neuroepidemiology 1998;17:2–9.

22. Erkinjuntti T. Clinicopathological study of vascular dementia. In: Prohovnik I, Wade J, Knezevic S, Tatemichi TK, Erkinjuntti T, eds. Vascular dementia. Current concepts. Chichester, UK: John Wiley and Sons; 1996:73–112.

23. Brun A. Pathology and pathophysiology of cerebrovascular dementia: pure subgroups of obstructive and hypoperfusive etiology. Dementia 1994;5:145–147.

24. Amar K, Wilcock G. Vascular dementia. BMJ 1996;312:227–231.

25. Wallin A, Blennow K. The clinical diagnosis of vascular dementia. Dementia 1994;5:181–184.

26. Pantoni L, Garcia JH. The significance of cerebral white matter abnormalities 100 years after Binswanger's report. A review. Stroke 1995;26:1293–1301.

27. Pantoni L, Garcia JH. Pathogenesis of leukoaraiosis: a review. Stroke 1997;28:652–659.

28. Englund E, Brun A, Alling C. White matter changes in dementia of Alzheimer's type. Biochemical and neuropathological correlates. Brain 1988;111:1425–1439.

29. Mielke R, Herholz K, Grond M, Kessler J, Heiss WD. Severity of vascular dementia is related to volume of metabolically impaired tissue. Arch Neurol 1992;49:909–913.

30. Garcia JH, Lassen NA, Weiller C, Sperling B, Nakagawara J. Ischemic stroke and incomplete infarction. Stroke 1996;27:761–765.

31. Erkinjuntti T, Haltia M, Palo J, Sulkava R, Paetau A. Accuracy of the clinical diagnosis of vascular dementia: a retrospective clinical and post-mortem neuropathological study. J Neurol Neurosurg Psychiatry 1988;51:1037–1044.

32. Rockwood K, Parhad I, Hachinski V, et al. Diagnosis of vascular dementia: Consortium of Canadian Centres for Clinical Cognitive Research consensus statement. Can J Neurol Sci 1994;21:358–364.

33. Erkinjuntti T. Clinical criteria for vascular dementia: The NINDS-AIREN criteria. Dementia 1994;5:189–192.

34. Wetterling T, Kanitz RD, Borgis KJ. The ICD-10 criteria for vascular dementia. Dementia 1994;5:185–188.

35. American Psychiatric Association. Diagnostic and statistical manual of mental disorders, 4th edition. Washington, DC: American Psychiatric Association; 1994.

36. World Health Organization. ICD-10 Classification of mental and behavioural disorders: diagnostic criteria for research. Geneva: World Health Organization; 1993.

37. Chui HC, Victoroff JI, Margolin D, Jagust W, Shankle R, Katzman R. Criteria for the diagnosis of ischemic vascular dementia proposed by the State of California Alzheimer's Disease Diagnostic and Treatment Centers. Neurology 1992;42:473–480.

38. Román GC, Tatemichi TK, Erkinjuntti T, et al. Vascular dementia: diagnostic criteria for research studies. Report of the NINDS-AIREN International Work Group. Neurology 1993;43:250–260.

39. Erkinjuntti T, Ostbye T, Steenhuis R, Hachinski V. The effect of different diagnostic criteria on the prevalence of dementia. N Eng J Med 1997;337:1667–1674.

40. Wetterling T, Kanitz RD, Borgis

KJ. Comparison of different diagnostic criteria for vascular dementia (ADDTC, DSM-IV, ICD-10, NINDS-AIREN). Stroke 1996;27:30–36.

41. Pohjasvaara T, Erkinjuntti T, Vataja R, Kaste M. Dementia three months after stroke. Baseline frequency and effect of different definitions of dementia in the Helsinki Stroke Aging Memory Study (SAM) cohort. Stroke 1997;28:785–792.

42. Erkinjuntti T, Inzitari D, Pantoni L, *et al.* Limitations of clinical criteria for the diagnosis of vascular dementia in clinical trials: is a focus on subcortical vascular dementia a solution? Ann N Y Acad Sci; in press.

43. Inzitari D, Erkinjuntti T, Wallin A, del Ser T, Romanelli M, Pantoni L. Subcortical vascular dementia as a specific target for clinical trials. Ann N Y Acad Sci; in press.

44. Erkinjuntti T. Vascular dementia: challenge of clinical diagnosis. Int Psychogeriatr 1997;9:51–58.

45. Lopez OL, Larumbe MR, Becker JT, *et al.* Reliability of NINDS-AIREN clinical criteria for the diagnosis of vascular dementia. Neurology 1994;44:1240–1245.

46. Verhey FR, Lodder J, Rozendaal N, Jolles J. Comparison of seven sets of criteria used for the diagnosis of vascular dementia. Neuroepidemiology 1996; 15:166–172.

47. Gold G, Giannakopoulos P, Montes-Paixao JC, *et al.* Sensitivity and specificity of newly proposed clinical criteria for possible vascular dementia. Neurology 1997;49:690–694.

48. Konno S, Meyer JS, Terayama Y, Margishvili GM, Mortel KF. Classification, diagnosis and treatment of vascular dementia. Drugs Aging 1997;11:361–373.

49. Erkinjuntti T. Types of multi-infarct dementia. Acta Neurol Scand 1987;75:391–399.

50. Cummings JL. Vascular subcortical dementias: clinical aspects. Dementia 1994;5:177–180.

51. Loeb C, Meyer JS. Vascular dementia: still a debatable entity? J Neurol Sci 1996;143: 31–40.

52. Sulkava R, Erkinjuntti T. Vascular dementia due to cardiac arrhythmias and systemic hypotension. Acta Neurol Scand 1987; 76:123–128.

53. Mahler ME, Cummings JL. The behavioural neurology of multi-infarct dementia. Alzheimer Dis Assoc Disord 1991;5:122–130.

54. Román GC. Senile dementia of the Binswanger type. A vascular form of dementia in the elderly. JAMA 1987;258:1782–1788.

55. Babikian V, Ropper AH. Binswanger's disease: a review. Stroke 1987;18:2–12.

56. Ishii N, Nishihara Y, Imamura T. Why do frontal lobe symptoms predominate in vascular dementia with lacunes? Neurology 1986;36:340–345.

57. Wallin A, Blennow K, Gottfries CG. Subcortical symptoms predominate in vascular dementia. Int J Geriatr Psychiatry 1991; 6:137–146.

58. Cummings JL. Fronto-subcortical circuits and human behavior. Arch Neurol 1993;50:873–880.

59. Garcia JH, Brown GG. Vascular dementia: neuropathologic alterations and metabolic brain changes. J Neurol Sci 1992; 109:121–131.

60. Pantoni L, Garcia JH, Brown GG. Vascular pathology in three cases of progressive cognitive deterioration. J Neurol Sci 1996; 135:131–139.

61. Lotz PR, Ballinger WE Jr, Quis-

ling RG. Subcortical arteriosclerotic encephalopathy: CT spectrum and pathologic correlation. AJNR Am J Neuroradiol 1986;7:817–822.

62. Janota J, Mirsen TR, Hachinski VC, Lee DH, Merskey H. Neuropathological correlates of leuko-araiosis. Arch Neurol 1989;46:1124–1128.

63. Révész T, Hawkins CP, du Boulay EPGH, Barnard RO, McDonald WI. Pathological findings correlated with magnetic resonance imaging in subcortical arteriosclerotic encephalopathy (Binswanger's disease). J Neurol Neurosurg Psychiatry 1989; 52:1337–1344.

64. Chimowitz MI, Estes ML, Furlan AJ, Awad IA. Further observations on the pathology of subcortical lesions identified on magnetic resonance imaging. Arch Neurol 1992;49:747–752.

65. Fazekas F, Kleinert R, Offenbacher H, et al. The morphologic correlate of incidental punctate white matter hyperintensities on MR images. AJNR Am J Neuroradiol 1991;12: 915–921.

66. Fazekas F, Kleinert R, Offenbacher H, et al. Pathologic correlates of incidental MRI white matter signal hyperintensities. Neurology 1993;43:1683–1689.

67. Awad IA, Johnson PC, Spetzler RF, Hodak JA. Incidental subcortical lesions identified on magnetic resonance imaging in the elderly. II. Postmortem pathological correlations. Stroke 1986;17:1090–1097.

68. Muñoz DG, Hastak SM, Harper B, Lee D, Hachinski VC. Pathologic correlates of increased signals of the centrum ovale on magnetic resonance imaging. Arch Neurol 1993;50:492–497.

69. Erkinjuntti T, Benavente O, Eliasziw M, et al. Diffuse vacuolization (spongiosis) and arteriolosclerosis in the frontal white matter occurs in vascular dementia. Arch Neurol 1996;53: 325–332.

70. Ho KL, Garcia JH. Neuropathology of the small blood vessels in selected diseases of the cerebral white matter. In: Pantoni L, Inzitari D, Wallin A, eds. The matter of white matter. Clinical and pathophysiological aspects of white matter disease related to cognitive decline and vascular dementia. Utrecht, The Netherlands: Academic Pharmaceutical Production; 2000:247–273.

71. Leifer D, Buonanno FS, Richardson EP Jr. Clinicopathologic correlations of cranial magnetic resonance imaging of periventricular white matter. Neurology 1990;40:911–918.

72. van Swieten JC, van Den Hout JHW, van Ketel BA, Hijdra A, Wokke JHJ, van Gijn J. Periventricular lesions in the white matter on magnetic resonance imaging in the elderly. A morphometric correlation with arteriolosclerosis and dilated perivascular spaces. Brain 1991; 114:761–774.

73. Marshall VG, Bradley WG Jr, Marshall CE, Bhoopat T, Rhodes RH. Deep white matter infarction: correlation of MR imaging and histopathologic findings. Radiology 1988;167:517–522.

74. Grafton ST, Sumi SM, Stimac GK, Alvord EC Jr, Shaw CM, Nochlin D. Comparison of postmortem magnetic resonance imaging and neuropathologic findings in the cerebral white matter. Arch Neurol 1991;48: 293–298.

75. Moody DM, Brown WR, Challa VR, Anderson RL. Periventricular venous collagenosis: association with leukoaraiosis. Radiol-

ogy 1995;194:469–476.

76. Scarpelli M, Salvolini U, Diamanti L, Montironi R, Chiaromoni L, Maricotti M. MRI and pathological examination of postmortem brains: the problem of white matter high signal areas. Neuroradiology 1994;36:393–398.

77. Sze G, De Armond SJ, Brant-Zawadzki M, Davis RL, Norman D, Newton TH. Foci of MRI signal (pseudolesions) anterior to the frontal horns: histologic correlations of a normal finding. AJNR Am J Neuroradiol 1986;7:381–387.

78. Jungreis CA, Kanal E, Hirsch WL, Martinez AJ, Moossy J. Normal perivascular spaces mimicking lacunar infarction: MR imaging. Radiology 1988;169:101–104.

79. Mäntyla R, Erkinjuntti T, Salonen O, et al. Variable agreement between visual rating scales for white matter hyperintensities on MRI. Comparison of 13 rating scales in a poststroke cohort. Stroke 1997;28:1614–1623.

80. Fisher CM. Lacunes, small deep cerebral infarcts. Neurology 1965;15:774–784.

81. Fisher CM. The arterial lesions: lacunes. Acta Neuropathol (Berl) 1968;12:1–15.

82. Fisher CM. Lacunar strokes and infarcts: a review. Neurology 1982;32:871–876.

83. Olsson Y, Brun A, Englund E. Fundamental pathological lesions in vascular dementia. Acta Neurol Scand Suppl 1996;168:31–38.

84. Braffman BH, Zimmerman RA, Trojanowski JQ, Gonatas NK, Hickey WF, Schlaepfer WW. Brain MR. Pathologic correlation with gross and histopathology. 1. Lacunar infarction and Virchow–Robin spaces. AJNR Am J Neuroradiol 1988;9:621–628.

85. Lammie GA, Brannan F, Wardlaw JM. Incomplete lacunar infarction (Type Ib lacunes). Acta Neuropathol (Berl) 1998;96:163–171.

86. Pantoni L. Incomplete lacunar infarction: an alternative hypothesis. Acta Neuropathol (Berl) 1999;97:322.

87. Inzitari D, Diaz F, Fox A, et al. Vascular risk factors and leukoaraiosis. Arch Neurol 1987;44:42–47.

88. Erkinjuntti T. Differential diagnosis between Alzheimer's disease and vascular dementia: evaluation of common clinical methods. Acta Neurol Scand 1987;76:433–442.

89. Johnson KA, Davis KR, Buonanno FS, Brady TJ, Rosen J, Growdon JH. Comparison of magnetic resonance and roentgen ray computed tomography in dementia. Arch Neurol 1987;44:1075–1080.

90. Bradley WG Jr, Waluch V, Yadley RA, Wycoff RR. Comparison of CT and MR in 400 patients with suspected disease of the brain and cervical spinal cord. Radiology 1984;152:695–702.

91. Brant-Zawadzki M, David PL, Crooks LE, et al. NMR demonstration of cerebral abnormalities: comparison with CT. AJR Am J Roentgenol 1983;140:847–854.

92. Zimmerman RD, Fleming CA, Lee BCP, Saint-Louis LA, Deck MDF. Periventricular hyperintensity as seen by magnetic resonance: prevalence and significance. AJNR Am J Neuroradiol 1986;7:13–20.

93. Salgado ED, Weistein M, Furlan AJ, et al. Proton magnetic imaging in ischemic cerebrovascular disease. Ann Neurol 1986;20:502–507.

94. Lechner H, Schmidt R, Bertha G, Justich E, Offenbacher H, Schneider G. Nuclear magnetic resonance image white matter lesions and risk factors for stroke in normal individuals. Stroke 1988;19:263–265.

95. Scheltens P, Erkinjuntti T, Leys D, *et al*. White matter changes on CT and MRI: an overview of visual rating scales. European Task Force on Age-Related White Matter Changes. Eur Neurol 1998;39:80–89.

96. Erkinjuntti T, Gao F, Lee DH, Eliasziw M, Merskey H, Hachinski VC. Lack of difference in brain hyperintensities between patients with early Alzheimer's disease and control subjects. Arch Neurol 1994;51:260–268.

97. Lopez OL, Becker JT, Jungreis CA, *et al*. Computed tomography – but not magnetic resonance imaging – identified periventricular white-matter lesions predict symptomatic cerebrovascular disease in probable Alzheimer's disease. Arch Neurol 1995;52:659–664.

98. Bokura H, Kobayashi S, Yamaguchi S. Distinguishing silent lacunar infarction from enlarged Virchow–Robin spaces: a magnetic resonance imaging and pathological study. J Neurol 1998;245:116–122.

99. Takao M, Koto A, Tanahashi N, Fukuuchi Y, Takagi M, Morinaga S. Pathologic findings of silent, small hyperintense foci in the basal ganglia and thalamus on MRI. Neurology 1999;52:666–668.

100. Wallin A, Blennow K. Heterogeneity of vascular dementia: mechanisms and subgroups. J Geriatr Psychiatry Neurol 1993;6:177–188.

101. Donnan GA, Yasaka M. Lacunes and lacunar syndromes. In: Ginsberg MD, Bogousslavsky J, eds. Cerebrovascular disease. Pathophysiology, diagnosis, and management. Malden, Massachussets, USA: Blackwell Science; 1998:1090–1102.

102. Millikan C, Futrell N. The fallacy of the lacune hypothesis. Stroke 1990;21:1251–1257.

103. Alex M, Baron EK, Goldenberg S, Blumenthal HT. An autopsy study of cerebrovascular accident in diabetes mellitus. Circulation 1962;25:663–673.

104. Furuta A, Ishii N, Nishihara Y, Horie A. Medullary arteries in aging and dementia. Stroke 1991;22:442–446.

105. Ostrow PT, Miller LL. Pathology of small artery disease. Adv Neurol 1993;62:93–123.

106. Brun A, Englund E. A white matter disorder in dementia of the Alzheimer type: a pathoanatomical study. Ann Neurol 1986;19:253–262.

107. Chamorro A, Pujol J, Saiz A, *et al*. Periventricular white matter lucencies in patients with lacunar stroke. A marker of too high or too low blood pressure? Arch Neurol 1997;54:1284–1288.

108. Van den Bergh R, van der Eecken H. Anatomy and embryology of cerebral circulation. Progr Brain Dis 1968;30:1–26.

109. Rowbotham GF, Little E. Circulation of the cerebral hemispheres. Br J Surg 1965;52:8–21.

110. Moody DM, Bell MA, Challa VR. Features of the cerebral vascular pattern that predict vulnerability to perfusion or oxygenation deficiency: an anatomical study. AJNR Am J Neuroradiol 1990;11:431–439.

111. Pantoni L, Garcia JH, Gutierrez JA. Cerebral white matter is highly vulnerable to ischemia. Stroke 1996;27:1641–1646.

112. Petito CK, Olarte JP, Roberts B, Nowak TS, Pulsinelli WA. Selective glial vulnerability following transient global ischemia in rat brain. J Neuropathol Exp Neurol 1998;3:231–238.

113. Nag S. Cerebral changes in chronic hypertension: combined permeability and immunohistochemical studies. Acta Neuropathol (Berl) 1984;62:178–184.

114. Pantoni L, Inzitari D, Pracucci G, *et al.* Cerebrospinal fluid proteins in patients with leucoaraiosis: possible abnormalities in blood–brain barrier function. J Neurol Sci 1993;115:125–131.

115. Akiguchi I, Tomimoto H, Suenaga T, Wakita H, Budka H. Alterations in glia and axons in the brains of Binswanger's disease patients. Stroke 1997; 28:1423–1429.

116. Chabriat H, Vahedi K, Iba-Zizen MT, *et al.* Clinical spectrum of CADASIL: a study of 7 families. Lancet 1995;346:934–939.

117. Sarti C, Pantoni L. CADASIL and other hereditary forms of vascular leukoencephalopathy. In: Pantoni L, Inzitari D, Wallin A, eds. The matter of white matter. Clinical and pathophysiological aspects of white matter disease related to cognitive decline and vascular dementia. Utrecht, The Netherlands: Academic Pharmaceutical Production; 2000:333–345.

118. Skehan SJ, Hutchinson M, MacErlaine DP. Cerebral autosomal dominant arteriopathy with subcortical infarcts and leukoencephalopathy: MR findings. AJNR Am J Neuroradiol 1995; 16:2115–2119.

119. Baudrimont M, Dubas F, Joutel A, Tournier-Lasserve E, Bousser MG. Autosomal dominant leukoencephalopathy and subcortical ischemic stroke: a clinicopathological study. Stroke 1993;24:122–125.

120. Ruchoux MM, Maurage CA. CADASIL: cerebral autosomal dominant arteriopathy with subcortical infarcts and leukoencephalopathy. J Neuropathol Exp Neurol 1997;56:947–964.

121. Joutel A, Corpechot C, Ducros A, *et al. Notch 3* mutations in CADASIL, a hereditary adult-onset condition causing stroke and dementia. Nature 1996; 383:707–710.

122. Markus HS, Barley J, Lunt R, *et al.* Angiotensin-converting enzyme gene deletion polymorphism. A new risk factor for lacunar stroke but not carotid atheroma. Stroke 1995;26: 1329–1333.

123. Amar K, MacGowan S, Wilcock G, Lewis T, Scott M. Are genetic factors important in the aetiology of leukoaraiosis? Results from a memory clinic population. Int J Geriatr Psychiatry 1998;13: 585–590.

124. Skoog I, Hesse C, Aevarsson O, *et al.* A population study of apoE genotype at the age of 85: relation to dementia, cerebrovascular disease, and mortality. J Neurol Neurosurg Psychiatry 1998;64:37–43.

125. Desmond DW, Erkinjuntti T, Sano M, *et al.* The cognitive syndrome of vascular dementia; implications for clinical trials. Alzheimer Dis Assoc Disord 1999;13(suppl 3):S21–S29.

126. Skoog I. Blood pressure and dementia. In: Hansson L, Birkenhäger WH, eds. Handbook of hypertension, vol 18. Assessment of hypertensive organ damage. Amsterdam: Elsevier Science BV; 1997:303–331.

127. Fischer P, Gatterer G, Marterer A, Simanyi M, Danielczyk W. Course characteristics in the differentiation of dementia of the Alzheimer type and multi-infarct

dementia. Acta Psychiatr Scand 1990;81:551–553.

128. Mölsä PK, Marttila RJ, Rinne UK. Long-term survival and predictors of mortality in Alzheimer's disease and multi-infarct dementia. Acta Neurol Scand 1995;91:159–164.

129. Chui HC, Gonthier R. Natural history of vascular dementia. Alzheimer Dis Assoc Disord 1999;13(suppl 3):S124–S130.

130. Pantoni L, Carosi M, Amigoni S, Mascalchi M, Inzitari D. A preliminary open trial with nimodipine in patients with cognitive impairment and leukoaraiosis. Clin Neuropharmacol 1996;19: 497–506.

131. Scheltens P, Barkhof F, Valk J. White matter lesions on magnetic resonance imaging in clinically diagnosed Alzheimer's disease. Evidence for heterogeneity. Brain 1992;115:735–748.

132. Erkinjuntti T, Bowler JV, DeCarli C, et al. Imaging of static brain lesions in vascular dementia: implications for clinical trials. Alzheimer Dis Assoc Disord 1999;13(suppl 3):S81–S90.

133. Meyer JS, Judd BW, Tawaklna T, Rogers RL, Mortel KF. Improved cognition after control of risk factors for multi-infarct dementia. JAMA 1986;256:2203–2209.

134. Forette F, Seux ML, Staessen JA, et al. Prevention of dementia in randomised double-blind placebo-controlled Systolic Hypertension in Europe (Syst-Eur) trial. Lancet 1998;352: 1347–1351.

135. SHEP Cooperative Research Group. Prevention of stroke by antihypertensive drug treatment in older persons with isolated systolic hypertension. Final results of the Systolic Hypertension in the Elderly Program (SHEP). JAMA 1991;265: 3255–3264.

136. Molnar FJ, Man-Son-Hing M, St John P, Brymer C, Rockwood K, Hachinski V. Subcortical vascular dementia: survey of treatment patterns and research considerations. Can J Neurol Sci 1998;25:320–324.

137. The Stroke Prevention in Reversible Ischemia Trial (SPIRIT) Study Group. A randomized trial of anticoagulants versus aspirin after cerebral ischemia of presumed arterial origin. Ann Neurol 1997;42: 857–865.

138. Pantoni L, Inzitari D, for the European Task Force on Age-Related White Matter Changes. New clinical relevance of leukoaraiosis. Stroke 1998;29: 543.

139. Erkinjuntti T. Cerebrovascular dementia. Pathophysiology, diagnosis and treatment. CNS Drugs 1999;12:35–48.

140. Meyer JS, Rogers RL, McClintic KL, Mortel KF, Lofti J. Randomized clinical trial of daily aspirin therapy in multi-infarct dementia: a pilot study. J Am Geriatr Soc 1989;37:549–555.

141. Richards M, Meade TW, Peart S, Brennan PJ, Mann AH. Is there any evidence for a protective effect of antithrombotic medication on cognitive function in men at risk of cardiovascular disease? Some preliminary findings. J Neurol Neurosurg Psychiatry 1997;62:269–272.

142. Schneider LS, Olin JT. Overview of clinical trials of hydergine in dementia. Arch Neurol 1994; 51:787–798.

143. Herrmann WM, Stephan K, Gaede K, Apeceche M. A multi-center randomized double-blind study on the efficacy and safety of nicergoline in patients with

multi-infarct dementia. Dementia Geriatr Cogn Disord 1997;8: 9–17.

144. Mielke R, Kittner B, Ghaemi M, *et al.* Propentofylline improves regional cerebral glucose metabolism and neuropsychological performance in vascular dementia. J Neurol Sci 1996; 141:59–64.

145. Marcusson J, Rother M, Kittner B, *et al.* A 12-month, randomized, placebo-controlled trial of propentofylline (HWA 285) in patients with dementia according to DSM III-R. Dementia Geriatr Cogn Disord 1997;8: 320–328.

146. Rother M, Erkinjuntti T, Roessner M, Kittner B, Marcusson J, Karlsson I. Propentofylline in the treatment of Alzheimer's disease and vascular dementia. Dementia Geriatr Cogn Disord 1998; 9(suppl 1):36–43.

147. Mielke R, Möller HJ, Erkinjuntti T, Rosenkranz B, Rother M, Kittner B. Propentofylline in the treatment of vascular dementia and Alzheimer-type dementia: overview of phase I and phase II clinical trials. Alzheimer Dis Assoc Disord 1998;12(suppl 2): S29–S35.

148. The European Pentoxifylline Multi-Infarct Dementia Study Group. European Pentoxifylline Multi-Infarct Dementia Study. Eur Neurol 1996;36:315–321.

149. Parnetti L, Ambrosoli L, Agliati G, *et al.* Posatirelin in the treatment of vascular dementia: a double-blind multicentre study vs placebo. Acta Neurol Scand 1996;93:456–463.

150. Le Bars PL, Katz MM, Berman N, Itil TM, Freedman AM, Schatzberg AF. A placebo-controlled, double-blind, randomized trial of an extract of Ginkgo biloba for dementia. North American EGb Study Group. JAMA 1997;278:1327–1332.

151. Pearsons CG, Danysz W, Quack G. Memantine is a clinically well tolerated NMDA receptor antagonist: a review of preclinical data. Neuropharmacology; in press.

152. Winblad B, Poritis N. Clinical improvement in a placebo-controlled trial with memantine in care-dependent patients with severe dementia (abstract). Neurobiol Aging 1998;19(suppl 4): S303.

153. Winblad B, Poritis N. Memantine in severe dementia. J Geriatr Psychiatry Neurol; in press.

154. Kittner B, Rossner M, Rother M. Clinical trials in dementia with propentofylline. Ann N Y Acad Sci 1997;826:307–316.

155. Rother M, Kittner B, Rudolphi K, Rossner M, Labs KH. HWA 285 (propentofylline): a new compound for the treatment of both vascular dementia and dementia of the Alzheimer type. Ann N Y Acad Sci 1996;777:404–409.

156. Pischel T. Long-term-efficacy and safety of propentofylline in patients with vascular dementia. Results of a 12 months placebo-controlled trial (abstract). Neurobiol Aging 1998;19(suppl 4): S182.

157. Welsch M, Nuglisch J, Krieglstein J. Neuroprotective effect of nimodipine is not mediated by increased cerebral blood flow after transient forebrain ischemia in rats. Stroke 1990;21(suppl IV):IV105–IV107.

158. de Jong GI, Jansen AS, Horvath E, Gispen WH, Luiten PGM. Nimodipine effects on cerebral microvessels and sciatic nerve in aging rats. Neurobiol Aging 1992;13:73–81.

159. de Jong GI, Traber J, Luiten PGM. Formation of cerebrovascular anomalies in the ageing

rats is delayed by chronic nimodipine application. Mech Ageing Dev 1992;64:255–272.

160. Pantoni L, Bianchi C, Beneke M, *et al*. The Scandinavian Multi-infarct dementia trial: a double-blind, placebo-controlled trial on nimodipine in multi-infarct dementia. J Neurol Sci; in press.

161. Pantoni L, Rossi R, Inzitari D, *et al*. Efficacy and safety of nimodipine in subcortical vascular dementia: a subgroup analysis of the Scandinavian multi-infarct dementia trial. J Neurol Sci; in press.

162. Pantoni L, Leys D, Fazekas F, *et al*. The role of white matter lesions in cognitive impairment of vascular origin. Alzheimer Dis Assoc Disord 1999;13(suppl 3): S49–S54.

6
Minimal cognitive impairment

Florence Pasquier

Introduction

Minimal cognitive impairment is a topical challenge. How should it be defined? Is it frequent? Is it an early stage of dementia? If so, what could predict the progression to dementia? How can the progression of the cognitive decline be prevented? Is minimal cognitive impairment related to memory (or cognitive) complaints? Are treatments available for mild cognitive impairment? As therapeutic strategies for Alzheimer's disease (AD) emerge, interest in identifying signs of cognitive decline as early as possible to prevent, delay or reverse the pathological process increases. In June 1999, a conference, 'Current Concepts in Mild Cognitive Impairment' was held to clarify the concept of MCI and refine its diagnostic criteria.[1] One of the main goals of the meeting was to bring MCI to the attention of generalist physicians, because they are the ones who are going to see patients with memory complaints first.

Definitions

Several terms have been used to define minimal cognitive impairment. They have in common that there should be no major repercussion on activities of daily living (ADL) and autonomy, unlike dementia. Memory is the most frequent cognitive function to be impaired with aging. Chronologically, the term 'benign senescent forgetfulness' was first used by Kral[2] to describe the memory complaints of retirement-home residents whom he studied. However, Kral never objectively distinguished between his 'normal' and his 'benign' patient groups.[3]

Age-associated memory impairment (AAMI) was then defined by Crook *et al.*[4] The specific criteria for AAMI include:

- age of at least 50 years;
- a gradual onset of memory dysfunction in daily life (e.g. difficulty remembering names, misplacing objects);
- subjective complaints, substantiated by psychometric evidence of

memory failure, as measured by performance at least 1 standard deviation (SD) below the mean established for young adults on a well-standardized test of secondary or recent memory (e.g. Logical Memory or Paired Associated subtests of the Wechsler Memory Scale);
- intact global intellectual function; and
- absence of dementia (e.g. a score less than 24 on the Mini Mental State Examination (MMSE)).

Subjects would be excluded if they had a definable disorder that might account for their condition (including psychiatric disturbances). These criteria include healthy elderly persons who complain of cognitive dysfunction.[3] The construct of AAMI has been criticized, especially on the main criteria (subjective complaints) because of the relatively poor correlation between memory complaints (or self-assessed memory functioning) and objective indices of performance, and on the objective cut-off (1 SD below the mean for young age groups), which may be overinclusive.[3] Furthermore, AAMI does not appear to describe any homogeneous group of individuals, and the neuropsychological methods used to diagnose AAMI are ambiguous.[5]

Some revisions of the AAMI criteria have been suggested,[6,7] and two further concepts were proposed: age-consistent memory impairment (ACMI) and late-life forgetfulness (LLF). ACMI applies for a reduced performance within 1 SD of the mean established for the respective age group on 75% or more of the tests administered, and LLF to denote test performance between 1 and 2 SD below the age-adjusted mean on 50% or more of the neuropsychological measures applied. Those patients who demonstrate mild cognitive deficits (relative to age peers) and related mild functional impairment are classified as 'cognitive impairment disorder, not otherwise specified', a category that would include mild cognitive impairment (MCI).

The term MCI was introduced by Jonker *et al.*[8] and Flicker *et al.*[9] The diagnosis of MCI is established by:

- a history indicative of intellectual decline;
- evidence of interference in higher order vocational, social and interpersonal tasks; and
- objective demonstration of cognitive impairment on one or more cognitive parameters, where both the cognitive deficits and the functional impairments remain relatively mild and do not cause sufficient impairment to qualify for a diagnosis of dementia.

This definition may vary. Flicker *et al.*[9] defined MCI as a Global Deterioration Scale (GDS)[10] score of 3. This score means that subjects have exhibited at least two of the following symptoms:

- getting lost when traveling to an unfamiliar location;
- a decline in work performance that is apparent to coworkers;
- word-finding deficit that is apparent to intimates;

- relatively little retention of material read in a passage or book;
- a decreased facility for remembering the names of newly introduced people;
- losing or misplacing an object of value; or
- a concentration deficit that is apparent upon clinical testing.

Memory deficit in these subjects is demonstrable but not superficially apparent. Zaudig[11] defined MCI as GDS stages 2–3 and Clinical Dementia Rating (CDR) stage 0.5.[12,13]

Some investigators believe that virtually all patients who have MCI have AD neuropathologically. Others note that, although many of these patients progress to AD, not all do, and consequently the distinction is important.[14] Petersen *et al.*[14] conducted a longitudinal study to produce a clinical characterization of subjects with MCI, and they claim that MCI constitutes a clinical entity that can be differentiated from healthy controls and patients with very mild AD. They made the diagnosis of MCI if the patient met the following criteria:

- memory complaint;
- normal activities of daily living;
- normal general cognitive function;
- abnormal memory for age; and
- undemented.

A CDR score of 0.5 is compatible both with MCI and with very mild dementia. However, subjects with MCI did not have a significant functional deficit since their mean CDR sum of boxes scores was 1.5, with most of the decline being accounted for by memory deficits, whereas patients with very mild AD had a mean CDR sum of boxes score of 3.3, which reflected impairment in functional domains.[14]

The primary distinction between controls and subjects with MCI is in the area of memory; other cognitive functions are similar. Since the memory decline is subjective, memory performance was considered abnormal when the scores were 1.5 SD below age- and education-matched control subjects, while general cognitive (verbal IQ, performance IQ) was within 0.5 SD of appropriate controls. Subjects with MCI and patients with very mild AD have similar memory performance, but patients with AD are more impaired in other cognitive domains, except in the Boston Naming Test. This finding is interpreted as indicating that either the linguistic function of naming is impaired early in the disease process or that this naming test actually assesses semantic memory and therefore is consistent with the other memory data. When a clinician sees a patient who has an impaired delayed recall performance or who has difficulty in benefiting from semantic cues during learning or recall in the setting of relatively preserved general cognition, the diagnosis of MCI should be entertained. Consideration of this diagnosis should lead to an extensive neuropsychiatric evaluation to determine whether a specific disorder (such as AD or a cerebrovascular pathology) is causing it. Subjects with MCI decline at a faster rate than controls but less rapidly than patients with mild AD.[14]

The cognitive decline that exceeds the decrement of age-matched peers may be the precursor of a more severe, progressive disorder. These disorders are not restricted to memory, and the term aging-associated cognitive decline (AACD) has been suggested.[3,15–18] Caine argued for the designation of such disorders in the fourth edition of the *Diagnostic and Statistical Manual of Mental Disorders* (DSM-IV): 'AACD is intended to capture the robust, objectively identified age-related decrement in cognitive processing abilities, including an array of intellectual function; these are not so severe as to significantly impair personal or vocational functioning. Individuals who experience this condition note occasional problems remembering names or appointments, may experience some greater difficulty solving complex problems, and often develop compensatory strategies to deal with these symptomatic but not impairing difficulties'.[3] AACD is an accepted term to use when reassuring patients that they do not have AD, and it also provides a descriptive label for those patients who might benefit from memory or cognitive enhancement through behavioral or pharmacological intervention. The exact standards for defining the limits of AACD are still not clear. According to Caine,[3] cognitive decline in the elderly can be considered dimensionally or hierarchically, involving AACD, MCI and dementia. AACD[15] is based on:

- the presence of a cognitive decline, reported by the subject or a reliable informant, for at least 6 months;
- objective evidence of abnormal performance in any principal domain of cognition (i.e. memory and learning, attention and concentration, thinking, language or visuospatial functioning – the abnormality is defined as a performance at least 1 SD below the age and education norms in well-standardized neuropsychological tests; and
- no evidence of any medical condition known to cause cerebral dysfunction.

A criterion that involves subjective complaints is unnecessary, contrary to the situation with AAMI. The selection of neuropsychological tests and the definition of reduced test performance are confounding variables. Particular tests are proposed in the AAMI criteria, whereas AACD criteria refer to domains of neuropsychological functioning without reference to certain tests. Neither the AAMI criteria nor the AACD criteria define the number of neuropsychological tests applied. Following both AAMI and AACD criteria, a reduced test performance is defined by a reduced performance in one or more tests. One may argue that the likelihood of meeting this criterion by chance increases when more tests are applied. In addition, none of the diagnostic criteria refers to the test–retest reliability of the neuropsychological tests used.[19]

AAMI and AACD have been compared in a sample of 111 community-dwelling participants who were not demented but who had informant evidence of cognitive decline.[18] Only 54% of participants with AAMI simultaneously met criteria for AACD, and those with AACD showed more extensive cognitive impairment than those with AAMI. This confirms that the prevalence of AACD is lower than that of AAMI.[16] This discrepancy comes from the fact that AAMI is defined as impairment with reference to young normal subjects, whereas AACD refers to impairment with respect to normal contemporaries. Because of a markedly lower prevalence rate, AACD might identify a more homogeneous group of elderly subjects who have a higher risk of developing dementia than subjects with AAMI.[16] AACD might be better than AAMI in differentiating those who have a genuine cognitive decline that might justify pharmacological intervention trials or those who should be observed in follow-up studies for the development of dementia.

Mild cognitive disorder (MCD) is a classification included in the research criteria for the *International Classification of Diseases*, tenth revision (ICD-10) by the World Health Organization.[20] This diagnosis is used only when there is an indication of a disease or condition that is known to cause cerebral dysfunction. It is intended to be applicable throughout adulthood and is not specific to the elderly, in contrast to AAMI.

Age-related cognitive decline (ARCD) is a related concept included in the DSM-IV. It is defined as 'an objectively identified decline in cognitive functioning consequent to the aging process that is within normal limits given the person's age'.[21]

The Canadian Study of Health and Aging identified a significant number of people over 65 years of age whose problems with memory and other areas of cognition were not sufficiently severe to meet the DSM-IIIR criteria for dementia; however these subjects were thought to be distinct from similarly aged, cognitively normal people. They were categorized as being 'cognitively impaired, not demented'.[22] The writing committee of the *Lancet* conference on dementias characterized the description and measurement of 'cognitive impairment, no dementia' (CIND) as one of the most important challenges in dementia epidemiology.[23] Circumscribed memory impairment is one subcategory; others are delirium, chronic alcohol and drug use, depression, psychiatric illness, mental retardation and 'other'.[24] The 'other' category was further split into a number of additional categories (cerebrovascular disease, general vascular, sociocultural, blind or deaf, Parkinson's disease, social isolation, multiple sclerosis, epilepsy and brain tumor).[22]

Devanand *et al.*[25] defined questionable dementia as follows:

- age over 40 years;
- intellectual impairment present for a minimum of 6 months and a maximum of 10 years; and

- diagnosis of 'not demented' or 'questionably demented' based on diagnostic evaluation (patients rated 'not demented' were required to have at least minimal evidence of cognitive impairment on clinical or neuropsychological evaluation; those judged to be totally normal were excluded (i.e. CDR of 0, a modified MMSE of 57 out of 57 and a normal age-adjusted performance on neuropsychological testing));
- a CDR of 0 (no dementia) or 0.5 (questionable dementia); and
- modified MMSE score over 30 (range, 0–57).

Patients with evidence of psychiatric or somatic disease were excluded.

Minimal cognitive impairment differs from normal aging: patients with these conditions have consistent structural changes in the brain and decreased regional cerebral blood flow.[26–29] On the other hand it seems desirable to avoid designation 'impairment' when describing the cognitive changes that occur in healthy elderly people.

Prevalence

There is variability in the literature, largely because of the use of different clinical criteria and neuropsychological measures and the small numbers of subjects.[30]

Prevalence estimates for AAMI, when the criteria have been applied in full, have ranged from 18.5% for those aged over 50 years (5.8% for the total population)[31] to 38.4% in a randomly selected sample of subjects aged 60–78 years.[32] In the Finnish study, age- and sex-specific prevalence rates were highest in the youngest group (those aged 60–64 years) and lowest in the oldest group (those aged 75–78 years). This may be a function of using the MMSE as the criterion for dementia.[33] At the 1.5-year follow-up, 36% of AAMI subjects no longer met the criteria of AAMI.[34] This may be attributable to improved affective state, to the practice effect in objective memory testing and to low reliability of subjective memory rating over long intervals.[34]

Hänninen et al.[16] found a prevalence rate of 26.6% for AACD in people aged 68–78 years. AACD is sensitive to the particular cognitive tests chosen by the investigators and especially to the number of tests (the number of subjects fulfilling the criteria increases with the number of tests). Memory tests are the most sensitive. The prevalence tended to be higher in men and in subjects with higher education, and it did not differ significantly in the various age groups. It is not so surprising that the best-educated subjects have a higher prevalence of AACD, and it may be consistent with the lower prevalence[35] and incidence[36] of dementia in well-educated patients: high educational level may delay the threshold of clinical dementia at a similar severity of cognitive impairment.

Twenty-six incident cases of MCD (4% of 612 subjects) were identified in a sample of elderly persons aged 70–97 years living in the community and followed up for 3–4 years.[37,38] The only predictor was age. This prevalence is close to that found in Spain with similar criteria,[39] raising the question of the validity of this construct.[37]

According to the Canadian Study of Health and Aging, 30% of Canadians over 65 have CIND, including 8% who had no obvious systemic contribution from psychiatric illnesses.[22] There were more than 17 subcategories of CIND. In a study on 202 subjects aged 60–64 years recruited from an interdisciplinary longitudinal study in Germany on adult development, the following prevalences were determined: 13.5% for AAMI, 6.5% for ACMI, 1.5% for LLF and 23.5% for AACD.[19] Taking a score at the modified mini mental test (3MS) of 78 as a threshold to characterize subjects with or without CIND, the Canadian Study of Health and Aging found a prevalence of CIND of 16.8% in subjects aged 65 years and over.[24] The most commonly identified subcategory of CIND was circumscribed memory impairment, accounting for 31.7% of all CIND cases. The prevalence of all types of dementia in this population was 8%.

Devanand *et al.*[25] found 127 patients with questionable dementia out of 828 (15%) new patients evaluated in their memory clinic over a 7-year period. Bowen *et al.*[40] found isolated memory loss in only 25 of 811 patients (3%) who presented with newly recognized cognitive impairment.

Complaints of memory difficulties

Complaints of memory difficulties are common in randomly assessed elderly populations, and they increase with increasing age and decreasing education.[41,42] Between 25[42,43] and 60%[44] of elderly people complain of memory trouble. The primary contributing factors to memory complaints are metamemory and affective status.[3] Metamemory refers to self-perceptions about one's memory capability and one's beliefs about memory abilities as related to a variety of processes, such as aging or memory rehearsal. Complaints of cognitive and memory declines are, in contrast, related to depressive mood and neurotic personality traits more than to a reduced test performance *per se*.[19,45–48] It is generally accepted that depressive symptoms may arise in a considerable number of patients with medical or neurological disorders. Therefore, one may hypothesize that depressive symptoms may also result from MCI in a subgroup of patients.[19] The fact that MCI comprises a subgroup with pronounced depressive symptoms is supported by Ritchie *et al.*[49] However, affective symptoms are associated with increasing subjective memory complaints among normal subjects who are not syndromically depressed.[41] Furthermore, cognitive complaints cannot be explained solely by depressive mood changes – subjects who have complaints and a reduced test performance exhibit a tendency to score even higher on depression scales than those who complain of cognitive decline but do not show reduced test performance.

Early studies did not show evidence of a correlation between subjective appraisal and objective performance on memory tests.[41,45,50,51] Subjective complaints of cognitive decline are much more frequent than objective cognitive impairment in the elderly (79.8% versus 26.6% in the Finnish study).[16] There is a relationship between self-evaluations of memory functioning and personal concerns about developing AD; adult children with living parents who have AD are more concerned about this than people who have no family history of dementia.[52]

A higher percentage of those who complain of memory trouble actually show decrements in recall performance.[42] Thirty-one per cent of the normal subjects and 47% of those with cognitive impairment had memory complaints in a study of non-demented, community-dwelling elderly subjects.[46] In a cross-sectional study of non-depressed and non-demented subjects aged 65–85 years and living in the community, those with complaints and memory-related problems performed more poorly on tests of memory-related functions. This relationship was strengthened after adjusting for age, sex and premorbid verbal intelligence, all of which related to complaint status and to performance on cognitive tests.[53] However, despite the fact that poorer performance on immediate recall and short-term memory is statistically associated with memory complaints, memory complaints do not have diagnostic validity in detecting cognitive impairment at the individual level and such complaints are not a substitute for measures of cognitive performance.[54] Relying solely on memory complaints would miss those in need and allocate resources to worried but cognitively healthy persons.[54]

Short-term follow-up of memory complaints (1 or 2 years) does not usually show a worsening in cognitive performance.[33] Flicker *et al.*[55] did not find a high risk of progressive cognitive deterioration during a follow-up period of 3–4 years in 59 healthy elderly subjects with memory complaints but no clinically apparent cognitive dysfunction. However, there was no control group and a test–retest effect was not controlled for in this study. The Gospel Oak study showed that, when followed up over a 2-year period, subjects with subjective memory impairment had a four-fold greater risk of developing dementia.[43] O'Brien *et al.*[56] found that 8.8% of patients with subjective memory complaints developed dementia at 3-year follow-up, a higher proportion than might have been expected. Taylor *et al.*[57] observed declines in performance of a verbal secondary episodic memory test that were roughly paralleled at the group level by a self-reported decline in everyday memory functioning. Moreover, several large longitudinal population studies on elderly subjects have shown that memory complaints at baseline could help to predict future dementia, especially in subjects with baseline cognitive impairment,[44,58,59] although another study did not.[47] In the PAQUID study, three groups of elderly people were recognized as being at high risk of dementia: subjects with self-perceived memory impairment who were consulting a family physician and who had either low memory performance (RR = 6.09) or normal memory performance (RR =.26) and subjects who had memory complaints but did not resort to a family physician despite a low memory performance (RR = 3.84).[44] A recent community-based follow-up study of the elderly has also shown that memory complaints were a relatively strong predictor of incident AD in older persons in whom cognitive impairment was not yet apparent. It suggested that older persons may be aware of a decline in cognition before mental status tests are able to detect a decline from premorbid functioning.[60]

Again, in a study of a population sample of women aged 70–79 at baseline that examined the incidence and prediction of dementia and cognitive decline over 5 years, both the individuals and the informants of those who subsequently demented were aware of decline 5 years earlier.[61] Tierney *et al.*[62] found that informants' perceptions, not patients' perception, contributed significantly to the prediction of AD.

Two items of subjective memory impairment are most likely to predict the development of dementia:[43]

- admission by subjects that they forget what they are attending to; and
- a feeling on the part of the subjects that their impaired memory is a problem.

The ratings of subjective memory complaints are inconsistent.[45] New memory complaints 1 year later may suggest the presence of significant impairment of memory or cognition better than subjective memory complaints at baseline can.[46]

Despite the lack of specificity and sensitivity of memory complaints,[63] it remains important to listen carefully to patients and their relatives at the primary care level as well as in the clinical setting, and not always to think that these complaints are due to depression. It should be noted that depression or depressive symptoms have been investigated and have usually been found to be a predictor of dementia.[64–69] or cognitive decline,[70] although the association between high depressive symptomatology and poor cognitive functioning may be cross-sectional.[71] Symptoms of depression and similar complaints may represent prodromal phases of dementia.[72,73] Anxiety symptoms are also common; they are often associated with depression and are significantly related to impairment in activities of daily living.[74]

Relationship between minimal cognitive decline and further cognitive decline

The clinical course of AAMI is heterogeneous, a fact that confirms the questionable reliability of this concept.[5,75] However, the major predictor of developing dementia in a 5-year follow-up study of healthy volunteers was the mental status score on entry into the study.[76]

In subjects with MCI (defined as a GDS rating of 3), 72% increased their GDS rating in the following 2 years and received the clinical diagnosis of dementia. Those whose GDS rating declined differed from others on tests of verbal and visuospatial recall and language at first evaluation.[9] The follow-up to 4 years of 76 consecutive subjects with MCI showed a conversion rate to dementia of 12% per year of each of the 4 years.[14] In comparison, more than 500 control subjects enrolled and followed up in the 10 years of the study tended to convert to MCI or AD at a rate of approximately 1–2% per year.[14] This is consistent with the findings of Tierney *et al.*,[77] who followed up 123 patients who had memory impairment but were not demented. Of these, 29 patients (24%) became demented within 2 years.

Fifty per cent of subjects with AACD progressed to dementia over 35 months of follow-up.[29]

An Australian study showed that after 3.3–4.2 years of follow-up, two of 25 subjects with MCD (aged 70–97 years) still met the criteria for MCD, three developed dementia, whereas 20 had no more MCD and no dementia. Recovery was largely attributable to the absence of complaint rather than to an improvement in test performance.[38] It was not demonstrated that a diagnosis of MCD carries an increased risk of subsequent dementia. It seems that MCD, 'a tentative construct being examined', has little coherence as a clinical syndrome, that it is more associated with anxiety depression than with observable cognitive impairment, and that its transient nature is not directly linked to recovery in cerebral dysfunction.[38] It has been suggested that, in a revision, consideration should be given to deleting criterion B (reported difficulty in cognitive function), on the grounds that subjective complaints in this domain are more likely to be a manifestation of mood disturbance.

The 2-year follow-up of 24 subjects with ARCD (mean age 62 years) found five subjects who presented with clinical evidence of dementia.[28]

Bowen *et al.*[40] followed up 23 subjects with isolated memory loss of unknown cause for a mean of 48 months (range, 12–85 months) and found that 10 patients (43%; 19% at 2 years) became demented compared with 18% in the comparison group. The mean time to a diagnosis of dementia was 3.77 years (95% CI, 2.99–4.56) in cases with isolated memory loss and 5.96 years (95% CI 5.60–6.31) in the comparison group. Neuropsychological test scores at intake did not predict which patients would progress to dementia.

As a whole, approximately 50% of subjects with minimal cognitive impairment will decline to dementia within 3 years and the remainder will have stable mild cognitive impairments that do not appear to progress. It may be that, if such patients are observed for long enough, they will decline, but few studies have gone beyond 2–3 years of follow-up. A first study supports this hypothesis – over a 7-year follow-up period, 11 of 16 subjects with 'questionable dementia' (CDR = 0.5) either had AD that was verified at autopsy or clinically progressed to a more advanced CDR stage in which the dementia was clearly evident.[78] More recently, Devanand *et al.* showed that, at follow-up (more than 1 year, mean 2.5 years), 31 of 75 patients (41.3%) with initially questionable dementia got a firm diagnosis of dementia, 33 (44%) were not demented, and 11 (14.7%) still had questionable dementia.[25] The cause of dementia in most patients was AD. Thus, follow-up is crucial for distinguishing between subjects with MCI and healthy subjects with long-standing poor memory function that may not progress. The persistent question in all these follow-up studies is, would the non-demented subjects also have met criteria for dementia with longer follow-up? Some authors do not have this conviction[25,28] but further studies are needed. There is, in any case, considerable heterogeneity in the outcome of minimal cognitive impairment,[49] as there is in AD and dementia.

Prediction of the progression of cognitive decline

Apart from age, delayed recall and several neuropsychological tests that correlated significantly with each other were the only clinical predictors of dementia.[25] The most cost-effective measure may be simple neuropsychological testing.[79] Several studies have indicated that impairment in delayed recall and mental control are good predictors of later development of AD.[77,80–86] Longitudinal studies indicate that the preclinical stage of AD is characterized by changes in cognitive abilities (especially verbal memory), which may predict the development of overt dementia.[87–94] Initial presentation of dementia may include isolated areas of memory impairment, and the NINCDS-ADRDA criteria allow a diagnosis of possible AD in the presence of a single gradually progressive severe cognitive deficit.[95] Memory loss is often the first symptom of dementia, and it is often the symptom that leads patients to consult a family physician[89,96] as well as being the problem that caregivers first notice and become concerned about.[40] In a general population sample, there was little evidence of cognitive decline during a 3.5-year period among persons who remain free of AD.[97]

Apolipoprotein E ε4 may predict a more rapid progression to AD,[98,99] but this is yet to be confirmed. Magnetic resonance imaging volumetric measurements of the hippocampal formation may also be useful,[101–104] as may computed tomography measures of medial temporal lobe atrophy,[105] whereas single photon emission computed tomography (SPECT) may be not so useful in predicting who will progress to dementia,[29] at least when the images are assessed by visual inspection. However, the rate of SPECT abnormality in one study was high[29] (64%, which is close to the rate of abnormal SPECT findings in probable AD). Previously, Celsis *et al.*[28] had shown in a smaller group of subjects with ARCD followed up for 2 years, that at study inclusion a pronounced temporoparietal asymmetry distinguished the five subjects that became demented from the 13 subjects who remained stable. Small *et al.*[27] showed, with a multiple regression analysis, that parietal asymmetry on positron emission tomography was a significant predictor of change in visuospatial memory in people with AAMI who were followed up for 3 years.

Vascular lesions may also be involved in the progression of cognitive decline,[106,107] although cerebrovascular disease was not predictive of diagnostic outcome in a follow-up study of questionable dementia.[25] However, in this study, neurological disorders, including stroke, were excluded.

Neuropathological substratum of minimal cognitive impairment

There is some evidence that pure amnestic syndrome of insidious onset may be a 'preclinical' stage of AD.[108,109] Senile plaques in the neocortex may not be part of normal aging but instead represent presymptomatic or unrecognized early symptomatic AD,[110] and minimal cognitive impairment may correspond to an early stage of AD according to the hierarchical progression of degenerative process.[111,112] In a study by Bowen *et al.*,[40] of the cases with initial isolated memory loss who progressed to dementia, two died and one had autopsy-confirmed AD, findings similar to those of Rubin *et al.*[78] Of the patients who did not progress to dementia, four died and the only autopsy showed no evidence of AD.

Treatment

Several pharmaceutical companies are initiating large randomized clinical trials in MCI. Crook has identified a number of possible treatment strategies and pointed out that many of the neurochemical deficits that underlie AAMI also underlie AD; therefore, many treatment strategies may merit exploration for both disorders.[113] A role for catecholamines in AAMI has been suggested.[114] Preliminary results with phosphatidylserine[115] and Ginko biloba extract[116] were promising. So far, no conclusive results have been found. Cotherapy of multiple neurochemical deficiencies may be required to achieve clinical benefit; when a combined loss of central norepinephrine (noradrenaline) and acetylcholine exists, it may be necessary to reach a certain balance between the respective replacement treatments, taking into account receptor sensitivity to transmitters, receptor responses to denervation, and activity of second messengers.[114] A 3-year study cosponsored by the National Institute of Aging and a pharmaceutical company is being conducted to compare high-dose vitamin E (to reduce oxidative damage of the brain), donepezil hypochloride and placebo in delaying or preventing the onset of AD in subjects with MCI.[1] Between 35 and 50% of subjects with MCI are expected to convert to AD in this period of time. Trials with other cholinesterase inhibitors are ongoing.

Conclusion

Minimal cognitive impairment including MCI is far from homogeneous, and diagnostic criteria should be specified. There is obvious inter-rater variability in the diagnosis of MCI or very mild AD. An appreciation of the consequence on daily living is subjective. Physicians who are convinced of the efficacy of cholinesterase inhibitors are inclined to diagnose early AD in countries where these drugs are available. It seems obvious that the more severe the MCI, the higher risk of developing dementia. Memory tests are the most appropriate way of detecting such patients.[105,117] The cognitive profile of subjects with MCI has to be examined further to detect those who are prone to develop dementia. Poor memory performance, particularly in delayed recall, may be a predictor of AD. Follow-up is crucial, since isolated memory impairment may be an early stage of AD that lasts for 4–6 years.[118–120] Imaging and biomarkers should also improve the accuracy of diagnosis of preclinical AD, a major issue of public health interest.

References

1. Friedrich MJ. Mild cognitive impairment raises Alzheimer disease risk. JAMA 1999;282: 621–622.

2. Kral VA. Senescent forgetfulness: benign and malignant. Can Med Assoc J 1962; 86:257–260.

3. Caine ED. Should aging-associated cognitive decline be included in DSM-IV? J Neuropsychiatr Clin Neurosci 1993; 5:1–5.

4. Crook T, Bartus RT, Ferris SH, et al. Age-associated memory impairment: proposed diagnostic criteria and measures of clinical change: report of a National Institute of Mental Health work group. Dev Neuropsychol 1986; 2:261–276.

5. Hanninen T, Soininen H. Age-associated memory impairment. Normal aging or warning of dementia? Drugs Aging 1997; 1:480–489.

6. Blackford RC, La Rue A. Criteria for diagnosing age-associated memory impairment: proposed improvements from the field. Dev Neuropyschol 1989;5: 295–306.

7. Derouesné C, Kalafat M, Guez D, Malbezin M, Poitrenaud J. The age-associated memory impairment construct revisited. Comments and recommendations of a French-Speaking Workgroup. Int J Geriat Psychiatry 1994;9:577–587.

8. Jonker C, Hooyer C. The Amstel Project: design and first findings. The course of mild cognitive impairment of the aged: A longitudinal 4-year study. Psychiatr J Univ Ottawa 1990;15: 207–211.

9. Flicker C, Ferris SH, Reisberg B. Mild cognitive impairment in the elderly: predictors or dementia. Neurology 1991;41: 1006–1009.

10. Reisberg B, Ferris SH, de Leon MJ, Crook T. The global deterioration scale for assessment of primary degenerative dementia. Am J Psychiatry 1982;139: 1136–1139.

11. Zaudig M. A new systematic method of measurement and diagnosis of 'mild cognitive impairment' and dementia according to ICD-10 and DSM-III-R criteria. Int Psychogeriatr 1992;4:203–219.

12. Berg L. Clinical Dementia Rating (CDR). Psychopharm Bull 1988; 24:637–639.

13. Morris JC. The Clinical Dementia Rating (CDR): current version and scoring rules. Neurology 1993;43:2412–2414.

14. Petersen RC, Smith GE, Waring SC, Ivnik RJ, Tangalos EG, Kokmen E. Mild cognitive impairment. Clinical characterization and outcome. Arch Neurol 1999; 56:303–308.

15. Levy R. Aging-associated cognitive decline. Working Party of the International Psychogeriatric Association in collaboration with the World Health Organization. Int Psychogeriatr 1994;6:63–68.

16. Hänninen T, Koivisto K, Reinikainen KJ, et al. Prevalance of ageing-associated cognitive decline in an elderly population. Age Ageing 1996;25:201–205.

17. Solfrizzi V, Panza F, Torres F, et al. High monounsaturated fatty acids intake protects against age-related cognitive decline. Neurology 1999;52:1563–1569.

18. Richard M, Touchon J, Ledesert B, Richie K. Cognitive decline in ageing: are AAMI and AACD distinct entities? Int J Geriatr Psychiatry 1999;14:534–540.

19. Schröder J, Kratz B, Pantel J, Minnemann E, Lehr U, Sauer H. Prevalence of mild cognitive impairment in an elderly community sample. J Neural Transm 1998(suppl);54:51–59.

20. World Health Organization. The ICD-10 classification of mental and behavioral disorders. Diagnostic criteria for research. Geneva: World Health Organization; 1993.

21. American Psychiatric Association. Diagnostic and statistical manual of mental disorders, 4th ed. Washington, DC: American Psychiatric Association; 1994.

22. Ebly EM, Hogan DB, Parhad IM. Cognitive impairment in the non-demented elderly. Results from the Canadian Study of Health and Aging. Arch Neurol 1995;52:612–619.

23. Writing committee, Lancet conference 1996. The challenge of the dementias; Lancet 1996; 347:1303–1307.

24. Graham JE, Rockwood K, Beattie BL, et al. Prevalence and severity of cognitive impairment

with and without dementia in an elderly population. Lancet 1997;349:1793–1796.

25. Devanand DP, Folz M, Gorlyn M, Moeller JR, Stern Y. Questionable dementia: clinical course and predictors of outcome. J Am Geriatr Soc 1997;45: 321–328.

26. Soininen HS, Partanen KC, Pitkänen A, *et al.* Volumetric MRI analysis of the amygdala and the hippocampus in subjects with age-associated memory impairment: correlation to visual and verbal memory. Neurology 1994;44:1660–1668.

27. Small GW, Okonek A, Mandelkern MA, *et al.* Apolipoprotein E type 4 allele and cerebral glucose metabolism in relatives at risk for familial Alzheimer's disease. JAMA 1995;273:942–947.

28. Celsis P, Agniel A, Cardebat D, Démonet JF, Ousset PJ, Puel M. Age related cognitive decline: a clinical entity? A longitudinal study of cerebral blood flow and memory performance. J Neurol Neurosurg Psychiatry 1997;62:601–608.

29. McKelvey R, Bergman H, Stern J, Rush C, Zahirney G, Chertlow H. Lack of prognosis significance of SPECT abnormalities in non-demented elderly subjects with memory loss. Can J Neurol Sci 1999;26:23–28.

30. Dawe B, Procter A, Philpot M. Concepts of mild memory impairment in the elderly and their relationship to dementia: a review. Int J Geriatr Psychiatry 1992;7:473–479.

31. Barker A, Jones R, Jennison C. A prevalence study of age-associated memory impairment. Br J Psychiatry 1995;167: 642–648.

32. Koivisto K, Reinikainen K, Hanninen T, *et al.* Prevalence of age-associated memory impairment in a randomly selected population from eastern Finland. Neurology 1995;45:741–747.

33. Larrabee GJ, McEntee J. Age-associated memory impairment: sorting out the controversies. Neurology 1995;45:611–614.

34. Helkala EL, Koivisto K, Hanninen T, *et al.* Stability of age-associated memory impairment during a longitudinal population-based study. J Am Geriatr Soc 1997;45:120–122.

35. Katzman R. Education and the prevalence of dementia and Alzheimer's disease. Neurology 1993;43:13–20.

36. Ott A, van Rossum CTM, van Harskamp F, van de Mheen H, Hofman A, Breteler MMB. Education and the incidence of dementia in a large population-based study: the Rotterdam study. Neurology 1999;52: 663–666.

37. Christensen H, Henderson AS, Jorm AF, Mackinnon AJ, Scott R, Korten AE. ICD-10 mild cognitive disorder: epidemiological evidence on its validity. Psychol Med 1995;25:105–120.

38. Christensen H, Henderson AS, Korten AE, Jorm AF, Jacomb PA, Mackinnon AJ. ICD-10 mild cognitive disorder: its outcome three years later. Int J Geriatr Psychiatry 1997;12:581–586.

39. Coria F, Gomez de Caso JA, Minguez L, Rodriguez-Artalejo F, Claveria LE. Prevalence of age-associated memory impairment and dementia in a rural community. J Neurol Neurosurg Psychiatry 1993;56:973–976.

40. Bowen J, Teri L, Kukull W, McCormick W, McCurry S, Larson E. Progression to dementia in patients with isolated memory loss. Lancet 1997;349:763–765.

41. O'Connor DW, Pollitt PA, Roth

M, *et al*. Memory complaints and impairment in normal, depressed, and demented elderly people identified in a community survey. Arch Gen Psychiatry 1990; 47:224–227.

42. Bassett SS, Folstein MF. Memory complaint, memory performance and psychiatric diagnosis: a community study. J Geriatr Psychiatry Neurol 1993; 6:105–111.

43. Tobiansky R, Blizard R, Livingston G, Mann A. The Gospel Oak Study stage IV: the clinical relevance of subjective memory impairment in older people. Psychol Med 1995;25:779–786.

44. Dartigues JF, Fabrigoule C, Letenneur L, Amieva H, Thiessard F, Orgogozo JM. Epidemiologie des troubles de la mémoire. Therapie 1997;52: 503–506.

45. Hanninen T, Reinikainen KJ, Helkala EL, *et al*. Subjective memory complaints and personality traits in normal elderly subjects. J Am Geriatr Soc 1994; 42:1–4.

46. Schofield PW, Jacobs D, Marder K, Sanon M, Stern Y. The validity of new memory complaints in the elderly. Arch Neurol 1997; 54:756–759.

47. Jorm AF, Christensen H, Korten AE, Hendersson AS, Jacomb PA, Mackinnon A. Do cognitive complaints either predict future cognitive decline or reflect past cognitive decline? A longitudinal study of an elderly community sample. Psychol Med 1997;27: 91–98.

48. Derouesné C, Lacomblez L, Thibault S, LePoncin M. Memory complaints in young and elderly subjects. Int J Geriatr Psychiatry 1999;14:292–301.

49. Ritchie K, Leibovici D, Ledesert B, Touchon J. A typology of subclinical senescent cognitive disorder. Br J Psychiatry 1996; 168:470–476.

50. Popkin SJ, Gallagher D, Thompson LW, *et al*. Memory complaint and performance in normal and depressed older adults. Exp Aging Res 1982;8:141–145.

51. Bolla KI, Lindgren KN, Bonaccorsy C, *et al*. Memory complaints in older adults: facts or fiction? Arch Neurol 1991;48: 61–64.

52. Cutler SJ, Hodgson LG. Anticipatory dementia: a link between memory appraisals and concerns about developing Alzheimer's disease. Gerontologist 1996;36:657–664.

53. Jonker C, Launer LJ, Hooijer C, Lindeboom J. Memory complaints and memory impairment in older individuals. J Am Geriatr Soc 1996;44:44–49.

54. Riedel-Heller SG, Matschinger H, Schork A, Angermeyer MC. Do memory complaints indicate the presence of cognitive impairment? Results of a field study. Eur Arch Psychiatry Clin Neurosci 1999;249: 197–204.

55. Flicker C, Ferris SH, Reisberg B. A longitudinal study of cognitive function in elderly persons with subjective memory complaints. J Am Geriatr Soc 1993;41:1029–1032.

56. O'Brien JT, Beats B, Hill K, Howard R, Sahakian B, Levy R. Do subjective memory complaints precede dementia? A three-year follow-up of patients with supposed 'benign senescent forgetfulness'. Int J Geriatr Psychiatry 1992;7:481–486.

57. Taylor JL, Miller TP, Tinklenberg JR. Correlates of memory decline: a 4-year longitudinal study of older adults with memory complaints. Psychol Aging 1992;7:185–193.

58. Schmand B, Jonker C, Hooijr C, Lindeboom J. Subjective memory complaints may announce dementia. Neurology 1996;46: 121–125.

59. Schofield PW, Marder K, Dooneief G, Jacobs DM, Sano M, Stern Y. Association of subjective memory complaints with subsequent cognitive decline in community-dwelling elderly individuals with baseline cognitive impairment. Am J Psychiatry 1997;154:609–615.

60. Geerlings MI, Jonker C, Bouter LM, Adèr HJ, Schmand B. Association between memory complaints and incident Alzheimer's disease in elderly people with normal baseline cognition. Am J Psychiatry 1999;156:531–537.

61. Brayne C, Best N, Muir M, Richards SJ, Gill C. Five-year incidence and prediction of dementia and cognitive decline in a population sample of women aged 70–79 at baseline. Int J Geriat Psychiatry 1997;12: 1107–1118.

62. Tierney MC, Szalai JP, Snow WG, Fisher RH. The prediction of Alzheimer disease. The role of patient and informant perceptions of cognitive deficits. Arch Neurol 1996;53:423–427.

63. Smith GE, Petersen RC, Ivnik RJ, Malec JF, Tangalos EG. Subjective memory complaints, psychological distress, and longitudinal change in objective memory performance. Psychol Aging 1996;11:272–279.

64. Devanand DP, Sano M, Tang MX, *et al.* Depressed mood and the incidence of Alzheimer's disease in the elderly living in the community. Arch Gen Psychiatry 1996;53:175–182.

65. Buntinx F, Kester A, Bergers J, Knottnerus JA. Is depression in elderly people followed by dementia? A retrospective cohort study based in general practice. Age Ageing 1996;25: 231–233.

66. Berger AK, Fratiglioni L, Forsell Y, Winblad B, Backman L. The occurrence of depressive symptoms in the preclinical phase of AD: a population-based study. Neurology 1999;53:1998–2002.

67. Ritchie K, Gilham C, Ledesert B, Touchon J, Kotzki PO. Depressive illness, depressive symptomatology and regional cerebral blood flow in elderly people with sub-clinical cognitive impairment. Age Ageing 1999;28: 385–391.

68. Palsson S, Aevarsson O, Skoog I. Depression, cerebral atrophy, cognitive performance and incidence of dementia. Population study of 85-year-olds. Br J Psychiatry 1999;174:249–253.

69. Van Reekum R, Simard M, Clarke D, Binns MA, Conn D. Late-life depression as a possible predictor of dementia: cross-sectional and short-term follow-up results. Am J Geriatr Psychiatry 1999;7:151–159.

70. Yaffe K, Blackwell T, Gore R, Sands L, Reus V, Browner WS. Depressive symptoms and cognitive decline in nondemented elderly women: a prospective study. Arch Gen Psychiatry 1999;56:425–430.

71. Dufouil C, Fuhrer R, Dartigues JF, Alperovitch A. Longitudinal analysis of the association between depressive symptomatology and cognitive deterioration. Am J Epidemiol 1996; 144:634–641.

72. Wetherell JL, Gatz M, Johansson B, Pedersen NL. History of depression and other psychiatric illness as risk factors for Alzheimer disease in a twin sample. Alzheimer Dis Assoc Disord 1999;13:47–52.

73. Chen P, Ganguli M, Mulsant BH, DeLoky ST. The temporal relationship between depressive symptoms and dementia: a community-based prospective study. Arch Gen Psychiatry 1999;56:261–266.

74. Teri L, Ferretti LE, Gibbons LE, *et al.* Anxiety of Alzheimer's disease: prevalence, and comorbidity. J Gerontol 1999;54:M348–M352.

75. Hänninen T, Hallikainen M, Koivisto K, *et al.* A follow-up study of age-associated memory impairment: neuropsychological predictors of dementia. J Am Geriatr Soc 1995;43:1007–1015.

76. Katzman R, Aronso M, Fuld P, *et al.* Development of dementing illness in an 80-year-old volunteer cohort. Ann Neurol 1989;25:317–324.

77. Tierney MC, Szalai JP, Snow WG, *et al.* Prediction of probable Alzheimer's disease in memory-impaired patients: a prospective longitudinal study. Neurology 1996;46:661–665.

78. Rubin EH, Morris JC, Grant EA, Vendegna T. Very mild senile dementia of the Alzheimer type: I. Clinical assessment. Arch Neurol 1989;46:379–382.

79. Black SE. Can SPECT predict the future for mild cognitive impairment? Can J Neurol Sci 1999;26:4–6.

80. Knopman DS, Ryberg S. A verbal memory test with high predictive accuracy for dementia of the Alzheimer type. Arch Neurol 1989;46:141–145.

81. Storandt M, Hill RD. Very mild senile dementia of the Alzheimer type. II Psychometric test performance. Arch Neurol 1989;46:383–386.

82. Tuokko H, Vernon-Wilkinson R, Weir J, Beattie BL. Cued recall and early identification of dementia. J Clin Exp Neuropsychol 1991;13:871–879.

83. Welsch K, Butters N, Hughes J, Mohs R, Heyman A. Detection of abnormal memory decline in mild cases of Alzheimer's disease using CERAD neuropsychological measures. Arch Neurol 1991;48:278–281.

84. Locascio JJ, Growdon JH, Corkin S. Cognitive test performance in detecting, staging and tracking Alzheimer's disease. Arch Neurol 1995;52:1087–1099.

85. Albert MS. Cognitive and neurobiologic markers of early Alzheimer's disease. Proc Natl Acad Sci U S A 1996;93:13547–13551.

86. Pasquier F. Early diagnosis of dementia: neuropsychology. J Neurol 1999;246:6–15.

87. Masur DM, Slivinski M, Lipton RB, Blau AD, Crystal HA. Neuropsychological prediction of dementia and the absence of dementia in healthy elderly persons. Neurology 1994;44:1427–1432.

88. Newman SK, Warrington EK, Kennedy AM, Rossor MN. The earliest cognitive change in a person with familial Alzheimer's disease: presymptomatic neuropsychological features in a pedigree with familial Alzheimer's disease confirmed at necropsy. J Neurol Neurosurg Psychiatry 1994;57:967–972.

89. Linn RT, Wolf PA, Bachman DL, *et al.* The preclinical phase of probable Alzheimer's disease. A 13-year prospective study of the Framingham cohort. Arch Neurol 1995;52:485–490.

90. Jacobs DM, Sano M, Dooneief G, Marder K, Bell KL, Stern Y. Neuropsychological detection and characterization of preclini-

cal Alzheimer's disease. Neurology 1995;45:957–962.

91. Howieson DB, Dame A, Camicioli R, Sexton G, Payami H, Kaye JA. Cognitive markers preceding Alzheimer's dementia in the healthy oldest old. J Am Geriatr Soc 1997;45:584–589.

92. Fabrigoule C, Rouch I, Taberly A, *et al.* Cognitive process in preclinical phase of dementia. Brain 1998;121:135–141.

93. Fox NC, Warrington EK, Seiffer AL, Agnew SK, Rossor MN. Presymptomatic cognitive deficits in individuals at risk of familial Alzheimer's disease. A longitudinal prospective study. Brain 1998;121:1631–1639.

94. Touchon J, Ritchie K. Prodromal cognitive disorder in Alzheimer's disease. Int J Geriatr Psychiatry 1999;14:556–563.

95. McKhann G, Drachman DA, Folstein MF, Katzman R, Price DL, Stadlan E. Clinical diagnosis of Alzheimer's disease: report of the NINCDS-ADRDA Work Group under the auspices of the Department of Health and Human Services Task Force on Alzheimer's disease. Neurology 1984;34:939–944.

96. McCormick W, Kukull W, van Belle G, Bowen J, Teri L, Larson E. Symptom patterns and comorbidity in the early stage of Alzheimer's disease. J Am Geriatr Soc 1994;42:517–521.

97. Wilson RS, Beckett LA, Bennett DA, Albert MS, Evans DA. Change in cognitive function in older persons from a community population. Arch Neurol 1999;56:1274–1279.

98. Tierney MC, Szalai JP, Snow WG, *et al.* A prospective study of the clinical utility of ApoE genotype in the prediction of outcome in patients with memory impairment. Neurology 1996;46:149–154.

99. Petersen RC, Smith GE, Ivnik RJ, *et al.* Apolipoprotein E status as a predictor of the development of Alzheimer's disease in memory-impaired individuals. JAMA 1995;273:1274–1278.

100. De Leon MJ, Convit A, George AE, *et al.* In vivo structural studies of the hippocampus in normal aging and in incipient Alzheimer's disease. Ann N Y Acad Sci 1996;777:1–13.

101. Jack CR, Petersen RC, Xu YC, *et al.* Medial temporal atrophy on MRI in normal aging and very mild Alzheimer's disease. Neurology 1997;49:786–794.

102. Fox NC, Freeborough PA, Brain atrophy progression measured from registered serial MRI: validation and application to Alzheimer's disease. J Magn Reson Imaging 1997;7:1069–1075.

103. Kaye JA, Swihart T, Howieson D, *et al.* Volume loss of the hippocampus and temporal lobe in healthy elderly persons destined to develop dementia. Neurology 1997;48:1297–1304.

104. Jack CR Jr, Petersen RC, Xu YC, *et al.* Prediction of AD with MRI-based hippocampal volume in mild cognitive impairment. Neurology 1999;52:1397–1403.

105. Wolf H, Grunwald M, Ecke GM, *et al.* The prognosis of mild cognitive impairment in the elderly. J Neural Transm Suppl 1998; 54:31–50.

106. Nagy Z, Esiri MM, Jobst KA, *et al.* The effects of additional pathology on the cognitive deficit in Alzheimer disease. J Neuropathol Exp Neurol 1997;56:165–170.

107. Snowdon DA, Greiner LH, Mortimer JA, *et al.* Brain infarction and the clinical expression of Alzheimer disease. The Nun Study. JAMA 1997;277:813–817.

108. Didic M, Ali Cherif A, Gambarelli D, Poncet M, Boudouresques J. A permanent pure amnestic syndrome of insidious onset related to Alzheimer's disease. Ann Neurol 1998;43:526–530.

109. Price JL, Morris JC. Tangles and plaques in nondemented aging and 'preclinical' Alzheimer's disease. Ann Neurol 1999;45: 358–368.

110. Morris JC, Storandt M, McKeel DW Jr, et al. Cerebral amyloid deposition and diffuse plaques in 'normal' aging: evidence for presymptomatic and very mild Alzheimer's disease. Neurology 1996;46:707–719.

111. Braak H, Braak E. Staging of Alzheimer's disease-related neurofibrillary changes. Neurobiol Aging 1995;16:271–278.

112. Delacourte A, David JP, Sergeant N, et al. The biochemical pathway of neurofibrillary degeneration in aging and Alzheimer's disease. Neurology 1999;52:1158–1165.

113. Crook TH III. Assessment of drug efficacy in age-associated memory impairment. Adv Neurol 1990;51:211–216.

114. McEntee WJ, Crook TH. Age-associated memory impairment: a role for catecholamines. Neurology 1990;40:526–530.

115. Crook TH, Tinklenberg J, Yesavage J, Petrie W, Nunzi MG, Massari DC. Effects of phophatidylserine in age-associated memory impairment. Neurology 1991;41:644–649.

116. Brautigam MRH, Blommaert FA, Verleye G, Castermans J, Jansen Steur ENH, Kleijnen J. Treatment of age-related memory complaints with Ginko biloba extract, a randomized double-blind placebo-controlled study. Phytomedicine 1998;5: 425–434.

117. Almkvist O, Basun H, Backman L, et al. Mild cognitive impairment: an early stage of Alzheimer's disease? J Neural Transm Suppl 1998;54:21–29.

118. Neary D, Snowden JS, Bowen DM, et al. Neuropsychological syndromes in presenile dementia due to cerebral atrophy. J Neurol Neurosurg Psychiatry 1986;49:163–174.

119. Grady CL, Haxby JV, Horwitz B, et al. Longitudinal study of the early neuropsychological and cerebral metabolic changes in dementia of the Alzheimer's type. J Clin Exp Neuropsychol 1988;10:576–596.

120. Haxby JV, Raffaele K, Gillette J, Schapiro MB, Rapoport SI. Individual trajectories of decline in patients with dementia of the Alzheimer type. J Clin Exp Neuropsychol 1992;14:575–592.

7
Functional aspects of dementia

Hartmut Lehfeld and Hellmut Erzigkeit

Introduction

Research into the functional disabilities of demented patients has increased substantially during the past decade owing to the establishment of impaired activities of daily living (ADL) as a diagnostic criterion of dementia.[1,2] Awareness of the importance of assessing ADL has been further stimulated by requirements drawn up by health authorities and work groups for clinical trials with antidementia compounds. To date, most of the published or proposed guidelines for dementia research acknowledge functional improvement as an essential criterion for the proof of treatment efficacy.[3–5]

However, until the late 1980s, the vast majority of functional assessment scales had not been specifically developed for application in the field of dementia. Consequently, these instruments were criticized for not measuring functional decline caused by the cognitive impairments that characterize dementing disorders. Furthermore, they were considered to lack sensitivity to change because they were developed to rate a patient's momentary status rather than change over the course of time.[6] This criticism was empirically supported by results from clinical studies in which ADL scales frequently did not prove sensitive enough to confirm the therapeutic benefits revealed by cognitive performance tests.[5,7,8] A lack of reliable and sensitive instruments designed especially for the functional assessment of patients suffering from mild cognitive impairment or early dementia has been pointed out.[9] Therefore, during the past 10 years, a series of scales that are also suggested for use in longitudinal studies has been developed for measuring functional problems specific to dementia. However, the psychometric properties of most of these scales, as well as their responsiveness to change, are still being evaluated.

In parallel with the development of new scales, efforts were undertaken to overcome conceptual and methodological shortcomings of traditional functional assessment instruments.[6,10] Thus, concise reviews of various aspects of functional disability and its measurement in demented patients have become available. For example, the theoretical framework and methodological problems of assessing functional competence have been outlined from a broader gerontological perspective[11,12] as well as with a focus on dementia.[13,14] Empirical studies of the association between cognitive and functional decline have been reviewed to summarize present knowledge on their relationship.[15] Furthermore, there are articles that highlight the strengths and weaknesses of different methodological approaches to the assessment of patients' functional capacities[16–18] as well as comparing instruments with regard to their application in specific settings.[19] Some of these papers also provide brief descriptions of newly developed dementia-specific ADL scales and review them on the basis of published data.[13,14,20]

Diagnostic criteria for dementia and the demands made by guidelines for clinical antidementia drug trials serve as the starting point of the present chapter. Diagnosis and evaluation of treatment effects require assessment of functional disabilities brought about by cognitive impairment. Therefore, it is relevant for clinicians to be familiar with factors other than cognition that interfere with everyday life. Next, strategies of detailed analyses into the relationship between cognition and functioning are outlined. These strategies can be used to increase the likelihood of measuring functional problems associated with cognitive impairment. Finally, various methodological approaches to the assessment of functional disabilities in demented patients are compared.

Functional assessment in diagnosis, staging and treatment evaluation of dementia

Current diagnostic criteria for dementia[2,21] require the existence of functional disabilities, which traditionally have been thought of as difficulties with independent execution of everyday activities. Annotated examples of compromised functions concern basic self-care activities such as dressing or bathing, more complex tasks that may require the capacity to operate technical devices or instruments (e.g. a telephone or a washing machine) and occupational or social functions.

In addition to being criteria for the diagnosis of dementia, functional deficits have also been suggested as markers of disease stages. For assessments of severity, diagnostic guidelines[22] as well as rating scales used for staging dementia[23] have adapted the concept of a hierarchical loss of everyday capacities developed by Katz et al.[24] and Lawton and Brody.[25] A hierarchical organization of function predicts that the more complex instrumental activities of daily living (IADL), such as managing finances, shopping or preparing food, will be impaired earlier in the natural history of dementia than basic self-care tasks (ADL). Furthermore, the ADL and IADL domains themselves are also assumed to be hierarchically organized, with the descending order of the original Katz Index of ADL being bathing, dressing, toileting, transferring, continence and feeding. A hierarchical model considerably facilitates the staging of the disease by listing ADL items according to their complexity. The underlying idea is that the ability to carry out a given activity implies the capacity to perform all activities of lesser difficulty, thus allowing for precise staging of individual patients. However, results from studies that have investigated the question of whether functional decline in dementia follows the assumed hierarchy are equivocal.[26–29] Nevertheless, disabilities concerning the more complex IADL functions have been shown to deteriorate before basic ADL in the course of dementia and, therefore, are considered to be of greater interest for the detection of early dementia and for screening purposes.[3,30]

Empirical studies have proved that standardized assessments of patients' functional capacities can be successfully used for early diagnosis and dementia screening. For example, a study that compared four informant-rated ADL scales found that all the scales identified even mild dementia cases adequately.[31] However, scales that assess complex social functions performed better than instruments that focus on disabilities of basic self-care. In a meta-analysis of screening studies, a questionnaire that asked for proxy ratings of patients' cognitive decline in everyday situations revealed similar sensitivity and specificity as a cognitive measure.[32] From this finding it was concluded that informant questionnaires work as well as cognitive performance tests in identifying early dementia. The usefulness and practicability of ADL assessment as a screening method was also indicated by results from an epidemiological survey that used a functional disability score derived from four IADL items.[33] Furthermore, especially in the border zone between normal aging and dementia, a combination of cognitive test scores and informant reports on patients' everyday functioning predicted the criterion diagnosis of dementia with higher accuracy than either measure alone.[34]

Besides diagnosis and staging, the assessment of functional impairment is also required for evaluating antidementia drugs within clinical studies.[3–5] In the evaluation of therapeutic efficacy, functional assessment scales are expected to provide evidence for the clinical relevance of improvement on cognitive performance tests.[4] The idea that ADL scales are superior to cognitive tests with regard to ecological validity and everyday relevance was already implicit in earlier guidelines and recommendations for drug trials in the field of dementia[35–37] and has also been supported by scale developers.[38] Today, improvement on the functional level is considered an integral part of proving the efficacy of any antidementia compound. Recently, a consensus was reached on the importance of measuring functionality as an outcome criterion for the evaluation of pharmacological treatments of dementia.[5]

However, as indicated in the criteria in the 10th edition of the *International*

Classification of Diseases (ICD-10) and the fourth edition of the *Diagnostic and Statistical Manual of Mental Disorders* (DSM-IV), in order for functional deficits to be diagnostically relevant they must be caused by cognitive impairment and not be due to other conditions. Similarly, a close link between cognitive test scores and the outcome of the functional assessment is desirable within clinical drug trials, and the guidelines stipulate that therapeutic improvement on the cognitive level should be confirmed by parallel improvement in everyday functioning. Therefore, empirical data on the association between cognition and everyday function deserve further attention.

Association between cognition and functioning

Empirical evidence for the close association between cognitive abilities and functional competence in dementia is available from regression analyses that revealed that dementia severity as assessed with the Mini Mental State Examination (MMSE) was the best predictor of everyday functioning.[39,40] Similarly, data from a 3-year follow-up study suggest that patients who deteriorate faster in their functional abilities also exhibit a steeper decline in cognitive performance.[41] However, correlation coefficients between cognitive and functional measures reported in literature mostly fall in the range of 0.4 to 0.6.[42–48] Although statistically significant, these values can not be considered exceedingly high. Therefore, additional factors besides cognition must be assumed to exert an influence on the functional capacities of dementia patients.

Depression

In a cross-sectional study, depression in addition to dementia was shown to be accompanied by greater functional disability than dementia alone.[49] In another longitudinal study, the adverse influence of depression on ADL capacities could be proved to cause a significant acceleration in functional decline.[50] A detailed analysis of different stages of dementia revealed that the severity of depressive symptoms and the extent of functional disability were associated in mildly impaired patients but not in moderately impaired patients.[51] As with the informant ratings used in these studies, the outcome of self-rated measures was also found to correlate with patients' depression.[44,45,47,52,53] However, it was not only depressive symptoms on the part of the patient that have been shown to exert an influence on the results of functional assessment tools; assessments of patients' everyday memory have also been found to be influenced by affective characteristics of the informants (e.g. anxiety, depression, feelings of burden).[44,54] As with most variables for which a significant association with functioning has been reported, some studies have produced conflicting results that do not support the impact of depression on ADL.[55,56]

Behavioral disturbances

Behavioral disturbances have been recognized as important concomitant symptoms of dementia. Consequently, a series of instruments for their measurement has been made available. In a longitudinal study that assessed the association between behavioral scales and functional assessments, it was found that functional decline in Alzheimer's disease could best be predicted not by cognition but by the behavioral problems that coexist with the dementia (e.g. hallucinations, paranoid ideation).[57] However, when the same instruments for measuring ADL and IADL competence but different scales for assessing behavioral pathology were used, a substantial impact of behavioral symptoms on patients' ADL could not be confirmed.[43,55]

Medical conditions not related to dementia

The influence of a number of medical conditions on IADL was assessed in a longitudinal study that included patients who did not show functional disability at their first visit.[58] It was found that each of the diseases diagnosed in these patients affects specific IADL capacities. For example, sensory impairments, which are frequently present in the elderly population, were shown to have a great impact on the ability to manage money or to use the telephone. Similarly, a study that assessed the reliability of diagnostic criteria of dementia pointed out that disability caused by dementia cannot be easily distinguished from physical infirmity.[59] The influence of comorbidity on everyday functioning was also revealed in a follow-up study in which improvements in ADL or IADL capacity were explained as occurring in consequence of intercurrent medical conditions.[41] However, the mere number of diseases in addition to dementia did not seem to be a decisive factor for reduced IADL capacities.[39]

Gender

Gender bias is a topic that has received a comparatively large amount of attention in the evaluation of functional measures. Everyday activities that are more complex than basic self-care tasks are heavily influenced by sociocultural standards. Therefore, the classical IADL scale by Lawton and Brody[25] was developed in an eight-item version for women and a five-item version for men. Doing laundry, housekeeping and preparing meals were not included in the male version. Consequently, it is difficult to draw direct comparisons between results obtained from male and female patients. From an investigation on longitudinal functional change in which raters were frequently uncertain whether men had ever carried out certain activities before the onset of dementia, it was concluded that more adequate IADL items need to be developed, especially for men.[60] In an ADL self-rated scale that contained the same set of items for both genders, more women than men reported disability and functional limitations.[61] The additional finding that women also showed poorer performance in physical tasks was taken as evidence for the accuracy of their self-reporting. However, in cases of disagreement between functional ratings and physical performance, men were found to under-report and women to over-report existing problems. Similar results are available from other investigations, which also showed that women stated that they had more ADL problems than men did.[62] On the other hand, in a review article, Avlund[11] cited studies that indicate female superiority in the performance of IADL tasks. This is in line with the findings from a sample of functionally impaired elderly people, which showed that men rated themselves as being more disabled than women.[26] However, no gender differences in informant reports on everyday activities could be observed in a several other studies.[43,63] Owing to their apparent relevance for functional assessment, effects of gender differences have already been taken into account in the construction phase of some newly developed ADL scales.[64,65]

Age

Studies that have assessed the influence of age on functioning in demented patients have also produced conflicting results. Whereas some investigators could not detect a significant correlation between the two variables[51] or did not find that a statistically significant amount of variance in functional disability was explained by age,[40] other authors report significant (but not large) effects of age on functioning.[43] Whereas in one study significant correlations between age and functional problems could be observed exclusively for basic ADL but not for IADL,[39] another study also indicated a significant correlation between age and IADL.[47] To explain the association between age and functional abilities, it has been suggested that the higher morbidity of older subjects is the causative factor of functional deterioration with age.[31]

Education

As with cognitive performance tests, the influence of education on functional measures must also be taken into account. Unlike self-care tasks, instrumental ADL have been found to be influenced by the duration of formal education.[40] This result was attributed to coping resources, which were assumed to be greater for better educated subjects who had experienced longer and more intense mental stimulation during their lifetime.

A similar conclusion was drawn from a study that suggested that there is a protective effect of education on functional abilities,[66] which has been discussed for dementia by other authors.[67,68]

Culture

There have been few studies comparing functional disabilities of dementia patients across cultures. International comparison studies focusing on differences in everyday tasks carried out by healthy elderly men and women have been briefly reviewed by Avlund;[11] this revealed great variations between countries. Nevertheless, a considerable number of functional assessment scales have been translated from their original versions into other languages for international usage. Of course, the translated scales were field tested in the target countries and psychometrically evaluated.[69-71] However, only a few instruments have been developed simultaneously in different languages (e.g. the DAD,[72] the B-ADL[64] and the ADL-IS).[65] In an international pilot study[73] that field tested an item pool of 141 informant-rated items, differences in ratings were observed for many items between the USA, Germany, Russia and Greece. In order to identify real differences between countries and to separate these differences from item or method bias, the plethora of factors described in the literature on cross-cultural testing must be taken into account.[74-77]

Disentangling conflicting results

At present, the strings of conflicting results from studies that have investigated the factors influencing functional abilities of demented patients need to be disentangled. A starting point may be to group together studies according to common features, e.g. the subjects investigated (community-dwelling subjects, inpatients), the source of information on patients' functional competence (a relative, a professional caregiver, the patient), the methods used to obtain this information (interview, questionnaire, performance test) or the exact activities that were assessed (ADL, IADL, ADL-related cognitive functions). In addition to the factors discussed above, it must be assumed that assessments are also affected by variables that have not yet been addressed in empirical studies, such as the motivation on the part of the patient to carry out a given activity, the opportunity to perform this activity or the economic situation that decides on the amount and the forms of support that are accessible to a patient.

It remains an unanswered question whether cognition and function in dementia would correlate perfectly if all non-cognitive factors that influence functional abilities could be eliminated or controlled for. Findings pertaining to this issue from a sample of dementia patients devoid of other psychiatric or medical problems suggest that global scores of cognitive functioning are poorer predictors of functional status in mild dementia than in moderate dementia.[42] Therefore, these authors concluded that functional loss and cognitive impairment are related but distinct aspects of dementia and that they call for separate assessments, a conclusion that other authors have also reached.[15,20]

Strategies to improve the correlation between cognitive and functional measures

A series of strategies have been considered for detailed analyses into the association between cognition and functioning. These could be used for strengthening correlations between results obtained from functional scales and cognitive test scores, which would be desirable for both diagnosis and the evaluation of treatment effects. When large samples are investigated, a convenient way to identify functional disability associated with the loss of cognitive capacities is also to assess other variables that potentially interfere with everyday competence and then to control statistically for their impact on ADL ratings. However, when assessing individual patients clinically, other routes must be taken. One appealing strategy is to ask the informant explicitly for the specific causes of the reported functional problems.[26] In order to identify functional disabilities that are closely related to cognitive impairment in the development of some dementia-specific ADL scales, an item pool was generated and then field-tested. Then, on the basis of empirical results, only those items that were strongly associated with the patients' cognitive status were selected for the final scale.[64,65] For future research, it has been suggested that the causes of functional disability should be more thoroughly assessed by breaking down ADL tasks into their subcomponents and investigating these subcomponents rather than global task performance.[14] If this approach is followed, every single step of an activity can be evaluated for its cognitive prerequisites.

To allow for more in-depth investigations into functional disability, activities can be scrutinized not only on the level of their subcomponents. Separate assessments have also been suggested for the motivational and the cognitive aspects of a task (e.g. for the initiative to begin an activity and the ability to remember the correct sequence of the involved steps).[72,78] However, this approach has been criticized for measuring cognitive impairment rather than functional disability, since it focuses on concepts, such as memory, that are undoubtedly of a cognitive nature.[12,13] Nevertheless, a distinction between instruments that assess a patient's functional abilities and scales that measure his or her cognitive performance in everyday situations cannot always be made precisely. For example, a scale that evaluates everyday memory, although it clearly pertains to cognition, may reveal important information about functional problems and their implications (e.g. by asking whether a patient forgets to turn off the oven before leaving the house).

At present, evidence about the contribution of different cognitive abilities to the performance of specific everyday tasks is limited. Therefore, recommendations have been made to analyse results obtained from functional scales on an item level rather than on a sum score level in order to establish clearer relationships between compromised areas of cognition and functional difficulties.[15] On an item level, it has been demonstrated that, for example, IADL tasks that require memory skills, such as remembering lists or handling money, are affected earlier in the course of dementia than highly overlearned activities.[41] This result is well in line with the widely held assumption that basic ADL and IADL differ in their relationship to cognition, with higher correlations to be found for the more complex IADL. From this point of view, the combination of ADL and IADL items in functional assessment scales becomes a questionable strategy for diagnostic purposes and for proving therapeutic efficacy, for which assessment of the cognition-linked functional disabilities is warranted. On the other hand, combined use of ADL and IADL items has the advantage of extending the range of applicability of a scale, thus allowing for discrimination within a broader spectrum of dementia severity. A number of studies have addressed the question of whether ADL and IADL items belong to the same dimension, which must be considered a prerequisite if a meaningful sum score from ADL and IADL items is to be computed. Results are contradictory in that some studies provide evidence for the unidimensionality of ADL and IADL items,[26,79] whereas other studies indicate that they must be considered as distinct concepts.[27,80]

Due to the growing importance of functional assessment in dementia, during the past 15 years a series of functional disability scales has been developed especially for use in demented patients. Because many of the traditional instruments were criticized for being too coarsely scaled to detect subtle changes in functioning,[81] most of their authors aimed at providing an instrument that not only satisfactorily assesses dementia-specific functional problems but is also responsive to longitudinal change. Table 7.1 gives a survey of some more recent dementia-specific scales. Not included are scales that mix functioning with other areas of assessment (e.g. behavior scales that only assess a single ADL task, preliminary scale versions that have been published). However, for other reasons, this selection is not entirely satisfactory. First, the list may be incomplete owing to the overwhelming amount of research on functional assessment within the past decade. Secondly, there are ADL scales available that cover the same domains of everyday life as those listed in Table 7.1.[82,83] However, since these scales were developed for a broader range of application than dementia, they cannot claim to be specific for the assessment of functional disabilities that characterize dementing disorders.

Table 7.1 Dementia-specific functional assessment scales. (Specifications given in the remarks column are taken from the original publication and do not preclude other scales from having the feature mentioned.)

Scale	No of Items	Format	What is assessed?	Scaling	Remarks
ADL-IS[65]	40	Informant rating (interview)	Frequency of difficulties	5-Point scale plus two additional categories (never performed, unknown)	Developed for international usage. Items selected after field testing a preliminary scale version
ADL-Situational Test[84]	4	Performance test (controlled and standardized environment)	Level of assistance needed and time to complete each task	5-Point scale (performance score)	Task segmentation, assessment of time needed to complete a task
B-ADL[64]	25	Informant rating (questionnaire)	Frequency of difficulties	10-Point scale (end-points: always, never) plus two additional categories (n/a, unknown)	Developed for international usage in mild to moderate dementia, 10-point scaling for the documentation of slight changes, field testing of a preliminary scale version
BADLS[63]	20	Informant rating (questionnaire)	Level of ability	4-Point scale plus one additional category (n/a)	Field testing of a preliminary scale version, sensitive to a wide range of ADL performance (complete independence to total dependence)
CSADL[85]	66	Informant rating (interview)	Dependency on others	4-Point scale plus one additional category (n/a)	Task segmentation (assessment of controlled and automatic aspects); also requires assessment of previous ability
DAD[72]	10	Informant rating (interview)	Ability to perform a task	2-Point scale plus one additional category (n/a)	Separate assessments of initiation, planning and organization and effective performance; French and English versions
DAFA[86]	10	Performance test (clinical outpatient setting)	Difficulty with task performance	4-Point scale	Scores subcomponents direct correspondence with FAQ items, application within a clinic-based setting
DAFS[87]	7	Performance test (laboratory setting)	Ability to fulfil task	Differs among items	Based on a hierarchical functional model; assessment of higher and lower order skills

DAQ[88]	50	Informant rating (professional's observations in controlled clinical settings)	Section 1: dependence Section 2: competence and interest	Section 1: visual analogue scale Section 2: 4-point scale plus one additional category (n/a)	Based on observation of routine performance; separate assessments of competence and interest; requires description of assistance needed
DS[89]	13	Informant rating (interview)	Needs of the patient	2-Point scale and 3-point scale	Focuses on needs of the patient; hence the scale is expected to predict service needs across the course of the disease
DSRS[90]	11	Informant rating (questionnaire)	Level of ability	4-Point scale to 8-point scale	First six items mirror CDR; developed for outpatient setting
FAQ[91]	10	Informant rating	Dependence	4-Point scale plus two additional categories (for activities not normally performed)	Suggested for the evaluation of borderline cognitive function scores
FAST[23]	16	Health-care professional	Functional disability	Score is the highest FAST stage	FAST stages reflect the characteristic progression of functional loss in AD, stages untestable patients in relative detail
IQCODE[67]	26	Informant rating (questionnaire)	Performance on everyday cognitive tasks	5-Point scale	Present performance is compared to performance 10 years earlier
IDDD[78]	33	Informant rating (interview)	Frequency of assistance	3-Point scale plus two additional categories (activity never performed, caregiver not able to judge)	Separate assessments for initiative and performance
PDS[92]	29	Informant rating (questionnaire)	Ability to perform task	Visual analogue scale	Developed in accordance with global clinical severity stagings of dementia
SAILS[93]	50	Performance test	Accuracy (all tasks) and time (timed tasks)	4-Point scale	From 10 subdomains, a motor score, a cognitive score, and a total score can be computed; SAILS can be used with patients who are too cognitively impaired to complete standard testing

Methods of functional assessment

The cognitive deficits of patients suffering from dementia render the validity of self-reports questionable. Therefore, self-rated instruments have not been developed for functional assessments (see Table 7.1), although the proxy versus patient report controversy is not yet considered settled.[94] At present, relatives or caregivers are judged to be the most valuable sources of information on patients' functional capacities. This is reflected by the fact that the majority of dementia-specific ADL scales rely on informant ratings, which are obtained either within an interview or by means of a questionnaire.

However, informant reports have been challenged by performance tests of ADL[16] that require direct observation of the patient while he or she carries out an activity in a test-like situation or in a natural environment. Rating scales were criticized for often failing to define precisely the activity under assessment or the available response categories. Consequently, little agreement has been found between different informants using rating instruments.[48,95] Therefore, the need for ADL items that assess clearly observable activities that allow for objective ratings has been stressed.[19,96]

Owing to their clear operationalizations, better reproducibility of results and greater sensitivity to change is expected for instruments that require direct observation of ADL.[16] Moreover, ADL performance tests that assess the patient while he or she carries out a task are considered to have greater face validity than indirect rating methods. Rating instruments have been criticized for not always specifying whether it is the capability to perform a task or the actual performance of the task that has to be evaluated.[11,81] Furthermore, assessments made by means of performance tests are considered to be less influenced by cognition, culture and education than those arrived at by rating tools.[16,87] Another advantage brought forward in favor of functional performance instruments is that they allow the time needed by the patient to complete a task to be measured – reduced speed of task performance may indicate beginning functional decline which could go undetected by rating scales.[47] Finally, because task performance becomes observable to a trained investigator, it is expected that direct assessment methods allow for a more detailed investigation into the nature of the functional difficulties than informant-rated tools.

However, direct observation methods depend on the motivation of the patient to perform the task when required to do so. Results may further be influenced by unfamiliar surroundings and the artificiality of the situation (i.e. performing everyday tasks under laboratory conditions). Generally, performance tests of ADL are more time-consuming than filling out questionnaires and have to be applied and scored by trained personnel. Furthermore, the relevance of an activity included in a performance test may be doubtful for patients who do not perform the required task regularly or who do not carry out the task at all. Adaptations made by the patient to his or her environment to facilitate task performance are also not reflected by performance-based measures.[16,17] Finally, the danger of injuries while carrying out the tasks in a performance test has been described.[16,19] Some of the studies that compare different approaches for assessing functional capacities in demented patients are outlined below.

Informant reports versus self-reports

Significant discrepancies between informant ratings and self-ratings were revealed in several studies in which caregivers rated patients' functional abilities more poorly than patients themselves did.[44,95–101] Furthermore, informant ratings proved to be more consistent and to correlate better with psychometric assessments of patients' cognitive status than patients' self-reports did.[44,45,52,98,99,102] As mentioned above, with self-ratings, a significant correlation reported frequently in the literature is that with depression.[44,45,47,52,53] Consequently, in longitudinal studies, patients' assessments of their own cognitive functioning in everyday situations were not found relevant for predicting cognitive deterioration.[52,103] However, as with ADL self-reports, caregivers' assessments have also been shown to be influenced by variables such as anxiety, depression, caregiver burden, age or their familial relationship to the patient.[44,48,54,104,105]

Encouraging results obtained with self-ratings of functional abilities have also been published. For example, deficits communicated by patients themselves have been successfully applied in studies that screen for early dementia.[33,53,106] Moreover, there is evidence that memory complaints should be taken into account as predictors of dementia,[107,108] and that ADL self-ratings are sensitive to change in demented patients who showed partial awareness of their functional decline.[99] Furthermore, many of the findings that revealed discrepancies between self-reports and proxy reports were obtained for subjects with a clinical diagnosis of dementia. For healthy persons, agreement between the two methods was found to be more acceptable.[98,99] In accordance with this, the severity of cognitive decline was shown to be a moderating factor for the concordance of the informant rated and the self-rated approach.[95,101]

The question that has not been conclusively answered pertains to the exact degree of cognitive decline to which self-reports can be considered a reliable method when used concurrently with informant ratings. Lehfeld et al.[109] assessed subjects in stages 1–5 of the Global Deterioration Scale (GDS)[110] and found excellent agreement between proxy ratings and self-ratings in stages 1 and 3. In stage 2, patients complained about subjectively noticed functional problems that could not be confirmed by their informants. Beyond GDS stage 3, significant differences in disability assessments became obvious between the two rating methods with patients under-reporting functional problems compared with their caregivers. Furthermore, studies indicate that agreement between both methods also depends on the complexity of the activities that have to be rated. In general, higher correlations were found for self-care activities and lower concordance rates for the more complex IADL.[101,111] Magaziner *et al.*[96] concluded from an investigation of cognitively mild impaired hip fracture patients that agreement between proxy ratings and self-ratings tends to be better for the observable and less private areas of functioning.

Informant reports versus performance tests

Comparisons between performance-based measures and informant-rated instruments in the assessment of ADL have revealed substantial correlations above 0.65 between the two methods.[87,104] However, a detailed analysis on an item level showed that correlations between patient performance in single ADL tasks and observer ratings of the same activity were not significant for four of the eight variables under comparison.[104] Additionally, the ADL performance test was found to assess patients' capacities more favorably than the proxy ratings. Besides this difference, informant reports were significantly associated with caregiver burden, unlike the performance measure. In another study, it could be shown that the strength of association between caregiver reports and performance tests of ADL differs for various tasks.[54] Therefore, it seems plausible to conclude that informant-rated scales and performance measures of everyday functioning do not assess the same construct. Performance tests are considered to address the functional limitations of a patient, whereas rating scales measure his or her functional disabilities, which also take the social context of an activity into account.

The over-reporting of patients' disabilities by proxies was confirmed in other studies.[86,96] However, in one of these studies,[96] this finding was restricted to basic ADL. For IADL, it was observed that proxies rated less need for assistance than was observed with the performance test. Contradictory findings indicate that, compared with a performance test, caregivers perceive patients as less disabled in both ADL and IADL functioning.[112] Zimmerman and Magaziner,[19] who reviewed the advantages and shortcomings of proxy reports and performance measures in nursing home settings, concluded that neither method can be viewed as a standard of reference. Instead, researchers must carefully consider the impact of the chosen instrument on study outcome and then make the appropriate selection of a tool.

Performance tests versus self-reports

As with the correspondence between informant reports and self-reports, the influence of cognitive impairment could also be demonstrated for the association between self-reporting and performance-based methods.[113] From the large proportion of patients who overestimated their functional ability in this study, which was carried out in a hospital setting, the authors concluded that the use of scales that require self-assessments may be problematic within institutional environments. Data from a study that investigated community-dwelling elderly subjects indicated that the results obtained in an ADL performance test were less influenced by depressive symptoms of the patients than ADL and IADL self-ratings, which was taken as evidence for the absence of a subjective component in the performance measure.[47] However, the presumed superiority of performance measures over self-report instruments has been challenged.[17] It was found that performance tests are not psychometrically superior (e.g. more reproducible or more sensitive to change), more acceptable for patients or easier to use or interpret than self-rated instruments. However, these results were obtained from a sample of cognitively non-impaired community-residing elderly subjects. Investigations that also included cognitively impaired subjects confirmed that self-rating instruments overestimate functional abilities as revealed by a performance measure.[86,113] Not surprisingly, correlations reported between self-rating measures and a functional performance test are only weak to moderate.[114] Therefore, authors who found discrepancies between different methods of assessment suggest that they pertain to different aspects of functional disability and recommend a combined usage of measures.[56,100,114]

Conclusions

To meet present diagnostic requirements, patients who are suspected on clinical grounds of having dementia should not only be assessed for impaired mental status but also for deteriorated everyday functioning. However, diagnostic criteria for dementia that have been criticized for a lack of operationalization[115] do not specify any assessment tools (either on the cognitive or the functional level) that could be used as an aid in the diagnostic process. For clinical studies that test the efficacy of anti-dementia drugs, some of the proposed guidelines encourage the application of newly developed dementia-specific ADL scales.[3,5] Consequently, for some of these scales, data from clinical drug trials have become available.[116–118] However, an instrument that can be considered a 'gold standard' has not yet emerged.

At the moment, much research into various aspects of functional assessment in dementia is being carried out. Owing to the increasing number of publications, not all studies pertaining to the topics addressed can be reviewed in the present chapter, which tries to provide an overview of some measurement issues. Starting from the requirement inherent in acknowledged standards for diagnosis and treatment evaluation to assess functional disability caused by cognitive impairment, the focus was on factors that have been shown to have a bearing on ADL assessments. Some of the strategies presented to strengthen the association between functioning and cognition have been used in the construction of dementia-specific assessment scales. Nevertheless, existing instruments that measure functional ability in dementia are heterogeneous in many respects, e.g. in what they assess (difficulties, dependency), the kind of questions included (ADL, IADL or a combination of both) and the number and range of specific activities. Furthermore, comparisons of several approaches (informant rating, self-rating, direct observation) revealed that results also depend on the chosen method and are therefore difficult to compare with each other.

The combined use of different instruments will be helpful for further validation efforts. In the same way, longitudinal analyses carried out on an item level must be considered beneficial for separating those ADL activities that are useful for staging dementia from tasks that are especially responsive to treatment. With regard to early detection, it is essential to identify difficulties with ADL tasks that can serve as early markers for dementia. Finally, another topic that, up to now, has not received much attention is the international validation of functional instruments. Surveys that answer the question of whether dementia affects functional abilities in the same way across cultures have not yet become available. However, it bears mentioning that it took decades of research to arrive at today's body of knowledge of cognitive performance tests, whereas studies into the functional aspects of dementia were only intensified some 15 years ago.

Acknowledgment

The authors would like to thank their Project Assistant, Eileen Lintz, for compiling references, editing and proof reading this article.

References

1. American Psychiatric Association. Diagnostic and statistical manual of mental disorders: DSM-III, 3rd ed. Washington DC: American Psychiatric Association; 1987.

2. World Health Organization. The ICD-10 classification of mental and behavioural disorders: clinical descriptions and guidelines. Geneva: World Health Organization, 1992.

3. Mohr E, Feldman H, Gauthier S. Canadian guidelines for the

development of antidementia therapies: a conceptual summary. Can J Neuro Sci 1995; 22:62–71.

4. CPMP Committee for Proprietary Medicinal Products. Note for guidance on medicinal products in the treatment of Alzheimer's disease. London: The European Agency for the Evaluation of Medicinal Products (EMEA), Human Medicines Evaluation Unit, 1997.

5. Gauthier S, Bodick M, Erzigkeit H, *et al.* Activities of daily living as an outcome measure in clinical trials of dementia drugs: position paper from the International Working Group on Harmonization of Dementia Drug Guidelines. Alzheimer Dis Assoc Disord 1997;11(suppl 3):6–7.

6. Feinstein AR, Josephy BR, Wells CK. Scientific and clinical problems in indexes of functional disability. Ann Intern Med 1986; 105:413–420.

7. Schmidt-Gollas N, Erzigkeit H. Ways of constructing a therapy sensitive scale for the assessment of ADL aspects of cognitively impaired elderly patients. In: Bergener M, Belmaker RH, Tropper MS, eds, Psychopharmacotherapy for the elderly: research and clinical implications. New York: Springer; 1993:119–131.

8. Ferris SH, Mackell JA, Mohs RC. A multicenter evaluation of new treatment efficacy instruments for Alzheimer's disease clinical trials: overview and general results. The Alzheimer's Disease Cooperative Study. Alzheimer Dis Assoc Disord 1997;11(suppl 2): S65–S69.

9. Erzigkeit H, Overall JE, Stemmler M, Steinwachs KC, Lehfeld H, Hulla FW. Assessing behavioral changes in antidementia therapy: perspectives of an international ADL project. In: Bergener M, Brocklehurst JC, Finkel SI, eds. Aging, health and healing. New York: Springer; 1995:359–374.

10. McDowell I, Newell C. Measuring health: a guide to rating scales and questionnaires. New York: Oxford University Press; 1987.

11. Avlund K. Methodological challenges in measurements of functional ability in gerontological research: a review. Aging 1997; 9:164–74.

12. Teresi JA, Lawton MP, Ory M, Holmes D. Measurement issues in chronic care populations: dementia special care. Alzheimer Dis Assoc Disord 1994;8(suppl 1):S144–S183.

13. Spector WD. Measuring functioning in daily activities for persons with dementia. Alzheimer Dis Assoc Disord 1997;11(suppl 6): 81–90.

14. Beck CK, Frank LB. Assessing functioning and self-care abilities in Alzheimer disease research. Alzheimer Dis Assoc Disord 1997;11(suppl 6):73–80.

15. Barberger-Gateau P, Fabrigoule C. Disability and cognitive impairment in the elderly. Disabil Rehabil 1997;19:175–193.

16. Guralnik JM, Branch LG, Cummings SR, Curb JD. Physical performance measures in aging research. J Gerontol 1989;44: M141–M146.

17. Myers AM, Holliday PJ, Harvey KA, Hutchinson KA. Functional performance measures: are they superior to self-assessments? J Gerontol 1993;48:M196–M206.

18. Magaziner J, Bassett SS, Hebel JR, Gruber-Baldini A. Use of proxies to measure health and functional outcomes in effectiveness research in persons with Alzheimer disease and related

disorders. Alzheimer Dis Assoc Disord 1997;11(suppl 6):168–174.

19. Zimmerman SI, Magaziner J. Methodological issues in measuring the functional status of cognitively impaired nursing home residents: the use of proxies and performance-based measures. Alzheimer Dis Assoc Disord 1994;8(suppl 1): S281–S290.

20. Gélinas I, Auer S. Functional autonomy. In: Gauthier S, ed. Clinical diagnosis and management of Alzheimer's disease. 2nd ed. London: Martin Dunitz; 1999:213–226.

21. American Psychiatric Association. Diagnostic and statistical manual of mental disorders: DSM-IV, 4th ed. Washington DC: American Psychiatric Association; 1994.

22. World Health Organization. The ICD-10 classification of mental and behavioural disorders: diagnostic criteria for research. Geneva: World Health Organization; 1993.

23. Reisberg B. Functional Assessment Staging FAST. Psychopharmacol Bull 1988;24: 653–659.

24. Katz S, Forst AB, Moskowitz RW, Jackson BA, Jaffe MW. Studies of illness in the aged. The index of ADL: a standardized measure of biological and psychosocial function. JAMA 1963;185: 914–919.

25. Lawton M, Brody E. Assessment of older people: self-maintaining and instrumental activities of daily living. Gerontologist 1969; 9:179–186.

26. Spector WD, Fleishman JA. Combining activities of daily living with instrumental activities of daily living to measure functional disability. J Gerontol B Psychol Sci Soc Sci 1998;53: S46–S57.

27. Thomas VS, Rockwood K, McDowell I. Multidimensionality in instrumental and basic activities of daily living. J Clin Epidemiol 1998;51:315–321.

28. Siu AL, Reuben DB, Hayys RD. Hierarchical measures of physical function in ambulatory geriatrics. J Am Geriatr Soc 1990; 38:1113–1119.

29. Lazaridis EN, Rudberg MA, Furner SE, Cassel CK. Do activities of daily living have a hierarchical structure? An analysis using the longitudinal study of aging. J Gerontol 1994;49: M47–M51.

30. Kay DWK. The diagnosis and grading of dementia in population surveys: measuring disability. Dementia 1994;5:289–294.

31. Juva K, Makela M, Erkinjuntti T, *et al*. Functional assessment scales in detecting dementia. Age Ageing 1997;26:393–400.

32. Jorm AF. Methods of screening for dementia: a meta-analysis of studies comparing an informant questionnaire with a brief cognitive test. Alzheimer Dis Assoc Disord 1997;11:158–162.

33. Barberger-Gateau P, Commenges D, Gagnon M, *et al*. Instrumental activities of daily living as a screening tool for cognitive impairment and dementia in elderly community dwellers. J Am Geriatr Soc 1992;40:1129–1134.

34. Wilder DE, Gurland BJ, Chen J, *et al*. Interpreting subject and informant reports of function in screening for dementia. Int J Geriatr Psychiatry 1994;9: 887–896.

35. Amaducci L, Angst J, Bech P, *et al*. Consensus conference on the methodology of clinical trials of 'nootropics', Munich, June 1989. Report of the Consensus Committee. Pharmacopsychiatry 1990;23:171–175.

36. Advisory Committees to the German Federal Health Office. Proof of efficacy of nootropics for the indication 'Dementia' (phase III): recommendations. Pharmacopsychiatry 1992;25:126–135.

37. Swash M, Brooks DN, Day NE, Frith CD, Levy R, Warlow CP. Clinical trials in Alzheimer's disease: a report from the Medical Research Council Alzheimer's Disease Clinical Trials Committee. J Neurol Neurosurg Psychiatry 1991;54:178–181.

38. Mackell JH, Ferris SH, Mohs RC, *et al.* Multicenter evaluation of new instruments for Alzheimer's disease clinical trials: summary of results. The Alzheimer's Disease Cooperative Study. Alzheimer Dis Assoc Disord 1997; 11(suppl 2):S65–S69.

39. Zanetti O, Bianchetti A, Frisoni GB, Rozzini R, Trabucchi M. Determinants of disability in Alzheimer's disease. Int J Geriatr Psychiatry 1993;8:581–586.

40. Hill RD, Bäckman L, Fratiglioni L. Determinants of functional abilities in dementia. J Am Geriatr Soc 1995;43:1092–1097.

41. Galasko D, Edland SD, Morris JC, Clark C, Mohs R, Koss E. The Consortium to Establish a Registry for Alzheimer's Disease CERAD. Part XI. Clinical milestones in patients with Alzheimer's disease followed over 3 years. Neurology 1995; 45:1451–1455.

42. Reed BR, Jagust WJ, Seab JP. Mental status as a predictor of daily function in progressive dementia. Gerontologist 1989;29: 804–807.

43. Teri L, Borson S, Kizak HA, Yamagishi M. Behavioral disturbance, cognitive dysfunction, and functional skill: prevalence and relationship in Alzheimer's disease. J Am Geriatr Soc 1989;37:109–116.

44. Jorm AF, Christensen H, Henderson AS, *et al.* Complaints of cognitive decline in the elderly: a comparison of reports by subjects and informants in a community survey. Psychol Med 1994;24:365–374.

45. Förstl H, Geiger-Kabisch C, Sattel H, *et al.* Die Selbst- und Fremdeinsschätzung klinischer Störungen bei der Alzheimer-Demenz: Ergebnisse eines strukturierten Interviews CAMDEX. Fortschr Neurol Psychiatr 1996;64:228–233.

46. Koss E, Patterson MB, Ownby R, *et al.* Memory evaluation in Alzheimer's disease: caregivers' appraisals and objective testing. Arch Neurol 1993;50:92–97.

47. Rozzini R, Frisoni GB, Bianchetti A, Zanetti O, Trabucchi M. Physical performance test and activities of daily living scales in the assessment of health status in elderly people. J Am Geriatr Soc 1993;41:1109–1113.

48. McLoughlin DM, Cooney C, Holmes C, Levy R. Carer informants for dementia sufferers: carer awareness of cognitive impairment in an elderly community-resident sample. Age Ageing 1996;25:367–370.

49. Pearson JL, Teri L, Reifler BV, Raskind MA. Functional status and cognitive impairment in Alzheimer's patients with and without depression. J Am Geriatr Soc 1989;37:1117–1121.

50. Ritchie K, Touchon J, Ledésert B. Progressive disability in senile dementia is accelerated in the presence of depression. Int J Geriatr Psychiatry 1998;13:459–461.

51. Fitz AG, Teri L. Depression, cognition, and functional ability in patients with Alzheimer's disease. J Am Geriatr Soc 1994; 42:186–191.

52. Tierney MC, Szalai JP, Snow WG, Fisher RH. The prediction of Alzeimer disease: the role of patient and informant perceptions of cognitive deficits. Arch Neurol 1996;53:423–427.

53. McGlone J, Gupta S, Humphrey D, Oppenheimer S, Mirsen T. Screening for early dementia using memory complaints from patients and relatives. Arch Neurol 1990;47:1189–1193.

54. Zanetti O, Geroldi C, Frisoni GB, Bianchetti A, Trabucchi M. Contrasting results between caregiver's report and direct assessment of activities of daily living in patients affected by mild and very mild dementia: the contribution of the caregiver's personal characteristics. J Am Geriatr Soc 1999;47:196–202.

55. Green CR, Marin DB, Mohs RC, *et al.* The impact of behavioral impairment on functional ability in Alzheimer's disease. Int J Geriatr Psychiatry 1999;14: 307–316.

56. Little AG, Hemsley DR, Volans PJ, Bergmann K. The relationship between alternative assessments of self-care ability in the elderly. Br J Clin Psychol 1986; 25:51–59.

57. Mortimer JA, Ebbitt B, Jun SP, Finch MD. Predictors of cognitive and functional progression in patients with probable Alzheimer's disease. Neurology 1992;42:1689–1696.

58. Furner SE, Rudberg MA, Cassel CK. Medical conditions differentially affect the development of IADL disability: implications for medical care and research. Gerontologist 1995;35:444–450.

59. O'Connor DW, Blessed G, Cooper B, *et al.* Cross-national interrater reliability of dementia diagnosis in the elderly and factors associated with disagree-ment. Neurology 1996;47: 1194–1199.

60. Green CR, Mohs RC, Schmeidler J, Aryan M, Davis KL. Functional decline in Alzheimer's disease: a longitudinal study. J Am Geriatr Soc 1993;41:654–661.

61. Merrill SS, Seeman TE, Kasl SV, Berkman LF. Gender differences in the comparison of self-reported disability and performance measures. J Gerontol A Bio Sci Med Sci 1997;52:M19–M26.

62. Avlund K, Schultz-Larsen K, Kreiner S. The measurement of instrumental ADL: content validity and construct validity. Aging (Milano) 1993;5:371–383.

63. Bucks R S, Ashworth DL, Wilcock GK, Siegfried K. Assessment of activities of daily living in dementia: development of the Bristol Activities of Daily Living Scale. Age Ageing 1996; 25:113–120.

64. Hindmarch I, Lehfeld H, de Jong P, *et al.* The Bayer Activities of Daily Living (B-ADL). Dementia Geriatr Cogn Disord 1998; 9(suppl 2):20–26.

65. Reisberg B, Finkel S, Overall J, *et al.* The Activities of Daily Living International Scale (ADL-IS). History and Progress. Eur Arch Psychiatry Clin Neurosci 1998;248(suppl 1):S4–S5.

66. Hill LR, Klauber MR, Salmon DP, *et al.* Functional status, education, and the diagnosis of dementia in the Shanghai survey. Neurology 1993;43: 138–145.

67. Jorm AF, Korten AE. Assessment of cognitive decline in the elderly by informant interview. Br J Psychiatry 1988;152:209–213.

68. Schmand B, Lindeboom J, Hooijer C, Jonker C. Relation between education and dementia: the role of test bias revisited. J Neurol Neurosurg Psychiatry 1995;59:170–174.

69. Böhm P, Peña-Casanova J, Hernández G, Sol JM, Blesa R. Clinical validity and utility of the interview for deterioration of daily living in dementia for Spanish-speaking communities. NORMACODEM Group. Int Psychogeriatr 1998;10:261–270.

70. Lam LC, Chiu HF, Li SW, *et al.* Screening for dementia: a preliminary study on the validity of the Chinese version of the Blessed–Roth Dementia Scale. Int Psychogeriatr 1997;9:39–46.

71. Fuh JL, Teng EL, Lin KN, *et al.* The Informant Questionnaire on Cognitive Decline in the Elderly (IQCODE) as a screening tool for dementia for a predominantly illiterate Chinese population. Neurology 1995;45:92–96.

72. Gélinas I, Gauthier L, McIntyre M, Gauthier S. Development of a functional measure for persons with Alzheimer's disease: the Disability Assessment for Dementia. Am J Occup Ther 1999;53:471–481.

73. Lehfeld H, Reisberg B, Finkel S, *et al.* Informant-rated activities-of-daily-living (ADL) assessments: result of a study of 141 items in the USA, Germany, Russia, and Greece from the International ADL Scale Development Project. Alzheimer Dis Assoc Disord 1997;11(suppl 4): 39–44.

74. Poortinga YH, Malpass RS. Making inferences from cross-cultural data. In: Lonner J, Berry JW, eds. Field methods in cross-cultural research. Cross-cultural research and methodology series, Vol 8. Beverly Hills, California, USA: Sage; 1986:17–46.

75. Lonner WJ. An overview of cross-cultural testing and assessment. In: Brislin RW, ed. Applied cross-cultural psychology. Cross-cultural research and methodology series, Vol 14.

Newbury Park: Sage; 1990: 56–76.

76. Bracken BA, Barona A. State of the art procedures for translating, validating and using psychoeducational tests in cross-cultural assessment. School Psychol Int 1991;12: 119–132.

77. Hambleton RK. Guidelines for adapting educational and psychological tests: a progress report. Eur J Psychol Assess 1994;10:229–244.

78. Teunisse S, Derix MMA, van Crevel H. Assessing the severity of dementia: patient and caregiver. Arch Neurol 1991;48: 274–277.

79. Suurmeijer TPBM, Doeglas DM, Moum T, *et al.* The Groningen Activity Restriction Scale for measuring disability: its utility in international comparisons. Am J Public Health 1994;84: 1270–1273.

80. Fitzgerald JF, Smith DM, Martin DK, Freedmann JA, Wolinsky FD. Replication of the multidimensionality of activities of daily living. J Gerontol 1993;48: S28–S31.

81. Applegate WB, Blass JP, Williams TF. Instruments for the functional assessment of older patients. N Engl J Med 1990; 322:1207–1214.

82. Kempen GIJM, Suurmeijer TPBM. The development of a hierarchical polychotomous ADL–IADL scale for noninstitutionalized elders. Gerontologist 1990;30:497–502.

83. Williams JH, Drinka TJK, Greenberg JR, *et al.* Development and testing of the Assessment of Living Skills and Resources (ALSAR) in elderly community-dwelling veterans. Gerontologist 1991;31:84–91.

84. Skurla E, Rogers, JC, Sunder-

land T. Direct assessment of activities of daily living in Alzheimer's disease. a controlled study. J Am Geriatr Soc 1988;36:97–103.

85. Patterson MB, Mack JL, Neundorfer MM, *et al*. Assessment of functional ability in Alzheimer disease: a review and a preliminary report on the Cleveland Scale for Activities of Daily Living. Alzheimer Dis Assoc Disord 1992;6:145–163.

86. Karagiozis H, Gray S, Sacco J, Shapiro M, Kawas C. The Direct Assessment of Functional Abilities (DAFA): a comparison to an indirect measure of instrumental activities of daily living. Gerontologist 1998;38:113–121.

87. Loewenstein DA, Amigo E, Duara R, *et al*. A new scale for the assessment of functional status in Alzheimer's disease and related disorders. J Geront 1989;44:114–121.

88. Oakley F, Sunderland T, Hill JL, *et al*. The Daily Activities Questionnaire: a functional assessment for people with Alzheimer's disease. Phys Occup Ther Geriatr 1992;102:67–81.

89. Stern RG, Mohs RC, Davidson M, *et al*. A longitudinal study of Alzheimer's disease: measurement, rate, and predictors of cognitive deterioration. Am J Psychiatry 1994;151:390–396.

90. Clark CM, Ewbank DC. Performance of the dementia severity rating scale: a caregiver questionnaire for rating severity in Alzheimer disease. Alzheimer Dis Assoc Disord 1996;10: 131–139.

91. Pfeffer RI, Kurosaki TT, Harrah CH, Chance JM, Filos S. Measurement of functional activities in older adults in the community. J Gerontol 1982;373:323–329.

92. DeJong R, Osterlund OW, Roy GW. Measurement of quality-of-life changes in patients with Alzheimer's disease. Clin Ther 1989;11:545–554.

93. Mahurin RK, DeBettignies BH, Pirozzolo FJ. Structured assessment of independent living skills: preliminary report of a performance measure of functional abilities in dementia. J Gerontol 1991;46:58–66.

94. Burgio L, Leon J. Using patient and proxy reports as outcome measures in Alzheimer disease research. Alzheimer Dis Assoc Disord 1997;11(suppl 6):179–180.

95. Østbye T, Tyas S, McDowell I, Koval J. Reported activities of daily living: agreement between elderly subjects with and without dementia and their caregivers. Age Ageing 1997;26:99–106.

96. Magaziner J, Zimmerman SI, Gruber-Baldini AL, Hebel JR, Fox KM. Proxy reporting in five areas of functional status: comparison with self-reports and observations of performance. Am J Epidemiol 1997;146: 418–428.

97. Kotler-Cope S, Camp CJ. Anosognosia in Alzheimer disease. Alzheimer Dis Assoc Disord 1995;9:52–56.

98. Ott BR, Lafleche G, Whelihan WM, *et al*. Impaired awareness of deficits in Alzheimer disease. Alzheimer Dis Assoc Disord 1996;10:68–76.

99. Kiyak HA, Teri L, Borson S. Physical and functional health assessment in normal aging and in Alzheimer's disease: self-reports vs family reports. Gerontologist 1994;34:324–330.

100. Rubenstein RZ, Schairer C, Wieland GD, Kane R. Systematic biases in functional status assessment in elderly adults: effects of different data sources. J Geront 1984;39:686–691.

101. Weinberger M, Samsa GP, Schmader K, *et al.* Comparing proxy and patients' perceptions of patients' functional status: results from an outpatient geriatric clinic. J Am Geriatr Soc 1992;40:585–588.

102. Neri M, Roth M, De Vreese LP, *et al.* The validity of informant reports in assessing the severity of dementia: evidence from the CAMDEX interview. Dementia 1998;9:56–62.

103. Flicker C, Ferris SH, Reisberg B. A longitudinal study of cognitive function in elderly persons with subjective memory complaints. J Am Geriatr Soc 1993;41: 1029–1032.

104. Mangone CA, Sanguinetti RM, Baumann PD, *et al.* Influence of feelings of burden on the caregiver's perception of the patient's functional status. Dementia 1993;4:287–293.

105. Magaziner J, Bassett SS, Hebel JR, Gruber-Baldini A. Use of proxies to measure health and functional status in epidemiologic studies of community-dwelling women aged 65 years and over. Am J Epidemiol 1996;143:283–292.

106. Myers AM. The clinical Swiss army knife: empirical evidence on the validity of IADL functional status measures. Med Care 1992;30:MS96–MS111.

107. Jonker C, Launer L, Hooijer C, *et al.* Memory complaints and memory impairment in older individuals. J Am Geriatr Soc 1996;44:93–94.

108. Schmand B, Jonker C, Hooijer C, Lindeboom J. Subjective memory complaints may announce dementia. Neurology 1996;46:121–125.

109. Lehfeld H, Kollmannsperger P, Erzigkeit H. SKT and ADL measures in the assessment of dementia severity. Eur Arch Psychiatry Clin Neurosci 1998; 248(suppl 1):S12.

110. Reisberg B, Ferris SH, de Leon MJ, Crook T. The Global Deterioration Scale for assessment of primary degenerative dementia. Am J Psychiatry 1982;139: 1136–1139.

111. Kivelä SL. Measuring disability: do self-ratings and service provider ratings compare? J Chron Dis 1984;37:115–123.

112. Zanetti O, Bianchetti A, Trabucchi M. The puzzle of functional status in mild and moderate AD: self-report, family report and performance-based (editorial). Gerontologist 1994;35:148.

113. Sager MA, Dunham NC, Schwantes A, Mecum L, Halverson K, Harlowe D. Measurement of activities of daily living in hospitalized elderly: a comparison of self-report and performance-based methods. J Am Geriatr Soc 1992;40:457–462.

114. Reuben DB, Valle LA, Hays RD, *et al.* Measuring physical function in community-dwelling older persons: a comparison of self-administered, interviewer-administered, and performance-based measures. J Am Geriatr Soc 1995;43:17–23.

115. Cummings JL, Khachaturian ZS. Definitions and diagnostic criteria. In: Gauthier S, ed. Clinical diagnosis and management of Alzheimer's disease. London: Martin Dunitz; 1999:3–15.

116. Raskind MA, Cyrus PA, Ruzicka BB, Gulanski BI. The effects of metrifonate on the cognitive, behavioral, and functional performance of Alzheimer's disease patients. J Clin Psychiatry 1999;60:318–325.

117. Burns A, Rossor M, Hecker J, *et al.* The effects of donepezil in Alzheimer's disease: results

from a multinational trial. Dementia Geriatr Cogn Disord 1999;10:237–244.

118. Rösler M, Anand R, Cicin-Sain A, *et al.* Efficacy and safety of rivastigmine in patients with Alzheimer's disease: international randomised controlled trial. BMJ 1999;318:633–638.

8
Neuropsychiatric manifestations of dementia

Yuri L Bronstein and Jeffrey L Cummings

Introduction

Alzheimer's disease (AD) is a progressive neurodegenerative disease with cognitive, neuropsychiatric and neurological manifestations. AD is the most common cause of age-related intellectual decline.[1] Clinical manifestations are attributed to a combination of specific neuropathological and neurochemical changes. In addition to intellectual decline, neuropsychiatric symptoms such as apathy, agitation, depression, anxiety, psychoses and disinhibition are frequently evident in patients with AD. A broad range of behavioral symptoms affects almost all patients with AD at some stage during the disease course. The neuropsychiatric symptoms in AD account for a significant amount of the distress experienced by patients and caregivers and are a major contributive factor in decisions to institutionalize patients.

In recent years, the significant progress that has been made in understanding the pathogenesis and pathophysiology of AD has led to the development of new therapeutic strategies and the introduction of several pharmacological agents that target cognitive as well as neuropsychiatric symptoms.

This review describes and characterizes non-cognitive symptoms of AD based on scales and inventories that have been developed and used in recent years. The development, validation and use of behavior assessment scales are critical to determining efficacy outcomes in clinical trials of new agents used in treating the multifaceted expression of AD. Longitudinal studies of behavioral manifestations in AD provide new information about the likely duration and persistence of neuropsychiatric symptoms and guide the optimal duration of treatment for specific subtypes of psychopathology. New insights into the biological basis of AD have been achieved using neuropathological, neurochemical, genetic and imaging techniques. Their correlation and relationship with neuropsychiatric symptoms in AD is discussed.

Recently, evidence has accumulated to suggest that cholinergic abnormalities play an important role in neuropsychiatric manifestations of AD, including delusions, apathy, aberrant motor behavior and disinhibition. The contribution of cholinergic deficiency to noncognitive symptoms of AD is outlined.

Comparison of behavioral changes in different neurodegenerative illnesses reveals specific neuropsychiatric profiles, which allows improved correlation of specific behavioral changes with specific brain circuitry and suggests targets for therapeutic manipulations. Comparative data about neuropsychiatric symptoms assessed with the Neuropsychiatric Inventory in dementia with Lewy Bodies (DLB), progressive supranuclear palsy (PSP) and corticobasal degeneration (CBD) are presented.

New data have emerged about treatment of the cholinergic abnormalities of AD. Beneficial psychotropic properties of cholinomimetic agents in AD and DLB are discussed, and advances in pharmacological and non-pharmocological therapy of behavioral target symptoms in AD are highlighted.

Spectrum of behavioral changes in AD

Patients with AD manifest a broad range of neuropsychiatric symptoms, including:

- personality alterations (e.g. irritability, apathy);
- anxiety;
- psychosis (e.g. delusions, hallucinations);
- agitation, mood changes (depression, euphoria and emotional lability);
- aberrant motor behavior (e.g. wandering, pacing); and
- neurovegetative alterations (e.g. appetite changes, sleep disturbance).

The prevalence of the various neuropsychiatric symptoms in AD patients is difficult to estimate, owing to a lack of consensus on the assessment instruments used and to selection bias in clinical samples.[2] Several rating scales have been developed to measure different aspects of neuropsychiatric manifestations, among them BEHAVE-AD,[3] Dementia Symptom Scale,[4] California Dementia Behavior Questionnaire,[5] the Consortium to Establish a registry for AD (CERAD) Behavioral Rating Scale for Dementia (C-BRSD),[6] Cohen-Mansfield Agitation Inventory,[7] Columbia University Scale for Psychopathology in Alzheimer's Disease (CUSPAD)[8] and Neuropsychiatric Inventory (NPI).[9]

Systematic assessment of behavioral disturbances in AD is a relatively recent research endeavor. In order to achieve reliable neuropsychiatric evaluation, the characteristics of rating scales must be considered; these characteristics include the sources of information, the psychometric properties, the contents of instrument, administration requirements and

Table 8.1 Attributes of rating scales used to assess neuropsychiatric symptoms in dementia.

Psychometric properties
Reliability
Validity

Source of information
Patient
Primary caregiver
Professional caregiver
Clinician observer

Content
Psychiatric symptoms
Single
Multiple
Dementia-specific behaviors
Behavioral and cognitive symptoms

Rating methods
Global ratings
Total score
Frequency of symptoms
Severity of symptoms

sensitivity to change (Table 8.1). Caregivers are often the principal observers of behavioral disturbances and are the principal informants for several scales and instruments used to assess non-cognitive symptoms. In a recent review, the caregiver was noted to be an informant for 13 of 16 (81%) of such instruments.[10]

The NPI was developed to assess neuropsychiatric symptoms in dementia patients.[9] This instrument assesses 12 neuropsychiatric disturbances commonly described in dementia patients: delusions, hallucinations, agitation, dysphoria, anxiety, apathy, irritability, euphoria, disinhibition, aberrant motor behavior, night-time behavioral disturbances, and appetite and eating abnormalities. The severity and frequency of each symptom are rated on the basis of scripted questions administered to the patient's caregiver. The NPI also assesses the amount of caregiver distress engendered by each of the symptoms. A total NPI score and a total caregiver distress score are calculated, in addition to the scores for the individual symptom domains. Inter-rater and test–retest reliability, content validity and concurrent validity of the NPI are established.[11] For institutionalized patients, the NPI-Nursing Home version (NPI-NH) has been introduced.[12] The NPI has been translated into many languages.

Recent studies using multidimensional assessments suggest that apathy is the most common neuropsychiatric disturbance, occurring in 72%

of AD patients.[13] The frontal–subcortical circuit that originates in the anterior cingulate gyrus mediates motivational expression.[14] Disruption of this circuit produces varying degrees of apathy, depending on the level of damage. Apathy results from damage to the medial prefrontal, anterior cingulate, and anterior temporal paralimbic areas.[15,16] Until recently, apathy was often treated as an aspect of depression. However, with the use of the NPI it was shown that apathy is distinct from depression in patients with neurodegenerative disorders.[17] Apathy was correlated with poorer cognitive function as measured by Mini Mental Status Examination (MMSE).[18] Kuzis *et al.*[19] studied neuropsychological correlates of apathy and depression in patients with AD. They found that patients with apathy had significantly lower scores on tests of verbal memory, naming, set-shifting and verbal fluency, suggesting more severe frontal lobe-related cognitive deficits in AD.

Clinical studies report prevalence rates for depression in patients with AD in the range of 0 to 87%, with a median of 41%. Mood changes are common, particularly minor depressive syndromes. Recent studies record a frequency of major depression of 0–10%;[20,21] other studies report a much higher frequency of depressive symptoms (up to 25–50%).[13] There is an emerging consensus that major depression is not common once the cognitive dysfunction is evident.[21] Dysphoria increases from over 10% in the mild stage of AD to more than 60% in severely impaired patients.[13] Suicide is rare in AD[22,23] and, when it occurs, it involves patients in early stages of the disease.

Delusions and hallucinations are common manifestations of AD and do not always occur together. Delusions affect 10–73% of AD patients. Rao and Lyketsos[24] reviewed the etiology, pathogenesis, risk factors and therapeutic options for delusions in AD. Among delusions, persecutory and theft themes prevail.[13,25] Delusions of theft are estimated to account for about 50% of all delusions. Half of the demented patients suspected that their primary caregivers are the thief.[26] AD patients have a tendency to experience brief delusional episodes,[27] although once delusions have occurred, they tend to recur.

Visual hallucinations are more frequent than auditory hallucinations in AD.[25] Although delusions increase as patients progress from mild to moderate AD, hallucinations decline in more severely impaired patients.[13]

Irritability is distinct from agitation. Irritability is defined in the NPI as rapid emotional fluctuations between frustration and impatience, with the patient becoming easily disturbed. Irritability correlates with agitation, dysphoria and disinhibition in AD patients.[13]

Aberrant motor behavior refers to apparently purposeless behaviors. Pacing with repetitive walking, rummaging through drawers and closets, packing and unpacking and endlessly rearranging or repetitively picking at clothing (carphologia) are typical examples. Aberrant motor behavior, although nearly certain to occur in moderately to severely impaired patients, is rare in patients in the early or mildly impaired stages of AD.

Anxiety is reported in 21–60% of AD patients. Anxiety has been shown to correlate with dysphoria and, in mildly impaired patients with agitation.[13]

Elation is uncommon in AD, occurring in 5–20% of patients.[13] It is more common in frontotemporal degeneration.

Agitation includes severe aberrant motor behavior, physical aggression or verbal abuse. These troublesome behaviors pose a significant clinical challenge. Agitation and aberrant motor behavior are the major behavioral manifestations that distinguish cortical dementia from subcortical dementia. Agitation has different behavioral correlates in AD as cognition declines.[13] In mildly impaired AD patients, agitation correlates with anxiety, irritability and disinhibition, whereas in moderately impaired patients, it correlates with delusions and hallucinations.

Neurovegetative symptoms are almost universal in AD, especially in advanced stages of the disease. Sleep and appetite disturbances are common. Occasionally, patients have periods of increased appetite and cravings for sweets. Most patients have a marked reduction in libido and sexual activity; a few have a period of increased sexual interest that resolves as the disease progresses.

Longitudinal course of neuropsychiatric alterations in AD

Longitudinal assessment suggests that most psychotic features and behavioral disturbances are associated with greater cognitive impairment. Devanand et al.[28] studied 235 patients with early probable AD for up to 5 years and used Markow analyses to predict the probability that a specific symptom would emerge. Misidentification, wandering or agitation, and physical aggression increased during follow-up. The likelihood of a new symptom developing was least for depressed mood with vegetative features and greatest for behavioral disturbance; it was intermediate for paranoid delusions and hallucinations.

Marin et al.[29] studied non-cognitive disturbances in patients with AD longitudinally, with a mean period of follow-up of more than 3 years. They used the non-cognitive subscale of the Alzheimer's Disease Assessment Scale (ADAC-noncog) to measure neuropsychiatric symptoms. This study found little evidence that non-cognitive disturbances worsen systematically over time. For the patient with mild to moderately severe AD, non-cognitive symptoms of depression, agitation and psychosis tended to be episodic, and the severity of behavioral disturbance at the first and second assessments were correlated significantly with one another. These authors inferred from these findings that an intervention to manage behavioral symptoms should probably be given only as long as the troublesome behaviors persist, and that it should be discontinued whenever the symptoms disappear for a period of time.

In another longitudinal study, Levy *et al.*[30] grouped neuropsychiatric symptoms in AD patients into three broader categories: depression, agitation and psychosis based on ADAS-noncog. About 25% of patients never developed behavioral problems during the observation period (1 year). Once symptoms occurred, patients were highly likely to experience a recurrence. Patients with multiple symptoms had higher recurrence rates. The investigation confirmed the findings of previous studies that psychosis was associated with a significantly more rapid cognitive decline. Women had more behavioral symptoms than men.

Relationship of neuropsychiatric changes to biological markers and pathology

There are several lines of evidence to support an important role of cholinergic system in the pathogenesis of the neuropsychiatric manifestations in AD, and these observations have therapeutic implications. AD is characterized by a cortical cholinergic deficiency. This cholinergic deficiency is due to cellular dysfunction in the nucleus basalis of Meynert, which is positioned strategically between the limbic afferent pathways and the neocortical efferent pathways.[31] Despite the profound presynaptic changes, the postsynaptic muscarinic receptors are relatively preserved in AD. The cholinergic deficit in AD is distributed unevenly; changes are more marked in areas that are relevant to behavior, such as the frontal and temporal lobes. Neuropsychological impairments characteristic of frontal and temporal dysfunction are present in AD patients who have psychosis, indicating that areas affected by cholinergic dysfunction are relevant to the observed behavioral changes.[32] Anticholinergic drugs induce psychosis, and AD patients are particularly prone to develop psychosis when they are given anticholinergics such as scopolamine, a finding that again links the cholinergic deficit to behavioral symptoms. The cholinergic function in AD contributes to depressive symptoms, agitation and personality alterations.[33]

The behavioral responses to cholinergic therapy in AD (discussed below) support a link between the cholinergic deficiency and neuropsychiatric symptoms in AD.[33,34]

Other neurotransmitter systems (the serotonergic and adrenergic systems) are abnormal in patients with AD. The locus ceruleus, which is the predominant source of noradrenergic projection neurons in the brain, is significantly damaged in AD. Russo-Neustadt and Cotman, who studied the distribution and concentration of adrenergic receptors in AD brains, obtained interesting results.[35] Aggressive AD patients had markedly increased concentrations of α-2 adrenergic receptors in the cerebellar cortex compared with non-aggressive patients with similar levels of cognitive deficit; there were also smaller but significant increases of β-1 and β-2 adrenergic receptors in the cerebellar cortex in aggressive AD patients compared with controls and nonagressive AD patients. These authors hypothesized that inhibitory influences of norepinephrine (noradrenaline) on Purkinje cells are preserved in agitated AD patients, in the face of cortical lesions known to be present in AD.

A recent study that examined the neuropathological correlates of agitation and physical aggression in AD revealed that AD patients with histories of unequivocal interpersonal violence had significantly higher neuron counts in the substantia nigra pars compacta than non-violent patients.[36] This observation implies that dopaminergic preservation may facilitate agitated behavior.

The apolipoprotein E (APOE) ε4 allele confers significant risk for AD and is associated with a greater amyloid burden in the brain. Several investigators have studied the relationship between APOE status and non-cognitive symptoms in AD. Ramachadran *et al.* assessed 46 AD patients and found a three-fold increase in depression and psychosis among AD patients with ε4 allele.[37] Murphy *et al.* assessed 77 AD patients and found that the total score on two psychiatric rating scales indicated more psychopathology in the group with ε4 allele.[38] Cacabelos *et al.* reported that disorientation, agitation and motor disorders were more common in patient with APOE 4/4, whereas anxiety and sleep disorders appeared more frequently with APOE 3/4 genotypes.[39] On the other hand, Holmes *et al.*,[40] Lyketos *et al.*[41] and Lopez *et al.*[42] found no association between ε4 allele and non-cognitive symptoms in patients with AD. Hirono *et al.*[43] and Levy *et al.*[44] using the NPI, found no relationship between ε4 dose and any of the 12 non-cognitive symptoms assessed with NPI, including psychosis, mood changes and personality alterations. The study by Levy *et al.* had a large population size ($n = 605$).

Overall, the issue of the relationship between the APOE genotype and neuropsychiatric disturbances in AD remains controversial, and differences in reported studies may be attributable to differences in methodological approaches and behavioral instruments.

Neuroimaging and behavioral changes in AD

In recent years, significant efforts have been made to explore the anatomical basis of behavioral abnormalities in dementia. Functional neuroimaging has advanced our understanding of neuroanatomical substrates of specific neuropsychiatric symptoms. Starkstein *et al.* found bilateral temporal hypoperfusion in delusional AD patients using technetium-99m *d,l* hexamethylpropelene amine oxime (^{99m}Tc-HMPAO) single-photon emission computed tomography (SPECT).[45] Kotrla *et al.* also used ^{99m}Tc-HMPAO SPECT and found that AD patients with delusions had greater degrees of hypoperfusion in the left frontal regions than in the right frontal regions, whereas delusional patients with hallucinations had bilateral parietal hypoperfusion.[46] Sultzer *et al.* using positron emission tomography (PET), showed that AD patients with psychosis had greater frontal hypometabolism, patients with agitation or disinhibition had greater frontal and temporal hypometabolism, and patients with anxiety or depression had greater parietal hypometabolism.[47]

Hirono *et al.*, using fluorodeoxyglucose-PET and the NPI in AD patients, found depression to be significantly correlated with bilateral hypometabolism in the superior frontal and left anterior cingulate cortices.[48] When these findings are combined with those of previous studies that showed bilateral anteromedial frontal and cingulate hypoperfusion in depressed Parkinson's disease patients,[49] these studies suggest that an anterior cingulate and dorsolateral frontal abnormality may mediate depression in patients with dementia.

Ott *et al.*, using ^{99m}Tc-HMPAO SPECT in AD patients, reported that apathy was correlated with right temporoparietal hypoperfusion.[50] Craig *et al.*, also using ^{99m}Tc-HMPAO SPECT and the NPI, noted a significant relationship between the level of apathy in AD patients and hypoperfusion of the anterior cingulate.[51] Differences in SPECT, behavioral assessment approaches and patient populations in these studies may account for these apparent discrepancies.

Since the introduction of magnetic resonance imaging (MRI), the presence of hyperintense white matter lesions (leukoaraiosis) has been noted. These changes can be divided into:

- those adjacent to the ventricles (periventricular hyperintensities); and
- those located in the deep white matter.

It has been shown that patients with AD have more extensive periventricular white matter hyperintensities than controls.[52] There is also growing evidence that changes in white matter are linked to depression late in life.[53,54] Few studies have assessed correlations between white matter changes and behavior disturbances in AD. Leukoaraiosis in AD was found to be associated with more severe apathy and extrapyramidal signs.[55] Barber *et al.* compared white matter lesions in DLB, AD, vascular dementia and normal aging.[56] Periventricular hyperintensities were positively correlated with age and were more severe in all dementia groups than in controls. In all patients with dementia, frontal white matter hyperintensities were associated with higher depression scores and occipital white matter hyperintensities were associated with an absence of visual hallucinations and delusions.

Response of neuropsychiatric changes to treatment

The principles of treatment of behavioral abnormalities in AD and other dementias have been outlined.[57–61] Before initiation of treatment, it is

Table 8.2 Guidelines for pharmacotherapy of neuropsychiatric symptoms in AD.

Before prescribing
Establish the most accurate profile of behavioral alterations
Minimize use of medications and seek non-pharmacological alternatives
Take careful medication history and note previous drug responses
Do not avoid pharmacotherapy just because of the age of the patient or the presence of AD

When prescribing
Choose specific target symptoms and carefully monitor the response to therapy
Provide easily understood verbal and written instructions both to patients and to caregivers
Start low and go slow
Know the pharmacology, side-effect profile and potential drug interactions
Avoid multiple drug regimens

After prescribing
Evaluate adherence to treatment instructions
Accept partial responses if more complete responses result in unacceptable side effects
Review drug regimens frequently, discontinue unnecessary drugs and simplify dose schedules
Monitor side effects regularly

important to evaluate for concomitant conditions such as intercurrent medical illness and concurrent medications that can produce side effects leading to psychopathology. Appropriate non-pharmacological intervention should be implemented.[62]

General considerations for pharmacological treatment are listed in Table 8.2. The pharmacological armamentarium used for the management of non-cognitive and behavioral problems in AD is broad (Table 8.3). Although the use of psychotropic medications is very common, the number of double-blind, placebo-controlled studies of psychotropic medications for control of neuropsychiatric abnormalities in AD remains remarkably small.[61]

In recent years, several studies have evaluated the effects of typical and atypical antipsychotic drugs that have been widely prescribed for patients with AD. The typical antipsychotic drugs may produce side effects such as extrapyramidal symptoms, and patients with DLB appear particularly susceptible to these adverse effects.[63] Devanand *et al.* compared low and high doses of haloperidol with placebo.[64] The low dose of haloperidol (0.5–0.75 mg/day) was no different from placebo. The high dose of haloperidol (2–3 mg/day) produced response rates of 55–60%, compared with placebo response rates of 25–30%. Unfortunately, 20% of patients developed moderate to severe extrapyramidal signs.

Table 8.3 Psychotropic medications used for the treatment of neuropsychiatric symptoms in AD.

Class of symptom	Medication	Usual daily dose
Delusions	Donepezil	10 mg (5–10 mg)
	Haloperidol	1 mg (0.5–3 mg)
	Fluphenazine	1 mg (1–5 mg)
	Thioridazine	75 mg (3–150 mg)
	Clozapine	50 mg (12.5–100 mg)
	Risperidone	1 mg (0.5–6 mg)
	Olanzapine	5 mg (5–20 mg)
	Quetiapine	50 mg (12.5–100 mg)
Agitation/aggression	Donepezil	10 mg (5–10 mg)
	Haloperidol	1 mg (0.5–3 mg)
	Trazodone	100 mg (100–400 mg)
	Risperidone	1 mg (0.5–6 mg)
	Olanzapine	5 mg (5–10 mg)
	Buspirone	15 mg (15–30 mg)
	Propranolol	120 mg (80–240 mg)
	Carbamazepine	400 mg (200–1200 mg)
	Divalproex	500 mg (250–3000 mg)
	Lorazepam	1 mg (0.5–6 mg)
Depression	Nortriptyline	50 mg (50–100 mg)
	Trazodone	100 mg (100–400 mg)
	Fluoxetine	40 mg (20–80 mg)
	Sertraline	50 mg (50–200 mg)
	Paroxetine	20 mg (10–50 mg)
	Citalopram	20 mg (10–30 mg)
	Venlafaxin	100 mg (50–300 mg)
	Nefazodone	400 mg (200–600 mg)
	Mirtazepine	15 mg (7.5–30 mg)
Anxiety	Oxazepam	30 mg (20–60 mg)
	Lorazepam	1 mg (0.5–6 mg)
	Buspirone	30 mg (15–45 mg)
	Propranolol	120 mg (80–240 mg)
Insomnia	Trazodone	100 mg (50–200 mg)
	Zolpidem	10 mg (5–10 mg)
	Temazepam	15 mg (15–30 mg)

The new atypical antipsychotic drugs such as clozapine, risperidone, olanzapine and quetiapine offer the theoretical advantage of reduced or minimal extrapyramidal side effects. Results from the first large, double-blind, placebo-controlled study of risperidone for psychoses and behavioral disturbances associated with dementia have been recently reported.[65] A total of 625 patients with fourth edition of the *Diagnostic and*

Statistical Manual of Mental Disorders (DSM-IV) diagnoses of AD (73%), vascular dementia (15%) or mixed dementia (12%) were included. The primary outcome measure was the BEHAVE-AD. All of the patients were institutionalized and most had severe dementia. Risperidone significantly improved symptoms of psychosis and aggressive behavior. The dose that produced maximum improvement without significant side effects was 1 mg/day. The most common dose-related side effects were somnolence, mild peripheral edema and extrapyramidal symptoms. A second large European trial confirmed that low doses of risperidone were well tolerated and reduced agitation in elderly patients with dementia.[66,67] A large open-label study of quetiapine for the control of psychosis in elderly patients with idiopathic and organic psychoses (50% of whom had AD) was recently reported.[68] Quetiapine in doses from 12.5 to 450 mg/day was associated with a reduction of psychotic symptoms with few side effects.

Clozapine therapy was found to be associated with significant improvement in psychosis in patients with Parkinson's disease in a large double-blind, placebo-controlled trial.[69]

Surprisingly, antidepressants, which are widely used in clinical practice, have not been rigorously studied in clinical trials in AD. A recent blinded, active-comparative study compared trazodone with haloperidol and found equal improvement in agitation, with a more benign side effect profile for the trazodone group.[70] A trial of citalopram, a serotonin reuptake inhibitor, showed that patients with AD achieved significant improvements in emotional bluntness, confusion and irritability.[71]

Recent studies have found that anticonvulsant agents such as carbamazepine and valproic acid are helpful in the treatment of agitation in AD patients.[72,73] The potential role of newer anticonvulsants (e.g. lamotrigine, gabapentin and topiramate) is not yet established.

Cholinomimetic agents

The use of cholinomimetic agents in the treatment of neuropsychiatric symptoms in AD represents a novel approach to behavior pharmacology.[33] Tacrine was the first cholinesterase inhibitor (CEI) to be approved for the treatment of AD. The first observations with tacrine were anecdotal and suggested that behavior disturbances improved in some patients.[74] A subsequent analysis of behavioral changes in a controlled study supported these observations.[75]

Xanomeline, a muscarinic agonist, reduced new instances of delusions and hallucinations as well as existing levels of the two behaviors.[76] The beneficial drug effects extended from delusions and hallucinations to agitation and physical aggressiveness.

The study of metrifonate was the first controlled trial with a planned analysis of behavioral data to verify the beneficial effect of a CEI on behavior.[77] The NPI was used as an instrument for assessing behavioral abnormalities. This study found that metrifonate improved hallucinations, agitation and apathy.

The spectrum of behavioral profiles may predict a patient's responses to CEI therapy.[78] The presence of more severe delusions, agitation, depression, anxiety, apathy, disinhibition and irritability as measured by NPI at baseline predicts a stronger response.

There are anecdotal reports and case studies of behavioral improvement with donepezil therapy in patients with DLB.[79]

Few clinical trials have assessed neurobehavioral changes in AD with disease-modifying agents. Some studies have reported moderate behavioral improvements with selegiline.[80–82] Total BRSD scores were reduced in patients who received combined vitamin E and selegiline therapy in a prolonged outpatient trial.[83] In contrast, no evidence in support of significant behavioral benefit has been found in other trials of selegiline in AD.[84,85]

Clinical trials are under way for other possible disease-modifying agents such as non-steroidal anti-inflammatory drugs, estrogen and progesterone. Preliminary reports of estrogen and progesterone indicate that these agents may be beneficial in reducing physical and sexual aggression in men.[58]

Neuropsychiatric disturbances in other neurodegenerative disorders

Movement disorders

The NPI has been used to characterize neuropsychiatric symptoms in patients with CBD and PSP.[86,87] Patients with CBD exhibited depression (73%), apathy (40%), irritability (20%) and agitation (20%), but few showed disinhibition, delusions, anxiety or aberrant motor behavior. Depression and irritability were more frequent and severe in CBD than in PSP. Patients with PSP had low scores on scales for agitation and anxiety and high scores on scales for apathy. Apathy in PSP was significantly associated with executive dysfunction.[86]

In a recent study, Litvan *et al.* compared neuropsychiatric symptoms in patients with hyperkinetic movement disorders (in Huntington's disease) and hypokinetic movement disorders (in PSP).[87] The NPI was used as the behavior assessment instrument in 29 patients with Huntington's disease and in 34 patients with PSP. Results of this study revealed no differences in total NPI scores. However, there was a double dissociation in behaviors – patients with Huntington's disease exhibited more agitation, irritability and anxiety, whereas patients with PSP exhibited more apathy. Depression was present in 41% of patients with Huntington's disease.

These authors suggested that differences in behavioral manifestations were due to involvement of different frontal–subcortical circuits.[88]

Several studies have investigated neuropsychiatric symptoms in patients with DLB. All of these studies have found that visual hallucinations occur significantly more frequently in DLB than in AD, and the presence of visual hallucinations is one of the cardinal symptoms required for diagnosis of DLB.[89] In a recent study, Ballard *et al.* assessed psychiatric morbidity in two groups – a clinical case register cohort (98 patients with DLB and 92 patients with AD) and 80 prospectively studied, neuropathologically confirmed cases (40 patients with DLB and 40 patients with AD).[90] The occurrence of psychiatric symptoms was reported over 1 month. Hallucinations, depression, delusions and delusional misidentification were all significantly higher for patients with DLB. The presence of psychiatric symptoms at presentation was a better discriminator between DLB and AD than occurrence over the course of dementia.

Visual hallucinations in DLB were studied in detail by Ballard *et al.*[27] They reported that visual hallucinations may be more likely to be multiple, to speak and to be persistent in DLB patients.

Hirono *et al.* used the NPI to assess neuropsychiatric features in patients with DLB and compared this with its use in patients with AD.[91] The frequency of misidentification delusions was significantly greater in the DLB group.

Frontotemporal dementia

Levy *et al.* used the NPI to compare the behavioral features of 22 frontotemporal dementia patients with that of 30 AD patients.[92] The frontotemporal dementia patients had significantly higher total scores and greater disinhibition, apathy, aberrant motor behavior and euphoria than the AD patients. The frontotemporal dementia patients had less depression than AD patients. Mendez *et al.* used the BEHAVE-AD scale to study behavioral differences between frontotemporal dementia and AD.[93] The results confirmed that patients with frontotemporal dementia tended to demonstrate disinhibition, manifested as verbal outbursts and inappropriate activity. They had more aggressiveness and less anxiety and depression. Patients who present for an initial dementia evaluation and who score high on the BEHAVE-AD are more likely to have frontotemporal dementia than AD.

Summary

AD has multiple manifestations and produces cognitive, behavioral and neurological abnormalities. Behavioral problems are common in AD and these disturbances often contribute to the morbidity, institutionalization and reduced survival of AD patients. In addition, neuropsychiatric symptoms adversely affect the psychological and physical well-being of caregivers. The behavioral disturbances are primary manifestations of brain dysfunction. Neurobiology of behavioral symptoms is being explored; neuropathological and neuroimaging studies suggest that specific brain structures, circuits and neurotransmitters are responsible for specific neuropsychiatric symptoms and profiles. Longitudinal studies allow transitional probability of behavioral disturbances to be estimated, which can be used for planning of treatment intervention.

Evidence has accumulated that the cholinergic deficiency of AD contributes to the neuropsychiatric disorders and cholinomimetic therapy ameliorates some of these abnormalities. Cholinergic agents exhibit disease-specific, broad-spectrum psychotropic effects. There is now a clear requirement in the design of clinical trials in AD for scales to measure behavioral symptoms to be included.

Functional neuroimaging provides insights into pathogenesis of neuropsychiatric symptoms and may potentially be used as a predictor of a therapeutic response for a specific agent.

Neuropsychiatric symptoms are common in other neurodegenerative diseases. Each disease has a specific neuropsychiatric symptom profile that corresponds to circuit-related pathology and neurotransmitter deficits. Instrumentation has evolved that allows reliable and valid assessment of neuropsychiatric symptoms in degenerative disorders. The NPI is the most commonly used in this research setting.

The ultimate goal of understanding the etiology and pathogenesis of AD is to be able to devise treatment. Combination therapies that delay the onset, slow the progression and improve the symptoms (including behavioral disturbances) promise to emerge.

Acknowledgements

This project was supported by a Geriatric Neurology Fellowship from the Department of Veterans Affairs (Dr Bronstein), a grant (AG10123) from the National Institute of Aging Alzheimer's Disease Research Center, a grant from the Alzheimer's Disease Research Center of California, and the Sidell–Kagan Foundation.

References

1. Cummings JL, Vinters HV, Cole GM, Khachaturian ZS. Alzheimer's disease: etiologies, pathophysiology, cognitive reserve, and treatment opportunities. Neurology 1998;51(suppl 1): S2–S17.

2. Borson S, Raskind MA. Clinical features and pharmacological treatment of behavioral symptoms of Alzheimer's disease. Neurology 1997;48(suppl 6):S17–S24.

3. Reisberg B, Borenstein J, Salob SP, et al. Behavioral symptoms in Alzheimer's disease: phenomenology and treatment. J Clin Psychiatry 1987;48(suppl):9–15.

4. Loveck DJ, Bylsma F, Folstein

MF. The dementia symptoms scale: a new scale for comprehensive assessment of psychopathology in Alzheimer's disease. Am J Geriatr Psychiatry 1994;2:60–74.

5. Victoroff J, Nielson K, Mungas D. Caregiver and clinician assessment of behavioral disturbances: the California dementia behavior questionnaire. Int Psychogeriatr 1997;9:155–174.

6. Tariot PN. Mack JL, Patterson MB, *et al.* The behavior rating scale for dementia of the consortium to establish a registry for Alzheimer's disease. Am J Psychiatry 1995;152:1349–1357.

7. Cohen-Mansfield J, Marx MS, Rosenthal AS. A description of agitation in a nursing home. J Gerontol 1989;44:M77–M84.

8. Bucht G, Adolfsson R. The Comprehensive psychopathological rating scale in patients with dementia of Alzheimer type and multiinfarct dementia. Acta Psychiatr Scand 1983;68:263–270.

9. Cummings JL, Mega M, Gray K, Rosenberg-Thompson S, Carusi DA, Gornbein J. The Neuropsychiatric Inventory: comprehensive assessment of psychopathology in dementia. Neurology 1994;44: 2308–2314.

10. Weiner MF, Koss E, Wild KV, *et al.* Measures of psychiatric symptoms in Alzheimer patients: a review. Alzheimer Dis Assoc Disord 1996;10:20–30.

11. Cummings JL. The Neuropsychiatric Inventory: assessing psychopathology in dementia patients. Neurology 1997;48(suppl 6): S1–S16.

12. Woods SW, Cummings JL, Hsu HA, *et al.* The use of the neuropsychiatric inventory in nursing home residents characterization and management; in press.

13. Mega M, Cummings JL, Fiorello T, Gornbein J. The spectrum of behavioral changes in Alzheimer's disease. Neurology 1996;46:130–135.

14. Mega MS, Cummings JL. The cingulate and cingulate syndromes. Trimble MR, Cummings JL, eds. Contemporary behavioral neurology. Boston: Butterworth–Heinemann; 1997:189–214.

15. Duffy JD. The neural substrates of motivation. Psychiatr Ann 1997;27:24–29.

16. Marin RS. Apathy: concept, syndrome, neural mechanisms, and treatment. Semin Clin Neuropsychiatry 1996;1:304–314.

17. Levy ML, Cummings JL, Fairbank LA, *et al.* Apathy is not depression. J Neuropsychiatry Clin Neurosci 1998;10:314–319.

18. Folstein MF, Folstein SE, McHugh PR. Mini-mental state: a practical method for grading the cognitive status of patients for the clinician. J Psychiatry Res 1975;12: 189–198.

19. Kuzis G, Sabe L, Tiberti C, Dorrego F, Starkstein SE. Neuropsychological correlates of apathy and depression in patients with dementia. Neurology 1999;52; 1403–1407.

20. Weiner MF, Edland SD, Lyszcynska H. Prevalence and incidence of major depression in Alzheimer's disease. Am J Psychiatry 1994;151:1006–1009.

21. Cummings JL, Ross W, Absher J, *et al.* Depressive symptoms in Alzheimer's disease: assessment and determinants. Alzheimer Dis Assoc Disord 1995;9:87–93.

22. Rohde K, Reskid ER, Raskid MA. Suicide in two patients with Alzheimer's disease. Am J Psychiatry 1995;43:187–189.

23. Ferris SH, Hofeldt GT, Carbone G, Masciandaro P, Troetel WM, Imbumbo BP. Suicide in two patients with a diagnosis of prob-

able Alzheimer's disease. Alzheimer Dis Assoc Disord 1999;13:88–90.

24. Rao V, Lyketsos CG. Delusions in Alzheimer's disease: a review. J Neuropsychiatry Clin Neurosci 1998;10:373–382.

25. Sala SD, Francescani A, Muggia S, Spinnler H. Variables linked to psychotic symptoms in Alzheimer's disease. Eur J Neurol 1998;5:553–560.

26. Hwang JP, Yang CH, Tsai SJ, Liu KM. Delusions of theft in dementia of the Alzheimer type: a preliminary report. Alzheimer Dis Assoc Disord 1997;11:110–112.

27. Ballard C, O'Brien J, Coope B, Fairbairn A, Abid F, Wilcock G. A prospective study of psychotic symptoms in dementia sufferers: psychosis in dementia. Int Psychogeriatr 1997;9:57–64.

28. Devanand OP, Jacobs DM, Tang MX, *et al.* The course of psychopathologic features in mild to moderate Alzheimer disease. Arch Gen Psychiatry 1997;54:257–263.

29. Marin DB, Green CR, Schmeidler J, *et al.* Noncognitive disturbances in Alzheimer's disease: frequency, longitudinal course, and relationship to cognitive symptoms. J Am Geriatr Soc 1997;45:1331–1338.

30. Levy ML, Cummings JL, Fairbanks LA, *et al.* Longitudinal assessment of symptoms of depression, agitation, and psychosis in 181 patients with Alzheimer's disease. Am J Psychiatry 1996;153:1438–1443.

31. Mesulam MM. The systems-level organization of cholinergic innervation in the human cerebral cortex and its alterations in Alzheimer's disease. Prog Brain Res 1996;109:285–297.

32. Cummings JL, Back C. The cholinergic hypothesis of neuropsychiatric symptoms in Alzheimer's disease. Am J Geriatr Soc 1998;6(suppl 1):64–78.

33. Cummings JL, Kaufer D. Neuropsychiatric aspects of Alzheimer's disease: the cholinergic hypothesis revised. Neurology 1996;47:876–883.

34. Cummings JL. Changes in neuropsychiatric symptoms as outcome measures in clinical trials with cholinergic therapies for Alzheimer disease. Alzheimer Dis Assoc Disord 1997;11(suppl 4):S1–S9.

35. Russo-Neustadt A, Cotman CW. Adrenergic receptors in Alzheimer's disease brain: selective increases in the cerebella of aggressive patients. J Neurosci 1997;17:5573–5580.

36. Victoroff J, Zarow C, Mack WJ, Hsu E, Chui HC. Physical aggression is associated with preservation of substantia nigra pars compacta in Alzheimer disease. Arch Neurol 1996;53:428–434.

37. Ramachadran G, Marder K, Tang M, *et al.* A preliminary study of apoliporotein E genotype and psychiatric manifestations of Alzheimer's disease. Neurology 1996;47:256–259.

38. Murphy GM Jr, Taylor J, Tinklenberg JR, Yesavage JA. The apolipoprotein E epsilon 4 allele is associated with increased behavioral disturbance in Alzheimer's disease. Am J Geriatr Psychiatry 1997;5:88–89.

39. Cacabelos R, Rodriguez B, Carrera C, Beyer K, Lao JI, Sellers MA. Behavioral changes associated with different apolipoprotein E genotypes in dementia. Alzheimer Dis Assoc Disord 1997;11(suppl 4):S27–S34.

40. Holmes C, Levy R, McLoughlin DM, Powell JF, Lovestone S. Apolipoprotein E: noncognitive symptoms and cognitive decline

in late onset Alzheimer's disease. J Neurol Neurosurg Psychiatry 1996;61:580–583.

41. Lyketsos CG, Baker L, Waren A, *et al*. Depression, delusions, and hallucinations in Alzheimer's disease: No relationship to apolipoprotein E genotype. J Neuropsychiatry Clin Neurosci 1997;9:64–67.

42. Lopez OL, Kamboh MI, Becker JO, Kaufer DI, DeKosky ST. The apolipoprotein E epsilon 4 allele is not associated with psychotic symptoms or extrapyramidal signs in probable Alzheimer's disease. Neurology 1997;49:794–797.

43. Hirono N, Mori E, Yasuda M, *et al*. Lack of effect of apolipoprotein E e4 allele on neuropsychiatric manifestations in Alzheimer's disease. J Neuropsychiatry Clin Neurosci 1999;11:66–70.

44. Levy ML, Cummings JL, Fairbanks LA, Sultzer DL, Small GW. Apolipoprotein E genotype and noncognitive symptoms in Alzheimer's disease. Biol Psychiatry 1999;45:422–425.

45. Starkstein SE, Vasquez S, Petracca G, *et al*. A SPECT study of delusions in Alzheimer's disease. Neurology 1994;44:2055–2059.

46. Kotrla KJ, Chacko RC, Harper RG, Jhingran S, Doody R. SPECT findings on psychosis in Alzheimer's disease. Am J Psychiatry 1995;152:1470–1475.

47. Sultzer DL, Mahler ME, Mandelkern MA, *et al*. The relationship between psychiatric symptoms and regional cortical metabolism in Alzheimer's disease. J Neuropsychiatry Clin Neurosci 1995;7:476–484.

48. Hirono N, Mori E, Ishii K, *et al*. Frontal lobe hypometabolism and depression in Alzheimer's disease. Neurology 1998;50:380–383.

49. Ring HA, Bench CJ, Trimble MR, Brooks DJ, Frackpwiak RS, Dolan RJ. Depression in Parkinson's disease. A positron emission study. Br J Psychiatry 1994;165:333–339.

50. Ott BR, Noto RB, Fogel BS. Apathy and loss of insight in Alzheimer's disease: a SPECT imaging study. J Neuropsychiatry Clin Neurosci 1996;8:41–46.

51. Craig HA, Cummings JL, Fairbanks L, *et al*. Cerebral blood flow correlates of apathy in Alzheimer's disease. Arch Neurol 1996;53:1116–1120.

52. Fazekas F, Kapeller P, Schmidt R, *et al*. The relation of cerebral magnetic resonance signal hyperintensities to Alzheimer's disease. J Neurol Sci 1996;142:121–125.

53. O'Brien JT, Ames D, Scwietzer I. White matter in depression and Alzheimer's disease: a review of magnetic resonance imaging studies. Int J Geriatr Psychiatry 1996;11:681–694.

54. Krishan KR, Hays JC, Blazer DG. MRI-defined vascular depression. Am J Psychiatry 1997;54:785–788.

55. Starkstein SE, Sabe L, Vazquez S, *et al*. Neuropsychological, psychiatric, and cerebral perfusion correlates of leukoaraiosis in Alzheimer's disease. J Neurol Neurosurg Psychiatry 1997;63:66–73.

56. Barber R, Scheltens P, Gholkar A, *et al*. White matter lesions on magnetic resonance imaging in dementia with Lewy bodies, Alzheimer's disease, vascular dementia, and normal aging. J Neurol Neurosurg Psychiatry 1999;67:66–72.

57. Cummings JL. Neuropsychiatric assessment and intervention in Alzheimer's disease. Int Psychogeriatr 1996;8:25–30.

58. Tariot PN. Treatment strategies for

agitation and psychoses in dementia. J Clin Psychiatry 1996;57(suppl 14):21–29.

59. Tariot PN. Treatment of agitation in dementia. J Clin Psychiatry 1999;60(suppl 8):11–20.

60. Maxiner S, Mellow AM, Tandon R. The efficacy, safety, and tolerability of antipsychotics in the elderly. J Clin Psychiatry 1999;60(suppl 8):29–41.

61. Raskind MA. Psychopharmacology of noncognitive abnormal behaviors in Alzheimer's disease. J Clin Psychiatry 1998;59(suppl 9):28–32.

62. Teri L, Logsdon RG, Uomoto J, McCurry SM. Behavioral treatment of depression in dementia patients: a controlled clinical trial. J Gerontol B 1997;52:159–166.

63. Schneider LS. Pharmacologic management of psychosis in dementia. J Clin Psychiatry 1999;60(suppl 8):54–60.

64. Devanand DP, Marder K, Micaels KS, et al. A randomized, placebo-controlled dose-comparison trial of haloperidol for psychosis and disruptive behaviors in Alzheimer's disease. Am J Psychiatry 1998;155:1512–1520.

65. Katz IR, Jeste DV, Mintzer JE, Clydee C, Napolitano J, Brecher M. Comparison of risperidone and placebo for psychosis and behavioral disturbances associated with dementia: a randomized, double-blind trial. Risperidone Study Group. J Clin Psychiatry 1999;60:107–115.

66. De Deyn PP, Rabheru K, Rasmussen A, et al. A randomized trial of risperidone, placebo, and haloperidol for behavioral symptoms of dementia. Neurology 1999;53:946–955.

67. Cummings JL, Knopman D. Advances in the treatment of behavioral disturbances in Alzheimer's disease. Neurology 1999;53:899–901.

68. McManus DQ, Arvantis LA, Kowalcyk BB. Quetiapine. A novel antipsychotic: experience in elderly patients with psychotic disorders. Seroquel 48 Study Group. J Clin Psychiatry 1999;60:292–298.

69. The Parkinson Study Group. Low-dose clozapine for the treatment of drug-induced psychosis in Parkinson's disease. N Engl Med 1999;340:757–763.

70. Sultzer DL, Gray KF, Gunay I, et al. A double-blind comparison of trazodone and haloperidol for treatment of agitation in patients with dementia. Am J Geriatr Psychiatry 1997;5:60–69.

71. Nyth AL, Gottfries CG, Lyby K, et al. A controlled multicenter clinical study of citalopram and placebo in elderly depressed patients with and without concomitant dementia. Acta Psychiatr Scand 1992;86:138–145.

72. Tariot PN, Erb R, Podgorski CA, et al. Efficacy and tolerability of carbamazepine for agitation and aggression in dementia. Am J Psychiatry 1998;55:54–61.

73. Porsteinsson A, Tariot PN, Erb R, et al. An open trial of valproate for agitation in dementia. Am J Geriatr Psychiatry 1997;5:344–351.

74. Kaufer DI, Cummings JL, Christine D, Effect of tacrine on behavioral symptoms in Alzheimer's disease: an open-label study. J Geriatr Psychiatry Neurol 1996;9:1–6.

75. Raskind MA, Sadowsky CH, Sigmund WR, Beitler PJ, Auster SB. Effect of tacrine on language, praxis, and noncognitive behavioral problems in Alzheimer's disease. Arch Neurol 1997;54:836–840.

76. Bodick NC, Offen WW, Levey AI, et al. Effects of xanomeline, a selective muscarinic receptor agonist, on cognitive function and

behavioral symptoms in Alzheimer's disease. Arch Neurol 1997;54:465–473.

77. Morris JC, Cyrus PA, Orazem J, *et al.* Metrifonate benefits cognitive, behavioral, and global function in patients with Alzheimer's disease. Neurology 1998;50:1222–1230.

78. Mega MS, Masterman DM, O'Connor SM, *et al.* The spectrum of behavioral responses to cholinesterase inhibitor therapy in Alzheimer disease. Arch Neurol 1999;56:1388–1393.

79. Kaufer DL, Catt KE, Lopez OL, DeKosky ST. Dementia with Lewy bodies: response of delirium-like features to donepezil. Neurology 1998;51:1512.

80. Goad DL, Davis CM, Liem P, *et al.* The use of selegiline in Alzheimer's patients with behavior problems. J Clin Psychiatry 1991; 52:342–345.

81. Tariot PN, Cohen RM, Sunderland T, *et al.* L-deprenyl in Alzheimer's disease. Preliminary evidence for behavioral change with monoamine oxidase B inhibition. Arch Gen Psychiatry 1987;44:427–433.

82. Lawlor BA, Aisen PS, Green C, Fine E, Schmeedidler J. Selegiline in the treatment of behavioural disturbance in Alzheimer's disease. Int J Geriatr Psychiatry 1997;12:319–322.

83. Sano M, Ernesto C, Thomas RG, *et al.* The Alzheimer's Disease Cooperative Study. A controlled trial of selegiline, alpha-tocopherol, or both as treatment for Alzheimer's disease. N Engl J Med 1997;336:1216–1222.

84. Freedman M, Rewilak D, Xerri T, *et al.* L-deprenyl in Alzheimer's disease: cognitive and behavioral effects. Neurology 1998;50: 660–668.

85. Tariot PN, Goldstein B, Podgorski CA, Cox C, Frambes N. Short-term administration of selegiline for mild-moderate dementia of the Alzheimer's type. Am J Geriatr Psychiatry 1998;6:145–154.

86. Litvan I, Mega MS, Cummings JL, Fairbank L. Neuropsychiatric aspects of progressive supranuclear palsy. Neurology 1996;47: 1184–1189.

87. Litvan I, Paulsen JS, Mega MS, Cummings JL. Neuropsychiatric assessment of patients with hyperkinetic and hypokinetic movement disorders. Arch Neurol 1998;55:1313–1319.

88. Mega MS, Cummings JL. Frontal–subcortical circuits and neuropsychiatric disorders. J Neuropsychiatry Clin Neurosci 1994;6:358–370.

89. McKeith IG, Galasko D, Kosaka K, *et al.* Consensus guidelines for the clinical and pathologic diagnosis of dementia with Lewy bodies (DLB). Neurology 1996;47: 1113–1124.

90. Ballard C, Holmes C, McKeith I *et al.* Psychiatric morbidity in dementia with Lewy bodies: a prospective clinical and neuropathological comparative study with Alzheimer's disease. Am J Psychiatry 1999;156:1039–1045.

91. Hirono N, Mori E, Imamura T, Shimomura T, Hashimoto M. Neuropsychiatric features in dementia with Lewy bodies and Alzheimer's disease. No To Shinkei 1998; 50:45–49.

92. Levy ML, Miller BL, Cummings JL, Fairbanks LA, Craig A. Alzheimer disease and frontotemporal dementias. Behavioral distinctions. Arch Neurol 1996;53: 687–690.

93. Mendez MF, Perryman KM, Miller BL, Cummings JL. Behavioral differences between frontotemporal dementia and Alzheimer's disease: a comparison of the BEHAVE-AD rating scale. Int Psychogeriatr 1998;10:155–162.

9
Cholinesterase inhibitors in the treatment of dementia

Serge Gauthier

Rationale for using cholinesterase inhibitors in dementia

The main reason for using cholinesterase inhibitors (CIs) in dementias such as Alzheimer's disease (AD) is the reduction in cortical and hippocampal choline acetyl transferase activity as documented in autopsy studies in the late 1970s.[1] A more recent report[2] suggests that the reduction in choline acetyl transferase activity occurs relatively late in the course of AD, a strong reason for studying the efficacy of cholinergic replacement therapy throughout the course of disease. The 'cholinergic hypothesis' assumes that many of the cognitive, functional and behavioral symptoms associated with AD are caused by a reduction in brain acetylcholine activity secondary to the loss of cholinergic neurons in the basal nucleus of Meynert and other nuclei that project to the hippocampus and mesial temporal region.[3] Although this reduction in cholinergic activity is not as important pathologically as diffuse synaptic loss in cortical associative areas,[4,5] it offers a target for symptomatic therapy until alternative therapies become available to restore and maintain synaptic integrity. Other dementias present cholinergic deficits similar to those that occur in AD, including Lewy body dementia,[6] mixed AD and vascular dementia,[7] and Gerstmann–Straussler dementia;[8] however, Pick's disease does not.[8,9] Since there are few published data available from randomized clinical trials using CIs in non-AD dementias, this chapter focuses on the safety and efficacy of CIs used as monotherapy in AD.

Natural history of AD and its effect on trial designs

AD is characterized by a progressive decline in cognitive and functional abilities in all stages, whereas mood and behavioral manifestations tend to peak and decrease in early and late stages respectively. This multidimensional aspect of AD has an impact on the type and duration of randomized clinical trials and in the selection of outcome measures.[10] Most of the published trials have enrolled patients with probable AD (as defined by a working group of the National Institute of Neurological and Communicative Disorders and Stroke)[11] in mild to moderate stages (operationally defined as Mini Mental State Examination (MMSE)[12] scores of 10–26, which corresponds to stages 3–5 on the Global Deterioration Scale).[13] So far, most placebo-controlled randomized clinical trials in AD have been of 3–6 months' duration. This represents between 3 and 6% of the disease duration if the average survival is taken to be 8 years.[14] The favored design is placebo-controlled parallel groups, and the most widely used primary outcome variables are the Alzheimer's Disease Assessment Scale (ADAS-cog)[15] and the Clinical Interview-Based Impression of Change (CIBIC-plus),[16] in answer to the Food and Drug Administration (FDA) guidelines in the USA, which asked for a dual outcome from a performance-based objective test instrument for cognition and an interview-based impression of change.[17] The Canadian and European regulatory guidelines have put additional emphasis on functional improvement or lesser decline of function.[18]

Ongoing studies are exploring a broader range of AD severity, such as mild cognitive impairment at one end of the spectrum and moderately severe AD at the other, with appropriate primary outcome variables such as time to conversion from mild cognitive impairment to diagnosable dementia. Other studies are looking at a broader spectrum of diagnosis, including probable–possible AD and mixed AD and vascular dementia, a situation that is closer to the reality of geriatric practice.

Published studies of CIs in AD

Tacrine

Tacrine (tetrahydroaminoacridine) was the first CI to be tested and clinically used in many countries. After the initial observations of a symptomatic benefit by Summers *et al.* in 1986,[19] multiple randomized clinical trials were performed, involving either small or large groups of patients, in a variety of designs, including single cross-over,[20] multiple cross-over,[21] and parallel groups with[22] or without[23,24] enrichment for 'responders'. Tacrine was approved for use in mild to moderate AD in the USA by the FDA in 1994. Its use has been seriously curtailed by the availability since 1997 of the second-generation CIs donepezil and rivastigmine. However, despite the practical issues of the short half-life of tacrine (meaning that four-times-daily administration was required), its gastrointestinal side effects (meaning that slow titration towards the therapeutic doses of 120–160 mg per day was required), and the reversible elevation in liver transaminases levels that it produced, many important facts were learned from this drug, particularly about long-term use and patterns of responders. Patients who were treated with tacrine at therapeutic doses for extended periods (2 years or more) needed nursing home care later than patients who could tolerate only a lower dose.[25]

A later analysis of efficacy data based on the MMSE and the ADAS-cog has shown that a delay of 6 weeks is required for the maximal cognitive improvement at the highest tolerated dose.[26] A meta-analysis of 12 randomized clinical trials confirmed both a measurable benefit that had been detected by the MMSE and the clinical impression of change, with no influence of age or severity of disease on therapeutic response.[27] An open-label study[28] and a later analysis[29] suggest a beneficial effect of tacrine on behavior.

Donepezil

Donepezil (E2020) was the second CI to be tested and it has been widely prescribed since 1997. After the initial randomized clinical trial, which demonstrated a statistically significant improvement in ADAS-cog after 12 weeks of treatment with doses of 5 mg daily (correlating with inhibition of red blood cell acetylcholinesterase activity),[30] trials of 15 weeks' duration[31] and 24 weeks' duration[32,33] have demonstrated that daily doses of both 5 mg and 10 mg are effective in improving cognition and global functioning. One of the 24-week studies[33] also showed a statistically significant reduction in the rate of loss of instrumental activities of daily living (ADL) at the 10 mg dose, using the modified Interview for Deterioration in Daily Living Activities in Dementia.[34] The symptomatic benefits are reversible after a 6-week wash-out period.

The long-term follow-up of patients treated with donepezil suggests a sustained therapeutic benefit, with a decline in ADAS-cog and Clinical Dementia Rating[35] that is parallel to groups of patients receiving no specific pharmacotherapy.[36] A 1-year placebo-controlled randomized clinical trial has been completed in five northern European countries; it showed improvements in cognition, global function and ADL.[37] Of particular interest was the fact that the MMSE scores were improved above baseline until week 36. An open-label retrospective study[38] of treatment-related behavioral assessments using the NeuroPsychiatric Inventory[39] as well as a prospective open-label treatment study[40] demonstrated improvement in behaviors and a reduction in caregiver distress.

There are no data to suggest which patients are more likely to improve on donepezil. A one-step titration from 5 mg to 10 mg/day with an interval of 4–6 weeks and a once-daily dosing schedule have facilitated its use by primary care practitioners as well as specialists.[41]

Rivastigmine

Rivastigmine (ENA 713) is the third CI to be made available in Europe since 1997. It will be marketed in the USA in early 2000. The initial dose-finding studies led to the large-scale ADENA program[42] to establish the safety and efficacy of lower doses (1–4 mg/day) versus higher doses (6–12 mg/day). Two 26-week pivotal studies[43,44] demonstrated a benefit from the higher doses on the primary outcome variables as well as on the decline of ADL as measured by the Progressive Deterioration Scale.[45] There is thus a clear dose–effect relationship for cognition, global impression of change, and ADL.

There are no data to suggest which patients are more or less likely to benefit from rivastigmine. Its use does require close collaboration between caregivers and clinicians, in order to find the best-tolerated and most effective dose for each individual patient.[46]

Metrifonate

Metrifonate is under regulatory review in the USA as the CI with the longest duration of action, through its active metabolite dichlorvos.[47] Results from randomized clinical trials of 12 weeks[48] and 26 weeks[49,50] of active treatment have shown efficacy on all primary outcomes. A pooled analysis of pivotal studies showed a clear dose–effect relationship for cognition,[51] ADL,[52] and behavior.[53] Metrifonate is administered once daily and has a good gastrointestinal tolerance. A reversible proximal limb weakness has been noted in some patients at high doses, and this side effect is likely to limit its use to the lower doses.

Galantamine

Galantamine is under regulatory review (except in Austria, where it is available as a regular prescription drug) as the CI with intrinsic nicotinic activity.[54] Data available from phase 2 randomized clinical trials show efficacy on cognition.[55] Galantamine could be used in two- or three-times daily regimen. It is as yet unclear if its dual CI and nicotinic actions will translate into higher or more sustained symptomatic benefit.

Comparison of CIs

There are as yet no published randomized clinical trials comparing different CIs within the same study population, and it is not possible to state whether there are true differences between the CIs in terms of efficacy profile in mild to moderately severe AD. Tolerance and ease of use are currently the major considerations when choosing between CIs (see below).

Pharmacogenetic considerations

A retrospective analysis of responder profiles suggest that apolipoprotein E (APOE) 4 carriers have less chance of improving on tacrine than other patients.[56] The proposed explanation for this difference is that APOE mutation is associated with a marked reduction in cholinergic activity and thus lessens the response to a CI such as tacrine. Another analysis in a large number of patients who were being treated with tacrine suggested that this pharmacogenetic effect is seen only in women, with men responding better overall to tacrine.[57] An open-label study confirmed that male sex increases response to tacrine or galatamine in the short term (3 months), but that a greater decrease in response occurs over 12 months in patients who do not carry an APOE4 mutation.[58] A report from France found that APOE4 carriers do better on tacrine with no differences between the sexes.[59] A meta-analysis of patients on metrifonate showed no influence of APOE genotype on response to treatment over 26 weeks.[60]

There are thus conflicting data as to the clinical validity and usefulness of APOE genotyping for the sole purpose of deciding whether or not an individual patient should be treated with a CI. Prospective studies are required to study further the important concept of pharmacogenetics, particularly because different classes of drugs for the treatment of dementia will be available in the future.

Pharmacoeconomic considerations

Pharmacoeconomic models in dementia, mainly derived from epidemiological studies,[61,62] have been built on cost of care for AD. The models had to take into account the relatively modest improvement above baseline for the average patient treated with a CI, in the order of 1–2 points on the MMSE, and carry that improvement over 6 months,[63] 2 years[64] and five years,[65,66] with the assumption (supported by open-label extension studies and wash-out data) that, despite the unchecked progression of the underlying disease, patients are better on sustained pharmacotherapy with CI than without them. All published cost analysis of CIs have been positive, including tacrine,[67,68] despite the need with tacrine therapy for blood monitoring for hepatotoxicity, which is not required with the second-generation CIs.

The issue of cost-effectiveness of CIs led to the First International Pharmacoeconomic Conference on Alzheimer's Disease under the auspices of the International Working Group for Harmonization of Dementia Drug Guidelines.[18] A positive outcome of the published models and of this meeting was the recognition of the need to incorporate caregiver burden, quality of life, and resource utilization into pre- and postmarketing drug development.[69] The evidence already available does suggest cost-neutrality or positive cost-effectiveness for the use of CIs in early to intermediate stages of AD.[70]

Clinical use considerations

Once CIs are approved by regulatory authorities and reimbursed by formulary bodies and other third-party payers, their appropriate use depends on the knowledge of the practicing clinician about differential diagnosis and on realistic expectations from patients, families and clinicians.[71] The first guidelines on the use of CIs came from a group of British old-age psychiatrists;[72] these were followed by a large number of regional[73] and national[74–76] consensus guidelines.

Certain common clinical features of CIs can be described. In terms of safety and tolerance, gastrointestinal side effects (nausea, vomiting, diarrhea, and anorexia) are dose-related but partially avoidable by a slower titration to therapeutic levels; they may be a limiting factor for the use of CIs in patients of small body weight. Cardiovascular side effects (symptomatic bradycardia, syncope) are not frequent, if caution is exercised in patients with sick sinus syndrome or other supraventricular conduction defects. Less common side effects include insomnia and exaggeration of depressive symptoms, which can be avoided by ingestion of CIs in the morning (with once-daily dosing) and treatment of depression before cholinergic therapy is started. The presence or absence of hepatic cytochrome P450 metabolism of CIs seem to have little importance with drugs commonly used in the management of AD (such as antidepressants, anticonvulsants, anxiolytics and neuroleptics), although it is important to be vigilant in documenting possible drug interactions in the liver and at the neuromuscular junction. The short-term (6-month) improvement in cognition and global functioning is similar between CIs. The benefit of ADL is best described as a slowing of decline rather than an actual improvement of specific ADLs, and there is some evidence for beneficial effects of CI on neuropsychiatric manifestations such as hallucinations and apathy. Longer-term effects (beyond 6 months) of CIs as monotherapy suggest a return to baseline of cognitive abilities at 9 months of uninterrupted therapy, followed by a decline that is parallel to untreated patients.

Responses to CIs in clinical practice have been described as:[77]

- obvious response, with return to hobbies and social activities, with or without improvement on MMSE scores;
- modest response, with a reduction in apathy and increased participation in conversation;
- no response, with clinical decline despite therapeutic doses.

Since it is not possible to predict which patients will improve significantly on CI therapy, it is recommended that a therapeutic trial should be offered to every patient in mild to moderate stages of AD after the diagnosis has been established and concomitant disorders have been treated; however, realistic expectations must be set, taking into account the past life experiences of the patient and the stage of the illness. A semistructured review of the various symptomatic domains of AD is suggested before therapy is initiated in order to assess the response to treatment, which may be a symptomatic improvement, stabilization of symptoms or a lesser decline in functioning. The Clinical Dementia Rating,[35] which systematically explores important domains (memory, orientation, judgement and problem solving, community affairs, ADL, hobbies, and personal affairs) may be a useful tool for the long-term follow-up of patients on CI therapy, as was demonstrated in the open-label, long-term follow-up of patients on donepezil.[36]

If a patient has no clinically detectable improvement despite receiving the maximal recommended or tolerated dose of a particular CI or if a patient has progressed to a severe stage of AD, the decision to withdraw treatment must be taken after discussion with the patient and his or her caregivers. If a patient rapidly deteriorates when the drug is stopped, it is preferable to start the medication again immediately.[78]

Perspectives on future use of CIs

CIs have so far been tested in randomized clinical trials only as monotherapy, and there is much interest in controlled studies using judicious drug combinations.[79] For instance, there are some data that suggest a potentiation effect of estrogens on CIs such as tacrine[80] and donepezil.[81] It will be also necessary to study prospectively the potential benefit of combinations of drugs, such as CIs with agents that may delay disease progression, e.g. non-steroidal anti-inflammatory drugs, selective estrogen receptor modulators and selective cyclo-oxygenase-2 inhibitors.[82] It is not, at present, recommended that any of these substances should be routinely added to a CI in clinical practice. On the other hand, when clinically indicated, antidepressants (such as selective serontonin reuptake inhibitors) and atypical neuroleptics (such as risperidone, olanzapine and quetiapine) can be combined with a CI clinically indicated.

Finally, comprehensive support and counseling programs have been shown to increase the time that a spouse or caregiver is able to give to caring for an AD patient at home,[83] and a combination of support programs from community and lay associations with disease-specific pharmacotherapy should prove the best therapeutic approach in mild to moderate stages of dementia.

Conclusions

Cholinergic therapy is now a component of the global management of AD. The value of CIs in the symptomatic therapy of AD has been established by randomized clinical trials and clinical experience for periods of 6–12 months. Beyond this period of time, a slowing of decline is a more realistic goal until safe and effect pharmacological combination therapies become available.

References

1. Davies P, Maloney AJF. Selective loss of central cholinergic neurons in Alzheimer's disease. Lancet 1976;2:1403.

2. Davis KL, Mohs RC, Marin E, *et al.* Cholinergic markers in elderly patients with early signs of Alzheimer's disease. JAMA 1999; 281:1401–1406.

3. Whitehouse PJ, Price DL, Clark AW, *et al.* Alzheimer's disease: evidence for selective loss of cholinergic neurons in the nucleus basalis. Ann Neurol 1981;10:122–126.

4. Terry RD, Masliah E, Salmon DP, *et al.* Physical basis of cognitive alterations in Alzheimer's disease: synaptic loss is the major correlate of cognitive impairment. Ann Neurol 1991;30:572–580.

5. DeKosky ST, Harbaugh RE, Schmitt FA, *et al.* Cortical biopsy in Alzheimer's disease: diagnostic accuracy and neurochemical, neuropathological, and cognitive correlations. Ann Neurol 1992; 32:625–632.

6. Langlais PJ, Thal L, Hansen L, *et al.* Neurotransmitters in basal ganglia and cortex of Alzheimer's disease with and without Lewy bodies. Neurology 1993;43: 1927–1934.

7. Kalaria RN, Ballard C. Overlap between pathology of Alzheimer disease and vascular dementia. Alzheimer Dis Assoc Disord 1999;13(suppl 3):S115–S123.

8. Wood PL, Nair NPV, Etienne P, *et al.* Lack of cholinergic deficit in the neocortex in Pick's disease. Prog Neuropsychopharmacol Biol Psychiatry 1983;7:725–727.

9. Yates CM, Simpson J, Maloney AFJ, Gordon A. Neurochemical observations in a case of Pick's disease. J Neurol Sci 1980;48: 257–263.

10. Gauthier S. Clinical trials and therapy. Curr Opin Neurol 1998;11: 435–438.

11. McKhann G, Drachman D, Folstein M, *et al.* Clinical diagnosis of Alzheimer's disease: report of the NINCDS–ADRDA workgroup. Neurology 1984;34:939–944.

12. Folstein MF, Folstein SE, McHugh PR. Mini Mental State: a practical method for grading the cognitive state of patients for the clinician. J Psychiatr Res 1975;12:189–198.

13. Sclan SG, Reisberg B. Functional Assessment Staging (FAST) in Alzheimer's disease: reliability, validity, and ordinality. Int Psychogeriatr 1992;4(suppl 1):55–69.

14. Barclay LL, Zemcov A, Blass JP, Sansone J. Survival in Alzheimer's disease and vascular dementia. Neurology 1985;35:834–840.

15. Rosen WG, Mohs RC, Davis KL. A new rating scale for Alzheimer's disease. Am J Psychiatry 1984;

141:1356–1364.

16. Schneider LS, Olin JT, Doody RS, *et al.* Validity and reliability of the Alzheimer's Disease Cooperative Study: clinical global impression of change. Alzheimer Dis Assoc Disord 1997;11(suppl 2):S22–S32.

17. Leber P. Guidelines for clinical evaluation of antidementia drugs. Washington, DC: US Food and Drug Administration, 1990.

18. Whitehouse P. Regulatory issues in anti-dementia drug development. In: Gauthier S, ed. Pharmacotherapy of Alzheimer's disease. London: Martin Dunitz; 1998: 57–74.

19. Summers WK, Majovski LV, Marsh GM, *et al.* Oral tetrahydroaminoacridine in long term treatment of senile dementia, Alzheimer type. N Engl J Med 1986;315:1241–1245.

20. Gauthier S, Bouchard R, Lamontagne A, *et al.* Tetrahydroaminoacridine–lecithin combination treatment in patients with intermediate-stage Alzheimer's disease. N Engl J Med 1990; 322:1272–1276.

21. Molloy DW, Guyatt GH, Wilson DB, *et al.* Effects of tetrahydroaminoacridine on cognition, function and behavior in Alzheimer's disease. Can Med Assoc J 1991;144:29–34.

22. Davis KL, Thal LJ, Gamzu ER, *et al.* A double-blind, placebo-controlled multicenter study of tacrine for Alzheimer's disease. N Engl J Med 1992;327:1253–1259.

23. Farlow M, Gracon SI, Hershey LA, *et al.* A controlled trial of tacrine in Alzheimer's disease. JAMA 1992; 268:2523–2529.

24. Knapp MJ, Knopman DS, Solomon PR, *et al.* A 30-week randomized controlled trial of high-dose tacrine in patients with Alzheimer's disease. JAMA 1994; 271:985–991.

25. Knopman D, Schneider L, Davis K, *et al.* Long-term tacrine (Cognex) treatment: effects on nursing home placement and mortality. Neurology 1996;47: 166–177.

26. Sands LP, Katz I, Schneider L. Assessing individual patients for cognitive benefits from acetylcholinesterase inhibitors. Alzheimer Dis Assoc Dis 1999;13: 26–33.

27. Qizilbash N, Whitehead A, Higgins J, *et al.* Cholinesterase inhibition for Alzheimer disease. A meta-analysis of the tacrine trials. JAMA 1998;280:1777–1782.

28. Kaufer DI, Cummings JL, Christine D. Effects of tacrine on behavioral symptoms in Alzheimer's disease: an open label study. J Geriatr Psychiatry Neurol 1996;9:1–6.

29. Raskind MA, Sadowsky CH, Sigmund WR, *et al.* Effects of tacrine on language, praxis and concognitive behavioral problems in Alzheimer's disease. Arch Neurol 1997;54:836–840.

30. Rogers SL, Friedhoff LT, the Donepezil Study Group. The efficacy and safety of donepezil in patients with Alzheimer's disease: results of a US multicenter, randomized, double-blind, placebo-controlled trial. Dementia 1996; 7:293–303.

31. Rogers SL, Doody RS, Mohs RC, *et al.* Donepezil improves cognition and global function in Alzheimer's disease. A 15-week, double-blind, placebo-controlled study. Arch Intern Med 1998; 158:1021–1031.

32. Rogers SL, Farlow MR, Doody RS, *et al.* A 24-week, double-blind, placebo-controlled trial of donepezil in patients with Alzheimer's disease. Neurology 1998;50:136–145.

33. Burns A, Rossor M, Hecker J, *et*

al. The effects of donepezil in Alzheimer's disease: results from a multinational trial. Dementia Geriatr Cogn Disord 1999; 10: 237–244.

34. Teunisse S, Derix M, van Crevel H. Assessing the severity of dementia and caregiver. Arch Neurol 1991;48:274–277.

35. Morris JC. The Clinical Dementia Rating (CDR): current version and scoring rules. Neurology 1993; 43:2412–2413.

36. Rogers SL, Friedhoff LT. Long-term efficacy and safety of donepezil in the treatment of Alzheimer's disease: an interim analysis of the results of a US multicenter open label extension study. Eur Neuropsychopharmacol 1998;8:67–75.

37. Winblad B, Engedal K, Soininen H, *et al.* Donepezil enhances global function, cognition and activities of daily living compared with placebo in a one-year, double-blind trial in patients with mild to moderate Alzheimer's disease. Ninth Congress IPA, 15–20 August 1999, Vancouver, Canada.

38. Mega MS, Masterman DM, O'Connor SM, *et al.* The spectrum of behavioral responses to cholinesterase inhibition therapy in Alzheimer's disease. Arch Neurol 1999;56:1388–1393.

39. Cummings JL, Mega M, Gray K, *et al.* The Neuropsychiatric Inventory: comprehensive assessment of psychopathology in dementia. Neurology 1994;44:2308–2314.

40. Kaufer DI, Catt K, Pollock BG, *et al.* Donepezil in Alzheimer's disease: relative cognitive and neuropsychiatric responses and impact on caregiver distress. Neurology 1998;50:A89.

41. Doody RS. Clinical profile of donepezil in the treatment of Alzheimer's disease. Gerontology 1999;45(suppl 1):23–32.

42. Anand R, Gharabawi G, Enz A. Efficacy and safety results of the early phase studies with Exelom (ENA-713) in Alzheimer's disease: an overview. J Drug Clin Pract 1996;8:1–8.

43. Corey-Bloom J, Anand R, Veach J for the ENA 713 B352 Study Group. A randomized trial evaluating the efficacy and safety of ENA 713 (rivastigmine tartrate), a new acetylcholinesterase inhibitor, in patients with mild to moderately severe Alzheimer's disease. Int J Geriatr Psychopharmacol 1998;1:55–65.

44. Rösler M, Anand R, Cicin-Sain A, *et al* on behalf of the B303 Exelon Study Group. Efficacy and safety of rivastigmine in patients with Alzheimer's disease: results of an international, 26-week, multicentre, randomised, placebo-controlled trial. BMJ 1999; 318: 633–638.

45. DeJong R, Osterlund O, Roy G. Measurement of quality-of-life changes in patients with Alzheimer's disease. Clin Ther 1989;1:545–554.

46. Schneider LS, Anand R, Farlow MR. Systematic review of the efficacy of rivastigmine for patients with Alzheimer's disease. Int J Geriatr Psychopharmacol 1998; 1(suppl 1):S26–S34.

47. Schmidt BH, Heinig R. The pharmacological basis for metrifonate's favourable tolerability in the treatment of Alzheimer's disease. Dementia Geriatr Cogn Disord 1998;9(suppl 2):15–19.

48. Cummings JL, Cyrus PA, Bieber F, *et al.* Metrifonate treatment of the cognitive deficits of Alzheimer's disease. Neurology 1998;50:1214–1221.

49. Morris JC, Cyrus PA, Orazem J, *et al.* Metrifonate benefits cognitive, behavioral and global function in patients with Alzheimer's disease. Neurology 1998;50:1222–1230.

50. Dubois B, McKeith I, Orgogozo JM, *et al.* A multicentre, randomized, double-blind, placebo-controlled study to evaluate the efficacy, tolerability and safety of two doses of metrifonate in patients with mild-to-moderate Alzheimer's disease: the MALT study. Int J Geriatr Psychiatry 1999;14:973–982.

51. Cyrus PA, Ruzicka BB, Gulanski B. The dose-related improvement by metrifonate of the cognitive performance of Alzheimer's disease patients. Neurology 1998; 50:A89.

52. Gélinas I, Gauthier S, Cyrus PA, *et al.* The efficacy of metrifonate in enhancing the ability of Alzheimer's disease patients to perform basic and instrumental activities of daily living. Neurology 1998;50:A91.

53. Cummings JL, Cyrus PA, Ruzicka BB, Gulanski B. The efficacy of metrifonate in improving the behavioral disturbances of Alzheimer's disease. Neurology 1998;50:A251.

54. Pontecorvo MJ. Clinical-development of galantamine: evaluation of a compound with possible acetylcholinesterase inhibiting and nicotine modulatory activity. Neurobiol Aging 1998;19:57.

55. Wilcock G, Wilkinson D. Galantamine hydrobromide: interim results of a group comparative, placebo-controlled study of efficacy and safety in patients with a diagnosis of senile dementia of the Alzheimer type. In: Iqbal K, Winblad B, Nishimura T, Takeda M, Wisniewski HM, eds. Alzheimer's disease: biology, diagnosis and therapeutics. Chichester, UK: John Wiley and Sons; 1997;661–664.

56. Poirier J, Delisle MC, Quirion R, *et al.* Apolipoprotein E4 allele as a predictor of cholinergic deficits and treatment outcome in Alzheimer's disease. Proc Natl Acad Sci USA 1995;92: 12260–12264.

57. Farlow MR, Lahiri DK, Poirier J, *et al.* Treatment outcome of tacrine therapy depends on apolipoprotein genotype and gender of the subjects with Alzheimer's disease. Neurology 1998;50: 669–677.

58. MacGowan SH, Wilcock GK, Scott M. Effect of gender and apolipoprotein E genotype on response to anticholinesterase therapy in Alzheimer's disease. Int J Geriatr Psychiatry 1998;13: 625–630.

59. Oddoze C, Michel BF, Bertézène P, *et al.* Apolipoprotein E epsilon 4 allele predicts a positive response to tacrine in Alzheimer's disease. Alzheimer Rep 1998;1: 13–16.

60. Farlow MR, Cyrus PA, Nadel A, *et al.* Metrifonate treatment of AD. Influence of APOE genotype. Neurology 1999;53:2010–2016.

61. Max W. Cost of illness of dementia. In: Wimo A, Jönsson B, Karlsson G, Winblad B, eds. Health economics of dementia. Chichester, UK; John Wiley and Sons; 197–206.

62. Hux MJ, O'Brien BJ, Iskedjian M, *et al.* Relation between severity of Alzheimer's disease and costs of caring. Can Med Assoc J 1998; 159:457–465.

63. Small GW, Donohue JA, Brooks RL. An economic evaluation of donepezil in the treatment of Alzheimer's disease. Clin Therapeutics 1998;20:838–850.

64. Newmann PJ, Hermann RC, Kuntz KM, *et al.* Cost-effectiveness of donepezil in the treatment of mild or moderate Alzheimer's disease. Neurology 1999;52:1138–1145.

65. Stewart A, Phillips R, Dempsey G. Pharmacotherapy for people

with Alzheimer's disease: a Markov-cycle evaluation of five years' therapy using donepezil. Int J Geriatr Psychiatry 1998; 13: 445–453.

66. O'Brien BJ, Goeree R, Hux M, *et al.* Economic evaluation of donepezil for the treatment of Alzheimer's disease in Canada. J Am Geriatr Soc 1999;47:570–578.

67. Lubeck DP, Mazonson PD, Bowe T. Potential effect of tacrine on expenditure for Alzheimer's disease. Med Interface 1994;7: 130–138.

68. Wimo A, Karlsson G, Nordberg A, Winblad B. Treatment of Alzheimer's disease with tacrine: a cost-analysis model. Alzheimer Dis Assoc Disord 1997;4:191–200.

69. Winblad B, Karlsson G, Jönsson, Wimo A. A proposed health economics research agenda for dementia. In: Wimo A, Jönsson B, Karlsson G, Winblad B, eds. Health economics of dementia. Chichester, UK; John Wiley and Sons; 4563–4565.

70. Knapp M, Wilkinson D, Wigglesworth R. The economic consequences of Alzheimer's disease in the context of new drug development. Int J Geriatr Psychiatry 1998;13:531–543.

71. Gauthier S. Managing expectations in the long-term treatment of Alzheimer's disease. Gerontology 1999;45(suppl 1):33–38.

72. Lovestone S, Graham N, Howard R. Guidelines on drug treatment for Alzheimer's disease. Lancet 1997;550:232–233.

73. Harvey RJ. A review and commentary on a sample of 15 UK guidelines for the drug treatment of Alzheimer's disease. Int J Geriatr Psychiatry 1999;14:249–256.

74. Rabins P, Blacker D, Bland W, *et al.* Practice guidelines for the treatment of patients with Alzheimer's disease and other dementias of late-life. Am J Psychiatry 1997;154(suppl):1–39.

75. Small GW, Rabins PV, Barry PP, *et al.* Diagnosis and treatment of Alzheimer's disease and related disorders. JAMA 1997;278: 1363–1371.

76. Patterson C, Gauthier S, Bergman H, *et al.* The recognition, assessment and management of dementing disorders: conclusions from the Canadian Consensus Conference on Dementia. Can Med Assoc J 1999;160(suppl 12): S1–S20.

77. Gauthier S. Do we have a treatment for Alzheimer's disease: yes. Arch Neurol 1999;56:738–739.

78. Francis PT, Palmer AM, Snape M, Wilcock GK. The cholinergic hypothesis of Alzheimer's disease: a review of progress. J Neurol Neurosurg Psychiatry 1999;66:137–147.

79. Murali Doraiswamy P, Steffens DC. Combination therapy for early Alzheimer's disease: what are we waiting for? J Am Geriatr Soc 1998;46:1322–1324.

80. Schneider LS, Farlow MR, Henderson VW, Pogoda JM. Effects of estrogen replacement therapy on response to tacrine in patients with Alzheimer's disease. Neurology 1996;46:1580–1584.

81. Relkin N, Orazem J, McRae T. The effect of concomitant donepezil and estrogen treatment on the cognitive performance of women with Alzheimer's disease. Neurology 1999;52(suppl 2): A397–A398.

82. Mayeux R, Sano M. Treatment of Alzheimer's disease. N Engl J Med 1999;341:1670–1679.

83. Mittelman MS, Ferris SH, Shulman E, Steinberg G, Levin B. A family intervention to delay nursing home placement of patients with Alzheimer's disease. JAMA 1996;276:1725–1731.

10
Hormonal therapies for Alzheimer's disease

Victor W Henderson and Bruce L Miller

Introduction

There are three major classes of hormones: peptides, amines, and steroids. Although many hormones affect brain function, this chapter is concerned only with members of the steroid class, which have been the recent focus of considerable neurological interest and which are the most immediately germane to current thought on therapy for Alzheimer's disease (AD).

Steroid hormones are synthesized from cholesterol, and all share a basic structure of three hexane rings and one pentane ring. It is convenient to divide the steroid hormones into gonadal, or sex, steroids, which are produced by reproductive tissues, and corticosteroids, which are produced by the adrenal cortex. Both naturally occurring steroids and their synthetic analogs are used in clinical practice.

Steroid hormones are small, lipophilic molecules, and in their unbound state they cross from the periphery into the central nervous system. Some steroids, such as pregnenolone, dehydroepiandrosterone and progesterone, can be synthesized within the nervous system; the term neurosteroids has been used to describe these compounds.[1] In addition, neurons that contain the enzyme aromatase[2] can form estradiol in situ from testosterone derived from peripheral sources.

Many steroid effects are dependent on interactions with high-affinity protein receptors located within the cell nucleus. Typically, the receptor–hormone complex, which may include additional regulatory proteins, binds to a region of the genome known as the hormone response element. Binding serves to regulate gene transcription and thus the formation of a specific protein product.[3] A high degree of regulatory complexity modulates the process by which the ligand–receptor complex ultimately affects transcription, which implies that there are numerous ways in which cell-specific estrogen effects are realized.

Several steroid hormones have been suggested for use in patients with AD. Among the gonadal steroids, both estrogens and androgens have been considered, with estrogens being the best studied. An androgenic precursor steroid, dehydroepiandrosterone, is also relevant to aging and AD. Finally, the glucocorticoid class of corticosteroids is of emerging interest. Preclinical and clinical data for all of the steroid hormones are incomplete, and therapeutic efficacy has yet to be convincingly demonstrated.

Estrogens

The principal natural estrogens, estradiol and estrone, are derived from cholesterol through testosterone and other androgenic intermediaries. The most important estrogen during a woman's reproductive years is estradiol, which is cyclically produced within the ovaries under the control of gonadotropins (luteinizing hormone and follicular stimulating hormone), which are released from the anterior lobe of the pituitary gland. Small quantities of estrogen also arise in peripheral target tissues from androgen precursors. After the menopause, ovarian production of estrogen ceases, although estrogens derived from peripheral conversion continue to circulate in low concentrations.

Estrogen affects the brain directly through interactions with receptors in the cell nucleus and putative receptors in the plasma membrane; other estrogen actions occur in the absence of receptors. There are two homologous nuclear receptors, referred to as α- and β-receptors. Neurons can express either of these two estrogen receptor types, and a few express both; many neurons express neither type. In the hippocampus and cerebral cortex, the β-receptor predominates.[4] There is a partial overlap in the distribution of neurons that contain estrogen receptors and those that contain receptors for androgen.[5]

Some estrogen effects on brain function (e.g. changes in ionic permeability or neurotransmitter release) occur too rapidly to require new protein synthesis. Many of these effects are attributed to estrogen interactions with receptors on the cell membrane.[6] Membrane receptors have yet to be biochemically characterized and may or may not differ from the classic intranuclear receptors.

Protective actions of estrogen are those that help maintain neuronal function in the face of injury. Some neuroprotective actions may have an impact on AD. In vitro, estrogen protects not only against oxidative stress[7] but also against other insults, including excitatory neurotoxins and ischemia.[8,9] Estrogen actions are also neurotrophic. In some neuronal systems, estrogen promotes the growth of nerve processes.[10,11] Within the hippocampus, estrogen mediates rapid changes in synaptic plasticity and enhances long-term potentiation,[12] a trans-synaptic process that is implicated in the encoding of new memories.

Estrogen has an impact on neurotransmitter systems that have been disrupted by the pathology of AD, including widely projecting neurons that use acetylcholine, noradrenaline, or serotonin.[13–16] An important pharmacological strategy in the therapy of AD is to boost levels of acetylcholine, which is involved in attention and memory.[17] Cholinergic neurons possess receptors for estrogen.[18] After experimental lesions, estrogen elevates markers of cholinergic activity[13,14] and, in oophorectomized rats, estrogen replacement prevents learning deficits induced by cholinergic (muscarinic) blockade.[19]

Estrogen levels decline dramatically after the menopause.[20] From the considerations summarized above, it is possible that postmenopausal estrogen treatment (commonly referred to as estrogen replacement therapy) could preserve or enhance neuronal function in women. Several studies suggest that estrogen therapy can reduce anxiety, improve mood and enhance subjective well-being,[21–23] but consequences of estrogen on cognition are controversial. One study suggested a positive correlation between levels of bioavailable estradiol and verbal memory scores but a negative correlation with spatial skills.[24] More generally, however, there appears to be little relationship between estrogen concentrations and the preservation of cognitive skills during normal aging, at least in the range of low values of serum estrogen that are found in postmenopausal women.[25] In larger observational studies, estrogen users are reported both to perform better than[26] or similarly to[27,28] non-users on cognitive tasks. Results of small, randomized, controlled clinical trials of healthy older women are also inconclusive. Some studies indicate an advantage for treated women on tasks designed to assess verbal memory or other cognitive skills,[29] but the absence of an estrogen effect is also reported.[30]

The hypothesis that estrogen therapy might benefit cognitive function in AD is supported by epidemiological evidence of an association between estrogen usage after the menopause and a lower risk of developing AD. Not all studies are positive,[31] but most recent case–control and cohort studies imply that estrogen use reduces the risk of developing AD by about one-half.[32–36]

In observational analyses of women with AD, estrogen use is associated with milder cognitive symptoms.[37,38] Results of small randomized clinical trials are less encouraging. In an early pilot study, 14 women with AD were given conjugated equine estrogens (1.25 mg/day) or placebo.[39] After 3 weeks, women in the active treatment arm improved significantly on each of three outcome measures: Mini Mental State Examination (from a score of 18 to a score of 22), a revised version of the Hasegawa Dementia Scale (from 17 to 21) and a screening test for dementia developed by the Japanese National Institute of Mental Health (from 12 to 14). The scores of women in the placebo group were essentially unchanged. A second pilot study assigned 12 women with dementia to either transdermal estradiol (50 μg/day) or placebo for 8 weeks.[40] Treated women improved significantly on a measure of verbal memory (assessed by delayed cued recall on a selective reminding task) and attention (assessed by the number of self-corrections in the interference condition of the Stroop color naming test). However, groups performed similarly on different measures of verbal memory and attention and on other aspects of cognition. Among estrogen-treated subjects, there was a significant correlation between delayed cued recall scores and serum estradiol levels. Most recently, a randomized, placebo-controlled trial involving 42 women with AD treated with either conjugated equine estrogens (1.25 mg/day) or oral placebo was conducted. After 16 weeks, there was no significant effect of treatment on measures of cognition (a difference favoring the placebo group of 1.3 points on the Alzheimer's Disease Assessment Scale cognitive subscale), global change, or functional status.[41]

Animal studies indicate that estrogen interacts with cholinergic neurotransmitter systems. An analysis of post hoc/data from a multicenter randomized controlled trial of a cholinomimetic drug (tacrine) revealed that a small proportion of women were receiving estrogen therapy at the time of initial randomization into active (tacrine) or placebo arms. After 30 weeks, estrogen users who were receiving active treatment performed significantly better on the primary cognitive outcome measure than women in the placebo group (a difference of about 6 points on the Alzheimer's Disease Assessment Scale cognitive subscale); for women who had been randomized to receive the active drug but who were not receiving estrogen, drug–placebo differences were smaller (about 2 points) and not statistically significant.[42] Findings imply that estrogen may interact with cholinergic systems to improve cognitive symptoms of women with Alzheimer's disease. However, estrogen use was not randomized in this study, and ongoing randomized controlled trials are now considering this important possibility in a prospective manner.

Androgens

The two major human androgens are testosterone and its metabolite dihydrotestosterone. Testosterone is converted to the more potent dihydrotestosterone by the enzyme 5α-reductase. Weaker androgens (e.g. dehydroepiandrosterone) are also present. In men, most testosterone is produced by the testes. Smaller quantities are made in the adrenal glands of both sexes and in the ovaries of women. Levels of circulating androgens are higher in men than women, but these compounds have important roles in both sexes. Androgens have protean functions and influence multiple target organs, including reproductive tissues, bone, muscle, blood, the cardiovascular system, adipose tissue and the brain. In the testes, androgens have an antiapoptotic effect, and some therapeutic and toxic effects of these steroids relate to their ability to stimulate cellular growth.[43] Compared with estrogens, clinical effects of androgens have been less well investigated, and research into central nervous system effects is in its infancy.

As with estrogen, systemic testosterone concentrations are modulated through the hypothalamic–pituitary axis. Gonadotropin-releasing hormone produced by the hypothalamus stimulates the release of luteinizing hormone from the pituitary gland, which in turn boosts testosterone production by the Leydig cells of the testes. In the blood, most testosterone is bound to sex-hormone-binding globulin and albumin. Release of luteinizing hormone is regulated through feedback inhibition by bioavailable testosterone. In healthy adult males, testosterone secretion shows a circadian pattern, with greatest levels occurring in the morning. With aging, diurnal fluctuations can disappear.

In rats, certain brain structures, including the hippocampus, are sexually dimorphic. Mammalian sex differences appear to be determined by early androgen exposures. For example, in comparison with normal prepubescent female rats, the granule cell layer of the dentate gyrus is larger in prepubescent male rats as well as in female rats that were exposed to testosterone in utero.[44] In male meadow voles, the role of androgens is suggested by a positive association between hippocampal volume and plasma testosterone levels.[45]

An understanding of the role of androgens in the brain is complicated by the fact that some actions of testosterone require aromatization of testosterone to estradiol. For example, hippocampal function of songbirds appears to be modulated by both androgens and estrogen.[46] However, the enzyme 5α-reductase is expressed in specific brain regions, including the hippocampus and the hypothalamus,[47] suggesting that androgen effects in these regions require conversion of testosterone to dihydrotestosterone and that the effects are therefore independent of estrogen.

An emerging literature documents direct and indirect effects of androgens on brain regions that are involved with memory, mood and cognition.[16] In female rats, estradiol increases the expression of genes that code for the 5-hydroxytryptamine (5-HT$_{2A}$) receptor and the serotonin transporter. These actions occur in the dorsal raphe nucleus of the brainstem and in regions of the forebrain that are involved with mood and cognition. Testosterone, but not dihydrotestosterone, also increases 5-HT$_{2A}$ receptor levels, implying that this particular effect of testosterone is mediated via aromatization to estradiol. Estrogen and testosterone (through its conversion to estrogen) also stimulate the expression of the arginine vasopressin gene in the bed nucleus of the stria terminalis. Olfactory memory requires intact function in this area, a finding that suggests a potential mechanism by which androgens can affect aspects of cognition.[16]

Additionally, a rich literature comparing cognitive performances of men with that of women implies a likely role for sex hormones in cognition in humans, in addition to gender-associated environmental influences.[48] For example, men tend to show better abilities in the area of spatial cognition whereas women tend to perform better on verbal tasks. The anatomical and physiological substrates for these differences are obscure, and it is unknown whether suspected responsible actions of implicated sex steroids occur in the perinatal period or in later developmental stages. It is important to note that there is no direct relationship between testosterone levels and spatial cognition in men. In one study of older men, testosterone supplementation improved spatial cognition, but this cognitive change may have been mediated by a reduction in the endogenous production of estradiol.[49]

Studies of patients with sex chromosome abnormalities imply that sex hormones alone do not fully account for sex differences in cognitive skills. Women with Turner's syndrome, a genetic disorder characterized by a single X chromosome, maintain low estrogen levels yet show relative strengths on verbal tasks. Paradoxically, hypogonadal males with Klinefelter's syndrome, which is characterized by an extra X chromosome, show verbal deficits but relative strength on visual tasks.[50]

The term 'andropause' has been used to describe symptoms that develop in elderly males as testosterone levels drop from the peak levels achieved during the third decade of life. The rate of decline is approximately 100 ng/dl per decade, with levels below 300 ng/dl sometimes taken as pathological. Using these criteria, a sizeable percentage of elderly men becomes hypogonadal during the aging process.[51] Some authors even speculate that androgen deficiency in women can contribute to loss of energy and to depression.[52]

Although it is not possible to draw a direct relation between androgen levels and psychological or cognitive symptoms in the elderly, there is a strong interest in determining whether replacing testosterone in men will reverse some of the stigmata of aging. Target areas include loss of muscle and bone mass, diminished libido, fatigue, depressed mood and memory deficits. Low serum levels of free testosterone are associated with diminished bone mineral density,[53] and androgen therapy may be protective. Additionally, administration of androgens to hypogonadal men tends to increase libido and mood.[54] However, few studies have yet demonstrated that androgens are safe and effective in the elderly. Potential side effects include increased incidence of prostate cancer, worsening of sleep apnea and increased serum viscosity.[55] Another potential concern is that androgens might precipitate untoward neuropsychiatric symptoms. In a short-term study of 20 younger male volunteers who were given a high dose of androgen, rating scores showed euphoria, increased energy and sexual arousal, but also irritability, mood swings, violent feelings, hostility, distractibility, forgetfulness and confusion.[56] Mania or hypomania developed in two (10%) subjects.

Finally, a small emerging literature suggests that testosterone might benefit the aging brain. In a large aging cohort, it was observed that men with higher serum levels of bioavailable testosterone had better scores on two psychometric measures (the Blessed Information–Memory–Concentration Test and long-term memory storage on the Buschke Selective Reminding Test). In general, low estradiol and high testosterone levels predicted better cognitive performance. Associations were both linear and non-linear, suggesting that an optimal level of sex hormones may exist for some cognitive functions.[57] In a randomized double-blind clinical trial that involved healthy older men, testosterone supplementation for 3 months resulted in significant enhancement of spatial cognition but had no effect on other cognitive measures.[49] Clinical studies of patients with AD remain anecdotal, although large randomized clinical trials are currently being conducted. However, hard data either supporting or refuting the use of androgens in AD are lacking, and much work is needed to determine whether androgen therapy will enhance quality of life, improve memory or protect the brain from the ravages of this illness.

Dehydroepiandrosterone and dehydroepiandrosterone sulfate

Dehydroepiandrosterone (DHEA), which is secreted primarily by the adrenal cortex, is an intermediary in the synthesis of androgens and estrogens. DHEA is in reversible equilibrium with its sulfate ester metabolite dehydroepiandrosterone sulfate (DHEA-S), which is the most abundant circulating steroid. Because DHEA-S circulates in much higher concentrations than DHEA, and because these two compounds are in reversible equilibrium with each other, measures of serum DHEA-S are commonly taken to reflect peripheral activity of both steroids.

DHEA is lipophilic and readily crosses the blood–brain barrier. There is a high correlation between cerebrospinal fluid and blood concentrations of DHEA and DHEA-S.[58] In addition to their peripheral formation, DHEA and DHEA-S have been isolated from the brain and are presumed to be manufactured in situ as neurosteroids.[1]

DHEA has weak androgenic properties. It is also a precursor to both androgens and estrogens, and in postmenopausal women very high oral doses of DHEA will increase circulating concentrations of these sex steroids.[59] Cross-sectional studies show dramatic, progressive declines in serum and spinal fluid concentrations of DHEA and DHEA-S throughout the entire adult life span.[58,60] Although the precise functions of these compounds are unknown, a variety of health benefits are ascribed to DHEA and DHEA-S, including enhancement of the immune system, cardiovascular protection and protection against cancer.

Neuronal survival in vitro is enhanced in the presence of DHEA or DHEA-S,[61] and administration of DHEA-S to aging mice is reported to improve memory retention.[62] In a large, elderly, population-based French cohort, higher DHEA-S concentrations were associated with maintenance of functional status.[63] No association between baseline DHEA-S levels and cognitive performance one and a half decades later was observed in a US retirement community cohort,[64] but a weak association between higher DHEA-S concentrations and maintenance of cognitive performance 2 years later was reported in a population-based Dutch cohort.[65] In a placebo-controlled, cross-over trial of DHEA (50 mg/day), healthy subjects reported an increase in well-being after 12 weeks of active drug.[66] However, a shorter but otherwise similar cross-over study in older men and women found no effect of the same DHEA dose on measures of well-being, mood, or cognitive performance.[67]

It is controversial whether plasma concentrations of DHEA-S are altered in AD or other forms of dementia. Lower concentrations are reported by some investigators[68,69] but not by others.[63,70,71] One study found no association between serum levels of DHEA-S and the duration of dementia symptoms or the extent of cognitive impairment among patients with AD.[70] No formal interventional trials have been reported for the use of DHEA in patients with AD.

Glucocorticoids

A variety of steroids are synthesized within the cortex of the adrenal glands. Corticosteroids include mineralocorticoids, which are produced in the outer portion of the adrenal cortex, and glucocorticoids, which, together with certain androgens such as dehydroepiandrosterone, are produced in the inner portion of the adrenal cortex. Glucocorticoids in particular are regulated by adrenocorticotrophic hormone, which is secreted by the anterior lobe of the pituitary gland, and corticotrophin releasing hormone, which is secreted by the hypothalamus. In humans, the principal glucocorticoid is cortisol. Glucocorticoid receptors, as well as mineralocorticoid receptors, are found within the hippocampus and other regions of the brain.

Glucocorticoids mediate the stress response and are potent immuno-suppressive and anti-inflammatory agents. It is hypothesized that inflammation may contribute to pathogenesis of AD.[72] Neuritic plaques in the brains of patients who have AD show evidence of activation of the classical complement pathway, inflammatory cytokines and acute-phase reactants, as well as activated microglial cells and astrocytes. A small co-twin study suggested a link between the use of corticosteroids or adrenocorticotrophic hormone and a reduced risk of AD,[73] and several epidemiological studies have shown associations between use of non-steroidal anti-inflammatory agents and lower risk.[74]

Little direct evidence indicates that glucocorticoids improve the symptoms of AD or slow progression of the disease, although a pilot study suggested that non-steroidal anti-inflammatory drugs might ameliorate the symptoms.[75] Glucocorticoids are associated with considerable systemic toxicity. In addition, prolonged exposure to endogenous glucocorticoids may actually impair cognitive function[76] or damage hippocampal neurons.[77] A 1-year multicenter study of prednisone (20 mg/day for 1 month followed by 10 mg/day for 11 months) in AD showed no cognitive benefit of steroid therapy (a non-significant difference of two points on the cognitive subscale of the Alzheimer's Disease Assessment Scale favored the placebo group.[78]

Summary and conclusion

Steroid hormones are of special interest for the treatment of dementia caused by AD. The brain has receptors both for gonadal steroids and for adrenal steroids, and these compounds affect brain function. Epidemiological studies suggest that postmenopausal estrogen therapy may help protect women against AD. Clinical trials in women with dementia, however, indicate that estrogen monotherapy is unlikely to improve the symptoms of AD substantially. Clinical trials of androgen for men with Alzheimer's disease are underway, but the results are not yet known. Serum levels of the weak androgen dehydroepiandrosterone decrease considerably during aging, but few clinical data suggest that treatment with this steroid improves the symptoms of AD. Finally, glucocorticoids have potent anti-inflammation properties, and inflammation may contribute to the pathological changes of AD. Clinical trial experience with glucocorticoids, however, fails to demonstrate a beneficial effect. In summary, although various steroid hormones hold theoretical promise for AD, available data do not justify their use in the treatment of dementia symptoms in this disorder.

References

1. Baulieu EE. Neurosteroids: of the nervous system, by the nervous system, for the nervous system. Recent Prog Horm Res 1997; 52:1–32.

2. Naftolin F, Horvath TL, Jakab RL, Leranth C, Harada N, Balhazart J. Aromatase immunoreactivity in axon terminals of the vertebrate brain. Neuroendocrinology 1996; 63:149–155.

3. Evans RM. The steroid and thyroid hormone receptor superfamily. Science 1988;249:889–895.

4. Shughrue PJ. Estrogen action in the estrogen receptor α-knockout mouse: is this due to ER-β? Mol Psychiatry 1998;3:299–302.

5. Wood RI, Newman SW. Androgen and estrogen receptors coexist within individual neurons in the brain of the Syrian hamster. Neuroendocrinology 1995;62:487–497.

6. Wong M, Thompson TL, Moss RL.

Nongenomic actions of estrogen in the brain: physiological significance and cellular mechanisms. Crit Rev Neurobiol 1996;10: 189–203.

7. Mooradian AD. Antioxidant properties of steroids. J Steroid Biochem Mol Biol 1993;45: 509–511.

8. Singer CA, Rogers KL, Strickland TM, Dorsa DM. Estrogen protects primary cortical neurons from glutamate toxicity. Neurosci Lett 1996;212:13–16.

9. Simpkins JW, Rajakumar G, Zhang YQ, et al. Estrogens may reduce mortality and ischemic damage caused by middle cerebral artery occlusion in the female rat. J Neurosurg 1997;87: 724–730.

10. Brinton RD, Tran J, Proffitt P, Montoya M. 17β-estradiol enhances the outgrowth and survival of neocortical neurons in culture. Neurochem Res 1997;22:1339–1351.

11. Shughrue PJ, Dorsa DM. Estrogen modulates the growth-associated protein GAP-43 (neuromodulin) mRNA in the rat preoptic area and basal hypothalamus. Neuroendocrinology 1993;57:439–447.

12. Foy MR, Henderson VW, Berger TW, Thompson RF. Estrogen and neural plasticity. Curr Dir Psychol Sci; in press.

13. Luine V. Estradiol increases choline acetyltransferase activity in specific basal forebrain nuclei and projection areas of female rats. Exp Neurol 1985;89: 484–490.

14. Gibbs RB, Pfaff DW. Effects of estrogen and fimbria/fornix transection on p75[NGFR] and ChAT expression in the medial septum and diagonal band of Broca. Exp Neurol 1992;116:23–39.

15. Sar M, Stumpf WE. Central noradrenergic neurones concentrate ^{3}H-oestradiol. Nature 1981;289: 500–502.

16. Fink G, Sumner BEH, McQueen JK, Wilson H, Rosie R. Sex steroid control of mood, mental state and memory. Clin Exp Pharmacol Physiol 1998;25:764–775.

17. Bartus RT, Dean RL, Beer B, Lippa AD. The cholinergic hypothesis of geriatric memory dysfunction. Science 1981; 217: 208–217.

18. Toran-Allerand CD, Miranda RC, Bentham WDL, et al. Estrogen receptors colocalize with low-affinity nerve growth factor receptors in cholinergic neurons of the basal forebrain. Proc Natl Acad Sci U S A 1992;89:4668–4672.

19. Fader AJ, Hendricson AW, Dohanich GP. Estrogen improves performance of reinforced T-maze alternation and prevents the amnestic effects of scopolamine administered systemically or intrahippocampally. Neurobiol Learn Memory 1998;69:225–240.

20. Trévoux R, De Brux J, Castanier M, Nahoul K, Soule JP, Scholler R. Endometrium and plasma hormone profile in the perimenopause and postmenopause. Maturitas 1986;8:309–326.

21. Fedor-Freybergh P. The influence of oestrogens on the wellbeing and mental performance in climacteric and postmenopausal women. Acta Obstet Gynecol Scand Suppl 1977;64:1–91.

22. Sherwin BB, Gelfand MM. Sex steroids and affect in the surgical menopause: a double-blind cross-over study. Psychoneuroendocrinology 1985;10:325–335.

23. Ditkoff EC, Crary WG, Cristo M, Lobo RA. Estrogen improves psychological function in asymptomatic postmenopausal women. Obstet Gynecol 1991;78:991–995.

24. Drake EB, Henderson VW, Stanczyk FZ, et al. Associations between circulating sex steroid hormones and cognition in normal

elderly women. Neurology 2000; 54:599–603.

25. Yaffe K, Grady D, Pressman A, Cummings S. Serum estrogen levels, cognitive performance, and risk of cognitive decline in older community women. J Am Geriatr Soc 1998;46:816–821.

26. Schmidt R, Fazekas F, Reinhart B, *et al.* Estrogen replacement therapy in older women: a neuropsychological and brain MRI study. J Am Geriatr Soc 1996;44: 1307–1313.

27. Szklo M, Cerhan J, Diez-Roux AV, *et al.* Estrogen replacement therapy and cognitive functioning in the Atherosclerosis Risk in Communities (ARIC) study. Am J Epidemiol 1996;144:1048–1057.

28. Barrett-Connor E, Kritz-Silverstein D. Estrogen replacement therapy and cognitive function in older women. JAMA 1993;269: 2637–2641.

29. Phillips SM, Sherwin BB. Effects of estrogen on memory function in surgically menopausal women. Psychoneuroendocrinology 1992; 17:485–495.

30. Polo-Kantola P, Portin R, Polo O, Helenius H, Irjala K, Erkkola R. The effect of short-term estrogen replacement therapy on cognition: a randomized, double-blind, cross-over trial in postmenopausal women. Obstet Gynecol 1998;91:459–466.

31. Brenner DE, Kukull WA, Stergachis A, *et al.* Postmenopausal estrogen replacement therapy and the risk of Alzheimer's disease: a population-based case-control study. Am J Epidemiol 1994;140:262–267.

32. Henderson VW, Paganini-Hill A, Emanuel CK, Dunn ME, Buckwalter JG. Estrogen replacement therapy in older women: comparisons between Alzheimer's disease cases and nondemented control subjects. Arch Neurol 1994;51:896–900.

33. Paganini-Hill A, Henderson VW. Estrogen replacement therapy and risk of Alzheimer's disease. Arch Intern Med 1996;156: 2213–2217.

34. Tang MX, Jacobs D, Stern Y, *et al.* Effect of oestrogen during menopause on risk and age at onset of Alzheimer's disease. Lancet 1996;348:429–432.

35. Kawas C, Resnick S, Morrison A, *et al.* A prospective study of estrogen replacement therapy and the risk of developing Alzheimer's disease: the Baltimore Longitudinal Study of Aging. Neurology 1997;48:1517–1521.

36. Waring SC, Rocca WA, Petersen RC, O'Brien PC, Tangalos EG, Kokmen E. Postmenopausal estrogen replacement therapy and risk of AD: a population-based study. Neurology 1999;52: 965–970.

37. Henderson VW, Watt L, Buckwalter JG. Cognitive skills associated with estrogen replacement in women with Alzheimer's disease. Psychoneuroendocrinology 1996;21:421–430.

38. Doraiswamy PM, Bieber F, Kaiser L, Krishnan KR, Reuning-Scherer J, Gulanski B. The Alzheimer's disease assessment scale: patterns and predictors of baseline cognitive performance in multicenter Alzheimer's disease trials. Neurology 1997;48:1511–1517.

39. Honjo H, Ogino Y, Tanaka K, *et al.* An effect of conjugated estrogen to cognitive impairment in women with senile dementia—Alzheimer's type: a placebo-controlled double blind study. J Jpn Menopause Soc 1993;1:167–171.

40. Asthana S, Craft S, Baker LD, *et al.* Cognitive and neuroendocrine response to transdermal estrogen in postmenopausal women with

Alzheimer's disease: results of a placebo-controlled, double-blind, pilot study. Psychoneuroendocrinology 1999;24:657–677.

41. Henderson VW, Paganini-Hill A, Miller BL, *et al.* Estrogen for Alzheimer's disease in women: randomized, double-blind, placebo-controlled trial. Neurology 2000;54:295–301.

42. Schneider LS, Farlow MR, Henderson VW, Pogoda JM. Effects of estrogen replacement therapy on response to tacrine in patients with Alzheimer's disease. Neurology 1996;46:1580–1584.

43. Sinha Hakim AP, Swerdloff RS. Hormonal and genetic control of germ cell apoptosis in the testis. Rev Reprod 1999;4:38–47.

44. Roof RL. The dentate gyrus is sexually dimorphic in prepubescent rats: testosterone plays a significant role. Brain Res 1999;610:148–151.

45. Galea LAM, Perrot-Sinal TS, Kavaliers M, Ossenkopp KP. Relations of hippocampal volume and dentate gyrus width to gonadal hormone levels in male and female meadow voles. Brain Res 1999;821:383–391.

46. Saldanha CJ, Clayton NS, Schlinger BA. Androgen metabolism in the juvenile oscine forebrain: a cross-species analysis at neural sites implicated in memory function. J Neurobiol 1999; 40: 397–406.

47. Poletti A, Martini L. Androgen-activating enzymes in the central nervous system. J Steroid Biochem Mol Biol 1999;69: 117–122.

48. Halpern DF. Sex differences in cognitive abilities. Hillsdale, New Jersey, USA: Lawrence Erlbaum; 1992.

49. Janowsky JS, Oviatt SK, Orwoll ES. Testosterone influences spatial cognition in older men. Behav Neurosci 1994;108:325–332.

50. Geschwind DH, Boone KB, Miller BL, Swerdloff RS. The neurobehavioral phenotype of Klinefelter's syndrome. Ment Retard Dev Dis; in press.

51. Tenover JL. Testosterone replacement therapy in older adult men. Int J Androl 1999;22:300–306.

52. Sands R, Studd J. Exogenous androgens in postmenopausal women. Am J Med 1995; 98(suppl 1A):76S-79S.

53. Center JR, Nguyen TV, Sambrook PN, Eisman JA. Hormonal and biochemical parameters in the determination of osteoporosis in elderly men. J Clin Endocrinol Metab 1999;84:3626–3635.

54. Anderson RA, Martin CW, Kung AWC, *et al.* 7α-methyl-19-nortestosterone maintains sexual behavior and mood in hypogonadal men. J Clin Endocrinol Metab 1999;84:3556–3562.

55. Basaria S, Dobs AS. Risks versus benefits of testosterone therapy in elderly men. Drugs Aging 1999;15:131–142.

56. Su TP, Pagliaro M, Schmidt PJ, Pickar D, Wolkowitz O, Rubinow DR. Neuropsychiatric effects of anabolic steroids in male normal volunteers. JAMA 1993;269: 2760–2764.

57. Barrett-Connor E, Goodman-Gruen D, Patay B. Endogenous sex hormones and cognitive function in older men. J Clin Endocrinol Metab 1999;84: 3681–3685.

58. Guazzo EP, Kirkpatrick PJ, Goodyer IM, Shiers HM, Herbert J. Cortisol, dehydroepiandrosterone (DHEA), and DHEA sulfate in the cerebrospinal fluid of man: relation to blood levels and the effects of age. J Clin Endocrinol Metab 1996;81:3951–3960.

59. Mortola JF, Yen SSC. The effects of oral dehydroepiandrosterone on endocrine–metabolic parame-

ters in postmenopausal women. J Clin Endocrinol Metab 1990;71: 696–704.

60. Orentreich N, Brind JL, Rizer RL, Vogelman JH. Age changes and sex differences in serum dehydroepiandrosterone sulfate concentrations throughout adulthood. J Clin Endocrinol Metab 1984; 59:551–555.

61. Bologa L, Sharma J, Roberts E. Dehydroepiandrosterone and its sulfated derivative reduce neuronal death and enhance astrocytic differentiation in brain cell cultures. J Neurosci Res 1987;17: 225–234.

62. Flood JF, Roberts E. Dehydroepiandrosterone sulfate improves memory in aging mice. Brain Res 1988;448:178–181.

63. Berr C, Lafont S, Debuire B, Dartigues JF, Baulieu EE. Relationships of dehydroepiandrosterone sulfate in the elderly with functional, psychological, and mental status, and short-term mortality: a French community-based study. Proc Natl Acad Sci USA 1996;93:13410–13415.

64. Barrett-Connor E, Edelstein SL. A prospective study of dehydroepiandrosterone sulfate and cognitive function in an older population: the Rancho Bernardo study. J Am Geriatr Soc 1994; 42:420–423.

65. Kalmijn S, Launer LJ, Stolk RP, et al. A prospective study on cortisol, dehydroepiandrosterone sulfate, and cognitive function in the elderly. J Clin Endocrinol Metab 1998;83:3487–3492.

66. Morales AJ, Nolan JJ, Nelson JC, Yen SSC. Effects of replacement dose of dehydroepiandrosterone in men and women of advancing age. J Clin Endocrinol Metab 1994;78:1360–1367.

67. Wolf OT, Neumann O, Hellhammer DH, et al. Effects of a two-week physiological dehydroepiandrosterone substitution on cognitive performance and well-being in healthy elderly women and men. J Clin Endocrinol Metab 1997;82:2363–2367.

68. Näsman B, Olsson T, Bäckström T, et al. Serum dehydroepiandrosterone sulfate in Alzheimer's disease and in multi-infarct dementia. Biol Psychiatry 1991; 30:684–690.

69. Yanase T, Fukahori M, Taniguchi S, et al. Serum dehydroepiandrosterone (DHEA) and DHEA-sulfate (DHEA-S) in Alzheimer's disease and in cerebrovascular dementia. Endocr J 1996;43:119–123.

70. Schneider LS, Hinsey M, Lyness S. Plasma dehydroepiandrosterone sulfate in Alzheimer's disease. Biol Psychiatry 1992;31: 205–208.

71. Legrain S, Berr C, Frenoy N, Gourlet V, Debuire B, Baulieu EE. Dehydroepiandrosterone sulfate in a long-term care aged population. Gerontology 1995;41: 343–351.

72. McGeer PL, McGeer EG. The inflammatory response system of brain: implications for therapy of Alzheimer and other neurodegenerative diseases. Brain Res Rev 1995;21:195–218.

73. Breitner JCS, Gau BA, Welsh KA, et al. Inverse association of anti-inflammatory treatment in Alzheimer's disease: initial results of a co-twin control study. Neurology 1994;44:227–232.

74. McGeer PL, Schulzer M, McGeer EG. Arthritis and anti-inflammatory agents as possible protective factors for Alzheimer's disease: a review of 17 epidemiologic studies. Neurology 1996;47:425–432.

75. Rogers J, Kirby LC, Hempelman SR, et al. Clinical trial of indomethacin in Alzheimer's disease. Neurology 1993;43: 1609–1611.

76. Lupien S, Lecours AR, Lussier I, Schwartz G, Nair NPV, Meaney MJ. Basal cortisol levels and cognitive deficits in human aging. J Neurosci 1994;14:2893–2903.

77. McEwen BS, Sapolsky RM. Stress and cognitive function. Curr Opin Neurobiol 1995;5:205–216.

78. Aisen PS, Davis KL, Berg JD, *et al.* A randomized controlled trial of prednisone in Alzheimer's disease. Neurology 2000;54:588–593.

11
Anti-inflammatory therapy for Alzheimer's disease

Paul S Aisen

Inflammation and Alzheimer's disease

Alzheimer's disease (AD) is a chronic, indolent, progressive neurodegenerative disorder. It is a disease of brain tissue without notable systemic features, particularly in the early phase of the disease. Insoluble proteinaceous material is deposited extracellularly (amyloid plaques) and intraneuronally (neurofibrillary tangles). There is a loss of synapses and neurotransmitters associated with these neuropathologic abnormalities, with resultant progressive cognitive deficits. From a clinical perspective, AD does not seem to be an inflammatory disorder. The cardinal features of inflammation – warmth, redness and pain – are not evident. The disease is not episodic, as is often the case in idiopathic inflammatory or autoimmune diseases such as rheumatoid arthritis, systemic lupus erythematosus and multiple sclerosis.

Nonetheless, it is absolutely clear that, although gross clinical evidence of inflammation may be lacking, inflammatory mediators participate at the cellular and molecular level in the pathophysiologic processes involved in AD. Much attention is now being directed to critical questions that arise:

- Do inflammatory processes represent a reaction to neurodegenerative events or do they play a more central, causative role?
- Which, if any, inflammatory processes contribute to neuronal dysfunction?
- Do some inflammatory mediators perform a neuroprotective role?

Inflammatory diseases such as rheumatoid arthritis can be effectively treated with anti-inflammatory and immunomodulatory drugs. Such therapy not only relieves symptoms and reduces clinical evidence of inflammation, it can also protect tissue from damage caused by inflammatory processes. In rheumatoid arthritis, a number of treatments have been proved to protect cartilage and bone from erosive damage and thus preserve joint function. If similar inflammatory mediators contribute to brain tissue damage in AD, the question arises whether anti-inflammatory or immunomodulatory treatment could preserve brain function.

Ultimately, the most important question is whether anti-inflammatory therapy can prevent the disease, reduce its incidence or slow its progression.

Inflammatory mediators in AD

Peripheral acute phase response in AD

The primary tools used to assess the activity and response to treatment of inflammatory disorders involve clinical assessment of inflammation. In AD, there are no clinical markers – there is no fever, erythema, pain or swelling. However, other tools to assess disease activity are available. In the practice of rheumatology, clinical assessment of inflammation is supplemented by laboratory markers of inflammation, notably the acute-phase response.

The acute-phase response represents a measurable systemic response to infection or inflammation.[1] Principally, this involves elevations of certain serum proteins, the acute-phase reactants. Among these are fibrinogen, C-reactive protein, serum amyloid A protein (SAA) and haptoglobin; elevation of each of these proteins results from increased hepatic synthesis. This increased synthesis is generally mediated by acute inflammatory cytokines, such as interleukin (IL)-1, IL-6 and tumor necrosis factor (TNF)-α, which are secreted mainly by activated mononuclear inflammatory cells. The oldest, simplest and most widely used measure of systemic inflammation, the erythrocyte sedimentation rate, reflects the increased aggregation and sedimentation of red blood cells in the presence of excess asymmetrical acute-phase proteins, particularly fibrinogen.

It is thought that the acute-phase response contributes to the host defense against infection, but in some cases in can be harmful. For example, the chronic elevation of SAA that accompanies inflammatory diseases such as rheumatoid arthritis can result in harmful tissue deposition in the form of secondary amyloidosis.

Consideration of the acute-phase response in AD may be important for at least two reasons:

- measurement of acute-phase proteins may provide a biomarker of harmful brain inflammation, a useful tool in the development of anti-inflammatory treatment strategies; and
- the acute-phase response may have pathophysiological importance and contribute to neuronal damage.

Acute-phase proteins include protease inhibitors that may contribute to abnormal processing of the amyloid precursor protein in AD. These proteins are also components of amyloid plaques, and just as SAA elevation complicating rheumatoid arthritis can lead to amyloid deposition in the kidney, the acute-phase response may contribute to amyloid deposition in the AD brain. It should be noted that amyloid precursor protein (APP), the source of amyloidogenic material in AD brain, and SAA are distinct proteins. Both may be considered to be acute-phase proteins regulated by inflammatory cytokines, and both may be important in amyloid deposition. But the deposits of secondary amyloidosis, which are related to SAA metabolism and deposition, are biochemically distinct from the deposits of APP-derived amyloid β peptide (Aβ) in the AD brain.

A number of laboratories have studied acute-phase proteins in AD. As discussed below, there is an acute-phase response in the AD brain, with upregulation and deposition of α1-antichymotrypsin, α2-macroglobulin and C-reactive protein. This inflammatory brain activity may be reflected by changes in blood levels of these acute-phase reactants. Studies of blood levels of acute-phase proteins in AD have yielded conflicting results. Several groups have reported elevations of α1-antichymotrypsin in blood in AD patients compared with age-matched controls,[2–6] but others have reported negative results.[7–9] Presumably, differences in patient selection, number of subjects and assay methodology explain the inconsistent findings.

There has been some hope that measurement of blood levels of acute-phase proteins, particularly α1-antichymotrypsin, would provide a method of titrating anti-inflammatory treatment. This has been included in pilot studies of glucocorticoids for AD,[10] but there has been no proof of the validity of this approach. Blood and cerebrospinal fluid measurement of cytokines have not yielded consistent findings.

Cerebral acute-phase response in AD

The primary constituent of the amyloid plaque, the major neuropathologic feature of AD, is Aβ, which is derived from APP. However, other proteins have been detected in these plaques, including the acute-phase proteins α1-antichymotrypsin[11,12] α2-macroglobulin[13–15] and C-reactive protein.[16] Presumably, acute-phase proteins are expressed in the AD brain in response to the inflammatory cytokines IL-1 and IL-6, which are also induced.[13,17] It has been suggested that IL-1 is a key element in a destructive inflammatory cycle that involves microglia, astrocytes and neurons, in which IL-1 promotes neuronal amyloid peptide generation and the activation of astrocytes to release neurotoxins such as S100-β; neuronal stress activates microglia to release more IL-1, continuing the cycle.[18] The association among IL-1-positive microglia, S100-β positive astrocytes and degenerating neurons supports this theory.[19]

Rodent studies support the theory that a cerebral acute-phase response may contribute to neurodegeneration in AD. Chronic neuroinflammation stimulated by intraventricular lipopolysaccharide infusion induces activation of microglia and astrocytes, upregulation of IL-1, TNF-α and APP, causing hippocampal neurodegeneration with cognitive impairment. Administration of non-steroidal anti-inflammatory drugs attenuates these responses.[20]

Transforming growth factor (TGF)-β is another cytokine that may be involved in the pathogenesis of AD; TGF-β is upregulated in the AD brain, and can increase the deposition of Aβ fibrils in hippocampal slice cultures.[21] However, these cytokines may also have a beneficial role. In certain conditions, TNF-α and TGF-β can have neuroprotective effects, reducing excitotoxic and oxidative damage to neurons.[22] Thus, it is not absolutely clear whether suppression of inflammatory cytokines and the cerebral acute phase response will be useful in the treatment of AD.

The complement system in the AD brain

The complement system includes a group of 14 plasma proteins, plus additional regulatory proteins, which represent an important component of the inflammatory response. The complement system can be activated by binding of the first component to immune complexes or by exposure of the third component to repeating polysaccharides, such as those that are found on bacterial coats. Activation of the complement system triggers a cascade that involves multiple complement components, resulting in release of the soluble fragments C3a and C5a, which are known as anaphylatoxins because they cause histamine release from mast cells and basophils. Ultimately, this cascade leads to generation of the membrane attack complex (MAC, or C5b-C9), which is capable of lysing membranes. C5a attracts and activates polymorphonuclear and mononuclear inflammatory cells, and thus is itself an important mediator of the inflammatory response. Inhibitors of complement activity, including C1 inhibitor and the membrane inhibitor of reactive lysis (CD59), provide a check on excessive complement-mediated effects.

Evidence suggests that complement activation accompanies the inflammatory response in AD.[23] Most of the components of the complement system are upregulated in the AD brain, and MAC has been demonstrated along membranes in the area of neuritic plaques.[24–27] In particular, the presence of MAC suggests that complement activation may directly contribute to cell loss in the AD brain. The presence of C1 and C4 and the absence of factor B and properdin suggests classical pathway activation, but evidence of immune complexes is generally lacking. However, there is evidence that C1q[28,29] or other complement components[30,31] may interact directly with Aβ peptide, resulting in activation of the complement cascade and also in increased aggregation and toxicity of the amyloid peptide.[32]

However, the role of complement in normal and diseased brain may be complex. Studies conducted in mice indicate that C5 protein or its derivatives may play an important neuroprotective role.[33] C5a receptors have been demonstrated not only on glia, but also on neurons.[34] Further experiments in mice indicate that C5a confers protection against excitotoxicity in vivo and in vitro, which suggests that C5a may be an important neuroprotectant. The mechanism of anaphylatoxin-mediated neuroprotection may involve neurotrophin release; it has been reported that C3a induces expression of nerve growth factor by microglia.[35] This has obvious, important implications for therapeutic strategies that target complement activation in AD – it is not clear whether the net effect of broad suppression of complement activation would be beneficial or harmful. Thus, the assumption that suppression of anaphylatoxin levels represents a therapeutic goal in AD,[36] as it is in the autoimmune disease systemic lupus erythematosus, may be erroneous. It may be that therapeutic maneuvers directed at the complement system must selectively target destructive elements such as MAC.

The role of microglia

Microglia are essentially tissue macrophages in brain. In the AD brain, microglia in white matter and grey matter express major histocompatability complex (MHC)-II antigens as well as β2 integrins. The former characteristic suggests that phagocytic microglia can act as antigen-presenting cells, although lymphocytes are difficult to demonstrate in the AD brain. These activated microglia are closely associated with neuritic plaques. Factors that may contribute to the accumulation and activation of microglia around plaques include amyloid peptide itself, anaphylatoxin released by complement activation and macrophage-colony stimulating factor released by neurons after binding of amyloid peptide to neuronal receptor for advanced glycation end-product.[37]

A number of contributing roles have been proposed for microglia with regard to AD pathology. Some are presumably detrimental, including synthesis of cytokines, acute-phase reactants, complement proteins and amyloid peptides, conversion of diffuse to fibrillar amyloid, generation of inflammatory prostanoids by cyclooxygenase,[38] and generation of nitric oxide,[39–41] superoxide[42] and other radicals.[43,44] The release of nitric oxide by microglia exposed to amyloid peptide may be mediated by binding of Aβ to the integrin MAC1.[40] Several laboratories have demonstrated the capacity of microglia to release neurotoxins;[45–47] this capacity suggests that these cells may be the major effectors of neuronal death in the AD brain.

However, there is also speculation that microglia perform useful functions in AD by limiting neuronal damage. Activated microglia secrete proteases that have the capacity to contribute to tissue damage, but they may also degrade harmful amyloid deposits.[48,49] A major function of microglia and other macrophage-like cells is phagocytosis; perhaps microglia that accumulate around amyloid plaques phagocytose and clear amyloid fibrils.[50,51] The recent report that immunization against amyloid peptide prevents amyloid deposition in transgenic mice includes evidence that plaques are cleared via microglial phagocytosis.[52] Finally, microglia synthesize nerve growth factor, the key neurotrophin that supports the survival of cholinergic neurons, in response to cytokines, C3a and amyloid peptide.[35]

Therefore, there is no consensus about the role of any of these three major components of inflammation in the AD brain. Various cell culture and animal systems, none of which fully and accurately models AD neuropathology, provide conflicting evidence about the role of the acute-phase response, complement activation and microglial activation. The data can be weighed and potential therapies can be selected, but only randomized, controlled clinical trials can establish efficacy of a specific anti-inflammatory intervention in the prevention or treatment of AD.

Epidemiology

Association between anti-inflammatory drugs and reduced risk of AD

Over a decade ago, it was first reported that it is unexpectedly rare for rheumatoid arthritis and AD to be diagnosed in the same person.[53] Subsequent studies that have analysed data from autopsies, clinic records and hospital discharges have corroborated this observation,[54] supporting the theory that treatment for rheumatoid arthritis (i.e. anti-inflammatory drugs) confers protection against the development of AD. Similarly, it has been reported that AD is uncommon in those with leprosy,[55] and in particular that amyloid deposition in brain is diminished in leprosy patients,[56] perhaps because the anti-inflammatory effects of the drug dapsone (a common treatment for leprosy) provide neuroprotection. Recent data call these observations into question, however.[57] Coupled with the demonstration of inflammatory processes in the AD brain, the reports spurred interest in anti-inflammatory therapy.

Many epidemiological studies have provided further evidence for a protective effect of anti-inflammatory treatment. In a study of 50 elderly twin pairs with at least one case of AD, previous use of glucocorticoids or adrenocorticotropic hormone was inversely associated with the onset of AD, and a similar but weaker trend was evident with previous use of non-steroidal anti-inflammatory drugs (NSAIDs) or aspirin.[58] A follow-up study of sibling pairs at high risk of AD indicated that sustained use of NSAIDs was associated with delayed onset and reduced risk of AD; unexpectedly, use of histamine H2 blocking drugs also seemed to offer protection.[59] Perhaps consistent with these findings, the use of NSAIDs by patients with AD enrolled in clinical trials was reported to be strikingly low compared with unselected elderly subjects;[60] more recent data showed that, among participants in AD clinical trials, concurrent use of anti-inflammatory drugs is associated with superior performance on cognitive assessments.[61] Data from the Canadian Study of Health and Aging, a population-based case-control study, indicated that a history of arthritis and previous use of NSAIDs were protective against AD.[62] The Rotterdam Study, another population-based survey, also provided data in support of reduced risk of AD among NSAID users.[63] Among patients followed by the Johns Hopkins Alzheimer's Disease Research Center, NSAID users had better scores on cognitive tests, and, importantly, showed a slower rate of cognitive decline.[64] Prospective data collected in the Baltimore Longitudinal Study of Aging demonstrated an inverse association between risk of AD and the duration of NSAID use.[65] It should be noted, however, that some studies have failed to confirm a protective effect of NSAIDs.[66–68]

Cellular and molecular targets of anti-inflammatory drugs in the AD brain

If, as the epidemiologic data suggests, anti-inflammatory drugs do confer protection against AD, what is the mechanism of this effect? What are the cellular and molecular targets of anti-inflammatory drugs in the AD brain?

NSAIDs inhibit cyclo-oxygenase (COX), the enzyme that begins the metabolic pathway from membrane-derived arachidonic acid to prostaglandins. Prostaglandins have diverse physiological functions, including roles in the regulation of vascular tone, platelet aggregability, protection of gastric epithelium against acid, and reproduction. Specific prostaglandins (PGs), such as PG_{E2} and PG_{I2}, are potent inflammatory mediators; the anti-inflammatory effect of NSAIDs has been attributed to inhibition of inflammatory PG generation, although other COX-independent mechanisms may be involved.[69] However, since classical NSAIDs block the generation of all PGs, toxic effects such as gastric ulceration and impaired renal blood flow regulation are unfortunately common. Indeed, NSAIDs, among the most widely used drugs, are a major cause of hospitalization and even mortality related to gastrointestinal bleeding.[70]

In the early 1990s, it was discovered that there are two isoforms of COX, with distinct physiologic functions.[71,72] COX-1 is constitutively expressed in many cell types, and it is involved in homeostatic mechanisms such as gastric cytoprotection and platelet aggregation. COX-2 is inducible in response to mitogens as well as inflammatory stimuli. Thus, induction of COX-2 is responsible for the generation of inflammatory prostaglandins at sites of inflammation. COX-2 induction can be inhibited by glucocorticoids.

Traditional NSAIDs generally inhibit COX-1 and COX-2 to a similar extent. But the arachidonic acid-binding sites of COX-1 and COX-2 are slightly different, and pharmaceutical companies have been able to develop selective COX-2 inhibitors that have similar anti-inflammatory potency to older NSAIDs but that appear to be much less likely to cause serious toxicity.[73] The recent approval by the Food and Drug Administration (FDA) in the USA of the first two selective COX-2 inhibitors, celecoxib and rofecoxib, has had a dramatic impact on the use of prescription anti-inflammatory drugs, both in the USA and elsewhere.

It seems likely that the mechanism of action of NSAIDs in the brain would be mediated by COX inhibition. Studies of COX expression in the brain have yielded surprising results. Both COX-1 and COX-2 are constitutively expressed in normal brain tissue[74–76] but COX-2 expression is primarily neuronal. COX-1 and COX-2 are found in neocortex and hippocampus, areas of neuronal loss in AD.[77–79]

The function of COX in normal brain remains unclear. Neuronal COX-2 is upregulated in response to a number of types of neuronal stress, including ischemia,[80,81] excitotoxicity[76] and amyloid toxicity,[77] and it may be involved in apoptosis.[82] There is evidence that the increase in neuronal COX-2 contributes to neuronal damage and that COX-2 inhibition may be neuroprotective.[83] In AD, COX-2 is upregulated in the hippocampus and the cortex.[77–79]

If COX-2 expression in the brain is primarily neuronal, is upregulated in response to neurodegenerative stress, and contributes to neuronal toxicity, neuronal COX-2 may be the target of NSAIDs in brain. This is a surprising conclusion – it had been assumed that anti-inflammatory drugs would primarily influence glial cells, particularly microglia. But direct neuronal activity is consistent with previous experiments that have demonstrated that COX inhibitors can protect neuronal-type cells in culture from amyloid toxicity in the absence of any glial cells.[84] Chronic NSAID exposure may directly protect brain neurons from neurodegenerative stress.

On the other hand, one study of autopsy brain specimens from non-demented subjects indicates that use of NSAIDs is associated with significant decrease in activated microglia;[85] this study is consistent with the theory that microglia are the target for the beneficial effect of NSAIDs with regard to AD. Consistent with this finding, indomethacin reduces the microglial response to intraventricular $A\beta$ infusion in rats.[86] Further, NSAID treatment reduces the neurotoxicity of a stimulated human monocyte line.[87]

Anti-inflammatory drug trials: methodological issues

The field of AD therapeutics came into its own only a few years ago, with the approval by the FDA in the USA of tacrine, a cholinesterase inhibitor. Tacrine, and newer cholinesterase inhibitors such as donepezil, rivastigmine and galantamine, represent primary, symptomatic therapy for AD. Treatment with these drugs improves cognitive function as measured by neuropsychological tests and improves clinical status as indicated by global assessment tools. The field has been galvanized by the arrival of these agents. However, although a major hurdle has been passed – AD is no longer an untreatable disease – the cholinesterase inhibitors have major limitations. They provide symptomatic benefit, improving cognitive function, but there is scant evidence that they modify the neurodegenerative disease process. Thus, despite therapy with cholinesterase inhibitors, the expected course of the disease is still inexorable deterioration.

Anti-inflammatory therapy represents one of the several approaches to modifying the disease process.[88] The hope is raised (based on the research findings discussed above) that anti-inflammatory drugs will slow the rate of neuronal loss, altering the downward slope of cognitive function.

Studies such as those described above have created optimism. But such studies can never be conclusive. Animal and cell culture models of the disease process have important limitations, so that experiments on these systems may not predict response in humans with the disease. Furthermore, epidemiologic studies cannot eliminate important issues of bias; the findings cannot be considered conclusive.

The only way of testing the inflammatory hypothesis is to conduct randomized, controlled clinical trials of anti-inflammatory drugs to prevent or slow the disease process. A number of such trials are under way. However, testing the efficacy of potential disease-modifying agents is much more difficult than establishing the efficacy of symptomatic treatments. Symptomatic drugs can be tested in short-term studies, measuring improvement in cognitive and clinical scores. No improvement is expected with disease-modifying interventions; rather, studies must include long observation periods (at least 1 year) so that slowing of deterioration can be documented.

Since trials of disease-modifying drugs must necessarily be long and include a large number of subjects (because of variability in progression rate on cognitive and clinical outcome measures), the resources required for each study are large. Guidance in drug selection from preclinical and epidemiologic studies is thus of paramount importance.

Drug selection for anti-inflammatory studies in AD

On the basis of descriptive studies of inflammatory features in the AD brain, an ideal anti-inflammatory drug for clinical trials should be broadly effective and active in suppressing a cytokine-driven acute-phase response, the activation of the complement cascade and the activity of microglial cells. A candidate drug should be tolerable for long-term use by elderly patients, and it should penetrate the brain.

The Alzheimer's Disease Cooperative Study (ADCS) group, a consortium of academic centers supported by the National Institute on Aging to conduct therapeutic trials in AD, selected the synthetic glucocorticoid prednisone, to be administered at a low dose, for its first multicenter, controlled trial of an anti-inflammatory drug for AD. This controversial selection was based on a number of considerations:

- glucocorticoids are the most powerful and broadly effective anti-inflammatory drugs available;
- long-term use of low-dose prednisone is well tolerated in the elderly, based on extensive clinical experience in the treatment of inflammatory diseases such as rheumatoid arthritis and polymyalgia rheumatica;
- low-dose prednisone suppresses peripheral acute-phase reactants in AD subjects;[10]
- low-dose prednisone suppresses plasma levels of the anaphylatoxin C3a in AD subjects;[36]
- short-term administration of low-dose prednisone to AD subjects has no adverse cognitive or behavioral effects;[10] and
- the feasibility of a large-scale trial of an NSAID was questionable in view of toxicity in the AD population.[89]

Based on pilot studies of prednisone in AD,[10] the treatment regimen for the multicenter trial consisted of an initial daily oral dose of 20 mg for 4 weeks, tapered to a maintenance dose of 10 mg daily for 1 year, followed by slow withdrawal over an additional 12 weeks. To minimize the likelihood of glucocorticoid toxicity, potential subjects with diabetes mellitus, positive skin tests for tuberculosis or radiographic evidence of osteoporotic vertebral fractures were excluded from the study. Additional safety precautions included the administration of calcium and vitamin D to all participants, ophthalmological monitoring and periodic spinal radiographs, in addition to regular physical examinations and laboratory testing.

A total of 138 subjects were enrolled at 22 sites and randomly assigned to receive prednisone or placebo. There were no serious adverse events related to treatment. The primary analysis, an intention-to-treat analysis of the 1-year change in the cognitive component of the Alzheimer's Disease Assessment Scale (ADAS-cog),[90] showed no significant difference between treatment groups.[90a] Secondary analyses, including completers-only analyses, similarly showed no significant effect of the intervention on cognitive function or clinical stage of disease as assessed by the Clinical Dementia Rating Scale (CDR).[91]

Several explanations have been suggested for the failure of the prednisone regimen to slow the rate of cognitive decline. First, the dose may have been too low; much higher doses are routinely used to treat inflammatory diseases of brain such as lupus cerebritis. However, data from the study suggest that higher doses are not feasible in this population. The low-dose regimen caused some decline in lumbar spine bone density despite calcium and vitamin D supplementation, and a few asymptomatic vertebral fractures were detected in the prednisone group. There were also several subjects with significant hyperglycemia. Finally, the prednisone-treatment group showed significant behavioral decline, as assessed by the Brief Psychiatric Rating Scale,[92] compared with the placebo group.

This adverse effect on behavior may have contributed to the failure to influence cognitive function favorably. Indeed, it is possible that glucocorticoid therapy has an adverse effect on hippocampal function, as has been demonstrated in rodents,[93] which may negate any beneficial effect on AD brain pathology. One recent study suggests, however, that the hippocampal neurodegeneration seen in rodents does not occur in primates with long-term exogenous glucocorticoid exposure.[94]

Recent studies suggest that the broad anti-inflammatory activity of glucocorticoids may have contributed to the failure of the prednisone study. Evidence suggests that some inflammatory mediators, such as anaphylatoxins[95] and TNF-α,[22] are actually neuroprotective. The demonstration that low-dose prednisone suppresses anaphylatoxin levels in AD[36] may thus provide evidence of a deleterious effect on the disease process.

The ADCS is now beginning a second trial of anti-inflammatory therapy. In selecting drug regimens for this trial, the above issues eliminated consideration of another glucocorticoid regimen. Interest in NSAID therapy for the prevention and treatment of AD has continued to grow, a major factor in the design of the new trial.

Toxicity remains a major block to a study of an anti-inflammatory dose of a traditional NSAID. One way of attempting to reduce NSAID toxicity is to add a cytoprotective agent to the treatment regimen. Misoprostol is a synthetic prostaglandin that has been proved to reduce the incidence of NSAID gastropathy. However, a recent report of a trial of diclofenac plus misoprostol indicated that this combination was not better tolerated than indomethacin in AD patients: the drop-out rate in this 25-week trial was 50% in the active drug group, and (not surprisingly) the results of the study were inconclusive.[96] It is unlikely that a study of a regimen that is tolerated by a minority of subjects over the course of 1 year of treatment will yield definitive results.

The ADCS has opted to study two NSAID-type regimens that are expected to have substantially less toxicity than the indomethacin and diclofenac regimens that have been reported. The first is rofecoxib, a new selective COX-2 inhibitor. As discussed above, COX-2 may be the target of action of NSAIDs in the AD brain, and COX-2 inhibitors appear to carry much reduced risk of serious gastrointestinal toxicity.

The second active drug regimen in the new ADCS trial is low-dose naproxen (200 mg twice daily). Naproxen is a non-selective COX inhibitor, and so at full doses has similar toxicity to indomethacin and diclofenac. If COX-1 is in fact an important target for NSAID action in AD, naproxen may be more effective than a selective COX-2 inhibitor. However, the dose studied is substantially less than a full anti-inflammatory dose; rather, it is the over-the-counter analgesic dose. Studies suggest that this regimen is reasonably well tolerated in the elderly,[97,98] although there are little data on long-term treatment. Systemic administration of naproxen suppresses COX activity in the brain of rodents,[99,100] indicating effective brain penetration. But will the low dose tested be sufficient to alter the AD process? The epidemiological studies suggest that casual use of NSAIDs obtained over the counter may be neuroprotective, supporting the study of a low-dose regimen.

The current ADCS trial has a design that is similar to the prednisone study. The primary outcome measure is the ADAS-cog, and the duration of treatment is 1 year. Secondary outcome measures include the CDR scale, the Neuropsychiatric Inventory,[101] the ADCS activities of daily living assessment[102] and measures of pharmacoeconomics and quality of life. Enrollment began in late 1999, and the study is expected to be completed in approximately 3 years.

Pharmaceutical companies are also investigating the utility of selective COX-2 inhibitors in the treatment of AD. Based on the idea that NSAIDs are effective but that their use in AD is limited by toxicity, and that selective COX-2 inhibitors may show similar benefit with much greater safety, companies that manufacture COX-2 inhibitors are investing in development of these agents for AD. Several large trials of selective COX-2 inhibitors to delay progression from mild cognitive impairment to AD diagnosis or slow the progression of established AD have been initiated in the past couple of years.

Other anti-inflammatory agents under investigation

Propentofylline is under study as a disease-modifying treatment for vascular dementia and AD.[103–105] Studies suggest that propentofylline slows, to a modest extent, the progression of both types of dementia; the benefit may be somewhat greater in the treatment of vascular dementia. The drug, a xanthine derivative, is a phosphodiesterase inhibitor that elevates intracellular cyclic adenosine monophosphate and cyclic guanosine monophosphate. The drug also inhibits adenosine reuptake, and its proposed mechanism of action includes suppression of microglial activation, perhaps via an adenosine-dependent mechanism.[106] There is also evidence that propentofylline has neurotrophic activity.

Hydroxychloroquine is an antimalarial agent that is commonly used in the treatment of rheumatoid arthritis and systemic lupus erythematosus. The mechanism of action of hydroxychloroquine is not fully understood. It is a lysosomotropic agent (i.e. it raises intralysosomal pH, inhibiting acid proteases);[107] there has been some controversy about whether such an effect will be beneficial[108–110] or harmful[111–114] with regard to AD. Hydroxychloroquine inhibits the release of inflammatory cytokines from stimulated monocytes,[115] which suggests that it may be useful in controlling microglial activity in AD. Hydroxychloroquine penetrates the blood–brain barrier to some extent,[116] and pilot studies demonstrate tolerability in AD (Aisen PS *et al.*, submitted).

A study of the efficacy of hydroxychloroquine in slowing the rate of cognitive decline in AD is under way in the Netherlands (van Gool WA, personal communication). A total of 168 patients with probable AD have been randomized to receive hydroxychloroquine 200 mg twice daily (reduced to once daily for subjects who weigh less than 65 kg) or matching placebo. The duration of treatment is 18 months. Primary outcome measures include the ADAScog and assessments of behavior and activities of daily living. There has been no serious drug toxicity reported to date. The last subject will complete the protocol in the middle of 2000.

Colchicine is a unique anti-inflammatory drug that may also be a candidate for use in the treatment or prevention of AD. The primary clinical use of colchicine is in the treatment and prophylaxis of gout, although it is also used in other inflammatory diseases such as complement-mediated cutaneous vasculitis.[117] Colchicine suppresses mononuclear cell activity and cytokine release,[118,119] which suggests it may have the potential to inhibit microglial function. Systemic administration of colchicine to animals results in some accumulation in the brain.[120–122]

Colchicine also has antiamyloidogenic effects. Chronic administration of colchicine is dramatically effective in preventing the deposition of amyloid complicating familial Mediterranean fever.[123,124] The drug also shows efficacy in animal models of amyloidosis[125–127] and perhaps in other human amyloidoses.[128] Colchicine (along with chloroquine) has been shown to reduce the delayed neurological deterioration, which is thought to be mediated by mononuclear phagocytes, that occurs after transient ischemia to the rabbit spinal cord.[129] Peripheral administration of colchicine protects against hippocampal neuron degeneration after transient carotid occlusion in the gerbil.[130] Colchicine also protects against ischemic hippocampal neurodegeneration in the rat.[131] On the other hand, colchicine is used in the laboratory as a neurotoxin; it is infused directly into the central nervous system to poison microtubules, with blockade of mitosis and axonal transport leading to neuronal destruction.[132] An open-label pilot study of colchicine in AD demonstrated that short-term administration is well tolerated in AD.[133]

Potent chemotherapeutic agents may also have a role in the treatment of AD. For example, cyclophosphamide, an alkylating agent used in the treatment of both malignancy and autoimmune disease, protects against late neuronal loss after transient global ischemia in the gerbil.[134] Anecdotal evidence suggests that cyclophosphamide may have efficacy in the treatment of AD.[135] One small, open-label trial also suggests clinical efficacy in AD.[136]

Immunophilin-binding agents such as cyclosporin A and tacrolimus (previously known as FK506) are immunosuppressant agents that inhibit T-cell function; they are primarily used in the prevention of transplant rejection. Their mechanism of action involves binding intracellular receptor proteins called immunophilins. The demonstration that immunophilins are more prevalent in neuronal tissues than in immune cells led to speculation that they may have non-immune-related functions.[137,138] Indeed, neurotrophic actions of immunophilin-binding drugs have been demonstrated in neuronal cell culture systems,[139] and tacrolimus reduces delayed hippocampal neuronal death after transient global ischemia in the gerbil.[140] Immunophilin-binding drugs inhibit the oxidative toxicity of amyloid peptides in vitro, further supporting their potential efficacy in AD.[141] The neurotrophic and immunosuppressive activities of these drugs can be uncoupled – non-immunosuppressive immunophilin-binding drugs with neurotrophic activity have been synthesized[142,143] for possible applications in the treatment of neurodegenerative diseases.

Conclusions

There are a large number of anti-inflammatory drugs that are candidates for testing in AD. Although studies of the most promising agents continue, it is important to improve our ability to select drugs for future studies. Epidemiological surveys may not provide much help in this regard – they provide no useful data on drugs that are not in widespread use. Animal studies, on the other hand, may be quite valuable. Transgenic models with AD-like cerebral amyloid plaques are currently used to screen drugs. Improvements in such models (perhaps by creating animals that carry amyloidogenic APP or PS1 mutations and also overexpress inflammatory mediators in the brain, so that the models include amyloid deposition, inflammatory activity and neurodegeneration) may allow efficacy studies of anti-inflammatory agents.

Immunogenetic studies may allow improved selection of subjects for anti-inflammatory drug prevention and treatment trials. There is some preliminary evidence that HLA genotype, which has an important influence on the incidence of many inflammatory and autoimmune diseases, has some influence on the neuropathology of AD. There may be a relationship between the HLA-A2 allele and age at disease onset.[144] Some evidence supports an effect of HLA-DR alleles on incidence of AD,[145] although a recent study failed to confirm this finding.[146] Since activated microglial cells, presumably controlling the inflammatory response in the AD brain, express HLA-DR surface molecules, it is plausible that HLA-DR genotype affects the AD inflammatory response. Indeed, the HLA-DR4 allele appears to influence glial activity in AD hippocampus.[147] HLA genotype may prove to be useful in predicting rate of progression and response to anti-inflammatory interventions.

Pilot screening trials in AD subjects should provide the best method for rapidly evaluating potential therapeutic drug candidates. However, because no symptomatic response to anti-inflammatory agents is expected, it will be necessary to develop biomarkers of destructive brain inflammation in AD. A useful biomarker should be elevated in AD subjects compared with controls, should correlate with clinical disease state and should respond to anti-inflammatory treatment; most importantly, the effect of treatment on the biomarker must predict the effect on the clinical course of AD. Attempts to date, including use of acute-phase proteins,[10] C3a,[36] plasma Aβ (Aisen PS, unpublished data) and neopterin (Hull *et al.*, submitted), have not been wholly successful, so further efforts are essential.

Nonetheless, the outlook is good. Large-scale industry and academic trials of anti-inflammatory drugs are under way, and basic research into inflammatory mechanisms in AD continues at a rapid pace. It is likely that in the near future anti-inflammatory therapy will become a component of the combination drug treatment of AD.

References

1. Kushner I. The acute phase response: from Hippocrates to cytokine biology. Eur Cytokine Net 1991;2:75–80.

2. Matsubara E, Hirai S, Amari M, *et al.* Alpha-1-antichymotrypsin as a possible biochemical marker for Alzheimer-type dementia. Ann Neurol 1990; 28:561–567.

3. Brugge K, Katzman R, Hill LR, Hansen LA, Saitoh T. Serological alpha 1-antichymotrypsin in Down's syndrome and Alzheimer's disease. 1992;32: 193–197.

4. Hinds TR, Kukull WA, Van Belle G, Schellenberg GD, Villacres EC, Larson EB. Relationship between serum alpha 1-antichymotrypsin and Alzheimer's disease. Neurobiol Aging 1994; 15:21–27.

5. Altstiel LD, Lawlor B, Mohs R, *et al.* Elevated alpha1-antichymotrypsin serum levels in a subset of nondemented first-degree relatives of Alzheimer's disease

patients. Dementia 1995;6:17–20.

6. Lieberman J, Schleissner L, Tachiki KH, Kling AS. Serum alpha 1-antichymotrypsin level as a marker for Alzheimer-type dementia. Neurobiol Aging 1995;16:747–753.

7. Pirttila T, Mehta PD, Frey H, Wisniewski HM. Alpha 1-antichymotrypsin and IL-1 beta are not increased in CSF or serum in Alzheimer's disease. Neurobiol Aging 1994;15:313–317.

8. Kuiper MA, Van Kamp GJ, Bergmans PLM, Scheltens P, Wolters EC. Serum alpha 1-antichymotrypsin is not a useful marker for Alzheimer's disease or dementia in Parkinson's disease. J Neurol Transm Park Dis Dement Sect 1993;6:145–149.

9. Lawlor BA, Swanwick GRJ, Feighery C, Walsh JB, Coakley D. Acute phase reactants in Alzheimer's disease. Biol Psychiatry 1996;39:1051–1052.

10. Aisen PS, Marin D, Altstiel L, et al. A pilot study of prednisone in Alzheimer's disease. Dementia 1996;7:201–206.

11. Abraham CR, Selkoe DJ, Potter H. Immunohistochemical identification of the serine protease inhibitor alpha-1 antichymotrypsin in the brain amyloid deposits of Alzheimer's disease. Cell 1988;52:487–501.

12. Rozemuller JM, Stam FC, Eikelenboom P. Acute phase proteins are present in amorphous plaques in the cerebral but not in the cerebellar cortex of patients with Alzheimer's disease. Neurosci Lett 1990;109:75–78.

13. Bauer J, Strauss S, Schreiter-Gasser U, et al. Interleukin-6 and alpha-2-macroglobulin indicate an acute phase response in Alzheimer's disease cortices. FEBS Lett 1991;285:111–114.

14. De Strooper B, Van Leuven F. α2-macroglobulin and suba-cute-phase responses in Alzheimer's disease. Immunol Today 1993;14:143–144.

15. Van Gool D, De Strooper B, Van Leuven F, Triau E, Dom R. Alpha2-macroglobulin expression in neuritic-type plaques in patients with Alzheimer's disease. Neurobiol Aging 1993; 14:233–237.

16. Iwamoto N, Nishiyama E, Ohwada J, Arai H. Demonstration of CRP immunoreactivity in brains of Alzheimer's disease: immunohistochemical study using formic acid pretreatment of tissue sections. Neurosci Lett 1994;177:23–26.

17. Vandenabeele P, Fiers W. Is amyloidogenesis during Alzheimer's disease due to an IL-1/IL-6-mediated 'acute phase response' in the brain? Immunol Today 1991;12:217–219.

18. Griffin WST, Sheng JG, Royston MC, et al. Glial–neuronal interactions in Alzheimer's disease: the potential role of a 'cytokine cycle' in disease progression. Brain Pathol 1998;8:65–72.

19. Sheng JG, Mrak RE, Griffin WST. Glial–neuronal interactions in Alzheimer disease: progressive association of IL-1Alpha+ microglia and S100Beta+ astrocytes with neurofibrillary tangle stages. J Neuropathol Exp Neurol 1997;56:285–290.

20. Hauss-Wegrzyniak B, Willard LB, Del SP, Pepeu G, Wenk GL. Peripheral administration of novel anti-inflammatories can attenuate the effects of chronic inflammation within the CNS. Brain 1999;815:36–43.

21. Harris-White ME, Chu T, Balverde Z, Sigel JJ, Flanders KC, Frautschy SA. Effects of transforming growth factor-beta

(isoforms 1–3) on amyloid-beta deposition, inflammation, and cell targeting in organotypic hippocampal slice cultures. J Neurosci 1998;18:10366–10374.

22. Mattson MP, Barger SW, Furukawa K, *et al*. Cellular signaling roles of TGFbeta, TNFalpha and betaAPP in brain injury responses and Alzheimer's disease. Brain Res Rev 1997; 23:47–61.

23. Pasinetti GM. Inflammatory mechanisms in neurodegeneration and Alzheimer's disease: the role of the complement system. Neurobiol Aging 1996;17: 707–716.

24. McGeer PL, Akiyama H, Itagaki S, McGeer EG. Activation of the classical complement pathway in brain tissue of Alzheimer patients. Neurosci Lett 1989; 107:341–346.

25. Shen Y, Li R, McGeer EG, McGeer PL. Neuronal expression of mRNAs for complement proteins of the classical pathway in Alzheimer brain. Brain Res 1997;769:391–395.

26. Webster S, Lue LF, Brachova L, *et al*. Molecular and cellular characterization of the membrane attack complex, C5b-9, in Alzheimer's disease. Neurobiol Aging 1997;18:415–421.

27. Yasojima K, Schwab C, McGeer EG, McGeer PL. Up-regulated production and activation of the complement system in Alzheimer's disease brain. Am J Pathol 1999;154:927–936.

28. Webster S, Bonnell B, Rogers J. Charge-based binding of complement component C1q to the Alzheimer amyloid beta-peptide. Am J Pathol 1997;150: 1531–1536.

29. Cribbs DH, Velazquez P, Soreghan B, Glabe CG, Tenner AJ. Complement activation by cross-linked truncated and chimeric full-length beta-amyloid. Neuroreport 1997;8: 3457–3462.

30. Watson MD, Roher AE, Kim KS, Spiegel K, Emmerling MR. Complement interactions with amyloid-beta1-42: a nidus for inflammation in AD brains. Amyloid. Int J Exp Clin Invest 1997; 4:147–156.

31. Bergamaschini L, Canziani S, Bottasso B, Cugno M, Braidotti P, Agostoni A. Alzheimer's beta-amyloid peptides can activate the early components of complement classical pathway in a C1q-independent manner. Clin Exp Immunol 1999;115: 526–533.

32. Webster S, Glabe C, Rogers J. Multivalent binding of complement protein C1Q to the amyloid beta-peptide (Abeta) promotes the nucleation phase of Abeta aggregation. Biochem Biophys Res Commun 1995;217: 869–875.

33. Tocco G, Musleh W, Sakhi S, Schreiber S, Baudry M, Pasinetti GM. Complement and glutamate neurotoxicity. Genotypic influences of C5 in a mouse model of hippocampal neurodegeneration. Mol Chem Neuropathol 1997;31:1–12.

34. Osaka H, McGinty A, Hoeepken UE, Lu B, Gerard C, Pasinetti GM. Expression of C5a receptor in mouse brain: role in signal transduction and neurodegeneration. Neuroscience 1999;88: 1073–1082.

35. Heese K, Hock C, Otten U. Inflammatory signals induce neurotrophin expression in human microglial cells. J Neurochem 1998;70:699–707.

36. Fagarasan MO, Sevilla D, Baruch B, Santoro J, Marin D, Aisen PS. Plasma C3a levels in

Alzheimer's disease. Alzheimer Res 1997;3:137–140.

37. Yan SD, Zhu HJ, Fu J, *et al.* Amyloid-beta peptide-receptor for advanced glycation end-product interaction elicits neuronal expression of macrophage-colony stimulating factor: a proinflammatory pathway in Alzheimer disease. Proc Natl Acad Sci U S A 1997; 94:5296–5301.

38. Slepko N, Minghetti L, Polazzi E, Nicolini A, Levi G. Reorientation of prostanoid production accompanies 'activation' of adult microglial cells in culture. J Neurosci Res 1997;49:292–300.

39. Akama KT, Albanese C, Pestell RG, Van Eldik LJ. Amyloid beta-peptide stimulates nitric oxide production in astrocytes through an NFkappaB-dependent mechanism. Proc Natl Acad Sci U S A 1998;95:5795–5800.

40. Goodwin JL, Kehrli ME Jr, Uemura E. Integrin Mac-1 and beta-amyloid in microglial release of nitric oxide. Brain Res 1997;768:279–286.

41. Hu JG, Akama KT, Krafft GA, Chromy BA, Van Eldik LJ. Amyloid-beta peptide activates cultured astrocytes: morphological alterations, cytokine induction and nitric oxide release. Brain Res 1998;785:195–206.

42. McDonald DR, Brunden KR, Landreth GE. Amyloid fibrils activate tyrosine kinase-dependent signaling and superoxide production in microglia. J Neurosci 1997;17:2284–2294.

43. Della Bianca V, Dusi S, Bianchini E, Dal Pra I, Rossi F. Beta-amyloid activates the O_2 forming NADPH oxidase in microglia, monocytes, and neutrophils. A possible inflammatory mechanism of neuronal damage in Alzheimer's disease. J Biol Chem 1999;274:15493–15499.

44. Johnstone M, Gearing AJ, Miller KM. A central role for astrocytes in the inflammatory response to beta-amyloid; chemokines, cytokines and reactive oxygen species are produced. J Neuroimmunol 1999;93:182–193.

45. Combs CK, Johnson DE, Cannady SB, Lehman TM, Landreth GE. Identification of microglial signal transduction pathways mediating a neurotoxic response to amyloidogenic fragments of beta-amyloid and prion proteins. J Neurosci 1999;19: 928–939.

46. Barger SW, Harmon AD. Microglial activation by Alzheimer amyloid precursor protein and modulation by apolipoprotein E. Nature 1997; 388:878–881.

47. Giulian D, Haverkamp LJ, Yu JH, *et al.* The HHQK domain of beta-amyloid provides a structural basis for the immunopathology of Alzheimer's disease. J Biol Chem 1998;273: 29719–29726.

48. Qiu WQ, Ye Z, Kholodenko D, Seubert P, Selkoe DJ. Degradation of amyloid beta-protein by a metalloprotease secreted by microglia and other neural and non-neural cells. J Biol Chem 1997;272:6641–6646.

49. Mentlein R, Ludwig R, Martensen I. Proteolytic degradation of Alzheimer's disease amyloid beta-peptide by a metalloproteinase from microglia cells. J Neurochem 1998;70: 721–726.

50. DeWitt DA, Perry G, Cohen M, Doller C, Silver J. Astrocytes regulate microglial phagocytosis of senile plaque cores of Alzheimer's disease. Exp Neurol 1998;149:329–340.

51. Paresce DM, Chung HY, Max-

field FR. Slow degradation of aggregates of the Alzheimer's disease amyloid beta-protein by microglial cells. J Biol Chem 1997;272:29390–29397.

52. Schenk D, Barbour R, Dunn W, *et al.* Immunization with amyloid-β attenuates Alzheimer-disease-like pathology in PDAPP mouse. Nature 1999;400:173–177.

53. Jenkinson ML, Bliss MR, Brain AT, Scott DL. Rheumatoid arthritis and senile dementia of the Alzheimer's type. Br J Rheumatol 1989;28:86–88.

54. McGeer PL, McGeer E, Rogers J, Sibley J. Anti-inflammatory drugs and Alzheimer disease. Lancet 1990;335:1037.

55. McGeer PL, Harada N, Kimura H, McGeer EG, Schulzer M. Prevalence of dementia amongst elderly Japanese with leprosy: apparent effect of chronic drug therapy. Dementia 1992;3:146–149.

56. Chui DH, Tabira T, Izumi S, Koya G, Ogata J. Decreased beta-amyloid and increased abnormal tau deposition in the brain of aged patients with leprosy. Am J Pathol 1994;145:771–775.

57. Endoh M, Kunishita T, Tabira T. No effect of anti-leprosy drugs in the prevention of Alzheimer's disease and beta-amyloid neurotoxicity. J Neurol Sci 1999;165:28–30.

58. Breitner JC, Gau BA, Welsh KA, *et al.* Inverse association of anti-inflammatory treatments and Alzheimer's disease: initial results of a co-twin control study. Neurology 1994;44:227–232.

59. Breitner JCS, Welsh KA, Helms MJ, *et al.* Delayed onset of Alzheimer's disease with nonsteroidal anti-inflammatory and histamine H2 blocking drugs.

Neurobiol Aging 1995;16:523–530.

60. Lucca U, Tettamanti M, Forloni G, Spagnoli A. Nonsteroidal antiinflammatory drug use in Alzheimer's disease. Biol Psychiatry 1994;36:854–856.

61. Doraiswamy PM, Bieber F, Kaiser L, Krishnan KR, Reuning-Scherer J, Gulanski B. The Alzheimer's disease assessment scale: patterns and predictors of baseline cognitive performance in multicenter Alzheimer's disease trials. Neurology 1997;48:1511–1517.

62. The Canadian Study of Health and Aging: risk factors for Alzheimer's disease in Canada. Neurology 1994;44:2073–2080.

63. Andersen K, Launer LJ, Ott A, Hoes AW, Breteler NMB, Hofman A. Do nonsteroidal anti-inflammatory drugs decrease the risk for Alzheimer's disease? The Rotterdam Study. Neurology 1995;45:1441–1445.

64. Rich JB, Rasmusson DX, Folstein MF, Carson KA, Kawas C, Brandt J. Nonsteroidal anti-inflammatory drugs in Alzheimer's disease. Neurology 1995;45:51–55.

65. Stewart WF, Kawas C, Corrada M, Metter EJ. Risk of Alzheimer's disease and duration of NSAID use. Neurology 1997;48:626–632.

66. Henderson AS, Jorm AF, Christensen H, Jacomb PA, Korten AE. Aspirin, anti-inflammatory drugs and risk of dementia. Int J Geriatr Psychiatry 1997;12:926–930.

67. Veld BAI, Launer LJ, Hoes AW, *et al.* NSAIDs and incident Alzheimer's disease. The Rotterdam Study. Neurobiol Aging 1998;19:607–611.

68. Beard CM, Waring SC, O'Brien PC, Kurland LT, Kokmen E. Non-

steroidal anti-inflammatory drug use and Alzheimer's disease: a case-control study in Rochester, Minnesota, 1980 through 1984. Mayo Clin Proc 1998;73: 951–955.

69. Abramson SB, Weissmann G. The mechanism of action of non-steroidal anti-inflammatory drugs. Arthritis Rheum 1989; 32:1.

70. Singh G, Ramey DR, Morfeld D, Shi H, Hatoum HT, Fries JF. Gastrointestinal tract complications of nonsteroidal anti-inflammatory drug treatment in rheumatoid arthritis. Arch Inter Med 1996;156:1530–1536.

71. Kujubu DA, Fletcher BS, Varnum BC, Lim RW, Herschman HR. TIS10, a phorbol ester tumor promoter-inducible mRNA from Swiss 3T3 cells, encodes a novel prostaglandin synthase/ cyclooxygenase homologue. J Biol Chem 1991;266: 12866–12872.

72. O'Banion MK, Winn VD, Young DA. cDNA cloning and functional activity of a glucocorticoid-regulated inflammatory cyclooxygenase. Proc Natl Acad Sci U S A 1992;89:4888–4892.

73. Vane JR, Botting RM. Anti-inflammatory drugs and their mechanism of action. Inflamm Res 1998;47(suppl 2):S78–S87.

74. Yamagata K, Andreasson KI, Kaufmann WE, Barnes CA, Worley PF. Expression of a mitogen-inducible cyclooxygenase in brain neurons: regulation by synaptic activity and glucocorticoids. Neuron 1993;11:371–386.

75. Kaufmann WE, Andreasson KL, Isakson PC, Worley PF. Cyclooxygenases and the central nervous system. Prostaglandins 1997;54:601–624.

76. Tocco G, Freire MJ, Schreiber SS, Sakhi SH, Aisen PS, Pasinetti GM. Maturational regulation and regional induction of cyclooxygenase-2 in rat brain: implications for Alzheimer's disease. Exp Neurol 1997;144: 339–349.

77. Pasinetti GM, Aisen PS. Cyclooxygenase-2 expression is increased in frontal cortex of Alzheimer's disease brain. Neuroscience 1998;87:319–324.

78. Ho L, Pieroni C, Winger D, Purohit DP, Aisen PS, Pasinetti GM. Regional distribution of cyclooxygenase-2 in the hippocampal formation in Alzheimer's disease. J Neurosci Res 1999;57:295–303.

79. Yasojima K, Schwab C, McGeer EG, McGeer PL. Distribution of cyclooxygenase-1 and cyclooxygenase-2 mRNAs and proteins in human brain and peripheral organs. Brain Res 1999;830:226–236.

80. Planas AM, Soriano MA, Rodriguez-Farr E, Ferrer I. Induction of cyclooxygenase-2 mRNA and protein following transient focal ischemia in the rat brain. Neurosci Lett 1995;200:187–190.

81. Nakayama M, Uchimura K, Zhu L, et al. Cyclooxygenase 2 promotes neuronal death after global ischemia in rat CA1 hippocampus. Soc Neurosci Abstr 1996;22:1670.

82. Ho L, Osaka H, Aisen PS, Pasinetti GM. Induction of cyclooxygenase (COX)-2 but not COX-1 gene expression in apoptotic cell death. J Neuroimmunol 1998;89:142–149.

83. Nakayama M, Uchimura K, Zhu RL, et al. Cyclooxygenase-2 inhibition prevents delayed death of CA1 hippocampal neurons following global ischemia. Proc Natl Acad Sci USA 1998;95:10954–10959.

84. Fagarasan MO, Aisen PS. Il-1 and anti-inflammatory drugs modulate Abeta cytotoxicity in PC12 cells. Brain Res 1996;723:231–234.

85. Mackenzie IRA, Munoz DG. Nonsteroidal anti-inflammatory drug use and Alzheimer-type pathology in aging. Neurology 1998;50:986–990.

86. Netland EE, Newton JL, Majocha RE, Tate BA. Indomethacin reverses the microglial response to amyloid beta-protein. Neurobiol Aging 1998;19:201–204.

87. Klegeris A, Walker DG, McGeer PL. Toxicity of human THP-1 monocytic cells towards neuron-like cells is reduced by non-steroidal anti-inflammatory drugs (NSAIDs). Neuropharmacology 1999;38:1017–1025.

88. Aisen PS, Davis KL. The search for disease-modifying treatment for Alzheimer's disease. Neurology 1997;48(suppl 6):S35–S41.

89. Rogers J, Kirby LC, Hempelman SR, et al. Clinical trial of indomethacin in Alzheimer's disease. Neurology 1993;43: 1609–1611.

90. Rosen WG, Mohs RC, Davis KL. A new rating scale for Alzheimer's disease. Am J Psychiatry 1984;141:1356–1364.

90a. Aisen PS, Davis KL, Berg JD, et al. A randomized controlled trial of prednisone in Alzheimer's disease. Alzheimer's Disease Cooperative Study. Neurology 2000;54:588–593.

91. Morris JC. The Clinical Dementia Rating (CDR): current version and scoring rules. Neurology 1993;43:2412–2414.

92. Overall JE, Gorham DR. Brief Psychiatric Rating Scale. Psychol Rep 1962;10:799–812.

93. Sapolsky RM, Krey LC, McEwen BS. Prolonged glucocorticoid exposure reduces hippocampal neuron number: implications for aging. J Neurosci 1985;5: 1222–1227.

94. Leverenz JB, Wilkinson CW, Wamble M, et al. Effect of chronic high-dose exogenous cortisol on hippocampal neuronal number in aged nonhuman primates. J Neurosci 1999;19: 2356–2361.

95. Osaka H, Mukherjee P, Aisen PS, Pasinetti GM. Complement-derived anaphylatoxin C5a protects against glutamate-mediated neurotoxicity. J Cell Biochem 1999;73: 303–311.

96. Scharf S, Mander A, Ugoni A, Vajda F, Christophidis N. A double-blind, placebo-controlled trial of diclofenac/misoprostol in Alzheimer's disease. Neurology 1999;53:197–201.

97. Gecsy M, Peltier L, Wolbach R. Naproxen tolerability in the elderly: a summary report. J Rheumatol 1987;14:348–354.

98. DeArmond B, Francisco CA, Lin JS, et al. Safety profile of over-the-counter naproxen sodium. Clin Ther 1995;17:587–601.

99. Abdel-Halim MS, Sjoquist B, Anggard E. Inhibition of prostaglandin synthesis in rat brain. Acta Pharmacol Toxicol 1978;43:266–272.

100. Ferrari RA, Ward SJ, Sobre CM, et al. Estimation of the in vivo effect of cyclooxygenase inhibitors on prostaglandin E2 levels in mouse brain. Eur J Pharmacol 1990;179:25–34.

101. Cummings J. The neuropsychiatric inventory: assessing psychopathology in dementia patients. Neurology 1997; 48(suppl 6):S10–S16.

102. Galasko D, Bennett D, Sano M, et al. An inventory to assess activities of daily living for clinical trials in Alzheimer's disease.

Alzheimer Dis Assoc Disord 1997;11(suppl 2):S33–S39.

103. Marcusson J, Rother M, Kittner B, *et al*. A 12-month, randomized, placebo-controlled trial of propentofylline (HWA 285) in patients with dementia according to DSM III-R. Dementia 1997;8:320–328.

104. Mielke R, Moeller HJ, Erkinjuntti T, Rosenkranz B, Rother M, Kittner B. Propentofylline in the treatment of vascular dementia and Alzheimer-type dementia: overview of phase I and phase II clinical trials. Alzheimer Dis Assoc Disord 1998;12(suppl 2): S29–S35.

105. Rother M, Erkinjuntti T, Roessner M, Kittner B, Marcusson J, Karlsson I. Propentofylline in the treatment of Alzheimer's disease and vascular dementia: a review of phase III trials. Dementia 1998;9(suppl 1):36–43.

106. Rudolphi KA, Schubert P. Modulation of neuronal and glial cell function by adenosine and neuroprotection in vascular dementia. Behav Brain Res 1997; 83:123–128.

107. DeDuve C, DeBarsy T, Poole B, Trouet A, Tulkens P, van Hoof F. Lysosomotropic agents. Biochemical Pharmacology 1974;23: 2495–2531.

108. Golde TE, Estus S, Younkin LH, Selkoe DJ, Younkin SG. Processing of the amyloid precursor for potentially amyloidogenic derivatives. Science 1992;155: 728.

109. Caporaso GL, Gandy SE, Buxbaum JD, Greengard P. Chloroquine inhibits intracellular degradation but not secretion of Alzheimer β/A4 amyloid precursor protein. Proc Natl Acad Sci U S A 1992;89:2252–2256.

110. Haass C, Koo EH, Mellon A, Hung AY, Selkoe DJ. Targeting of cell-surface beta-amyloid precursor protein to lysosomes: alternative processing into amyloid-bearing fragments. Nature 1992;357:500–503.

111. Tsuzuki K, Kukatsu R, Takamaru Y, *et al*. Amyloid beta protein in rat soleus muscle in chloroquine-induced myopathy using end-specific antibodies for Abeta40 and Abeta42: immunohistochemical evidence for amyloid beta protein. Neurosci Lett 1995;202:77–80.

112. Mielke JG, Murphy MP, Maritz J, Bengualid KM, Ivy GO. Chloroquine administration in mice increases beta-amyloid immunoreactivity and attenuates kainate-induced blood–brain barrier dysfunction. Neurosci Lett 1997;227:169–172.

113. Oyama F, Murakami N, Ihara Y. Chloroquine myopathy suggests that tau is degraded in lysosomes: implication for the formation of paired helical filaments in Alzheimer's disease. Neurosci Res 1998;31:1–8.

114. Chua T, Tran T, Yang F, Beech W, Cole GM, Frautschy SA. Effect of chloroquine and leupeptin on intracellular accumulation of amyloid-beta (Abeta) 1-42 peptide in a murine N9 microglial cell line. FEBS Lett 1998;436:439–444.

115. Sperber K, Quraishi H, Kalb TH, Panja A, Stecher V, Mayer L. Selective regulation of cytokine secretion by hydroxychloroquine: inhibition of interleukin 1 alpha (IL-1–à) and IL-6 in human monocytes and T cells. J Rheumatol 1993;20:803–808.

116. Berliner RW, Earle DPJ, Taggart JV, *et al*. Studies on the chemotherapy of the human malarias. VI. The physiological disposition, antimalarial activity, and toxicity of several derivatives of 4-amino quinoline. J Clin Invest 1948;27:98–107.

117. Chang YH, Silverman SL, Paulus HE. Colchicine. In: Paulus HE, Furst DE, Droomgoole, eds. Drugs for rheumatic disease. New York: Churchill Livingstone; 1987;431.

118. Li ZY, Davis GS, Mohr C, Nain M, Gemsa D. Inhibition of LPS-induced tumor necrosis factor-alpha production by colchicine and other microtubule disrupting drugs. Immunobiology 1996;195:624–639.

119. Peters-Golden M, McNish RW, Davis JA, Blackwood RA, Brock TG. Colchicine inhibits arachidonate release and 5-lipoxygenase action in alveolar macrophages. Am J Physiol Lung Cell Mol Physiol 1997;271:L1004–L1013.

120. Bennett EL, Alberti MH, Flood JF. Uptake of [3H]colchicine into brain and liver of mouse, rat, and chick. Pharmacol Biochem Behav 1981;14:863–869.

121. Drion N, Lemaire M, Lefauconnier JM, Scherrmann JM. Role of P-glycoprotein in the blood–brain transport of colchicine and vinblastine. J Neurochem 1996; 67:1688–1693.

122. Evrard PA, Ragusi C, Boschi G, Verbeeck RK, Scherrmann JM. Simultaneous microdialysis in brain and blood of the mouse: extracellular and intracellular brain colchicine disposition. Brain Res 1998;786:122–127.

123. Zemer D, Pras M, Sohar E, Modon M, Cabili S, Gafni J. Colchicine in the prevention and treatment of amyloidosis of familial Mediterranean fever. N Engl J Med 1986;314:1001–1005.

124. Zemer D, Livneh A, Langevitz P. Reversal of the nephrotic syndrome by colchicine in amyloidosis of familial Mediterranean fever. Ann Intern Med 1992; 116:426.

125. Shirahama T, Cohen AS. Blockage of amyloid induction by colchicine in an animal model. J Exp Med 1974;140:1102–1107.

126. Kisilevsky R, Boudreau L, Foster D. Kinetics of amyloid deposition. II. The effects of dimethylsulfoxide and colchicine therapy. Lab Invest 1983;48:60–67.

127. Wolach B, Gotfried M, Jedeikin A, Lishner M, Brossi A, Ravid M. Colchicine analogues: effect on amyloidogenesis in a murine model and, in vitro, on polymorphonuclear leukocytes. Eur J Clin Invest 1992;22:630–634.

128. Escalante A, Ehresmann GR, Quismorio FP. Regression of reactive systemic amyloidosis due to ankylosing spondylitis following the administration of colchicine. Arthritis Rheum 1991;34:920–922.

129. Giulian D, Robertson C. Inhibition of mononuclear phagocytes reduces ischemic injury in the spinal cord. Ann Neurol 1990;27:33–42.

130. Pratt J, Roux M, Henneguelle E, Stutzmann JM, Laduron PM. Neuroprotective effects of colchicine in the gerbil model of cerebral ischaemia. Neurosci Lett 1994;169:114–118.

131. Kimura M, Saji M. Protective effect of a low dose of colchicine on the delayed cell death of hippocampal CA1 neurons following transient forebrain ischemia. Brain Res 1997;774: 229–233.

132. Mundy WR, Tilson HA. Neurotoxic effects of colchicine. Neurotoxicology 1990;11:539–547.

133. Aisen PS, Marin D, Fusco M, Baruch B, Ryan T, Davis KL. A pilot study of colchicine in Alzheimer's disease. Alzheimer's Res 1996;2:153–156.

134. Williams LR, Oostveen JA, Hall ED, Jolly RA, Satoh PS, Petry TW. Cyclophosphamide is neuroprotective in a gerbil model of

transient severe focal cerebral ischemia: correlation with effects of tirilazad mesylate (U-74006F). J Neurotrauma 1996;13:103–113.

135. Keimowitz RM. Dementia improvement with cytotoxic chemotherapy: a case of Alzheimer disease and multiple myeloma. 1997;54:485–488.

136. Leszek J, Gasiorowski K. Therapeutic efficacy of cyclophosphamide in Alzheimer's disease. Alzheimer Res 1996;2:43–46.

137. Steiner JP, Dawson TM, Fotuhi M, *et al.* High brain densities of the immunophilin FKBP colocalized with calcineurin. Nature 1992;358:584–587.

138. Dawson TM, Steiner JP, Lyons WE, Fotuhi M, Blue M, Snyder SH. The immunophilins, FK506 binding protein and cyclophilin, are discretely localized in the brain: relationship to calcineurin. Neuroscience 1994;62:569–580.

139. Ankarcrona M, Dypbukt JM, Orrenius S, Nicotera P. Calcineurin and mitochondrial function in glutamate-induced neuronal cell death. FEBS Lett 1996;394:321–324.

140. Tokime T, Nozaki K, Kikuchi H. Neuroprotective effect of FK506, an immunosuppressant, on transient global ischemia in gerbil. Neurosci Lett 1996;206:81–84.

141. Osaka H, Aisen PS, Pasinetti GM. Immunophilin binding drugs reduce amyloid-mediated oxidative stress. Alzheimer Rep 1998;3:1–4.

142. Steiner JP, Connolly MA, Valentine HL, *et al.* Neurotrophic actions of nonimmunosuppressive analogues of immunosuppressive drugs FK506, rapamycin and cyclosporin A. Nature Med 1997;3:421–428.

143. Steiner JP, Hamilton GS, Ross DT, *et al.* Neurotrophic immunophilin ligands stimulate structural and functional recovery in neurodegenerative animal models. Proc Natl Acad Sci U S A 1997;94:2019–2024.

144. Payami H, Schellenberg GD, Zareparsi S, *et al.* Evidence for association of HLA-A2 allele with onset age of Alzheimer's disease. Neurology 1997;49: 512–518.

145. Curran M, Middleton D, Edwardson J, *et al.* HLA-DR antigens associated with major genetic risk for late-onset Alzheimer's disease. NeuroReport 1997;8: 1467–1469.

146. Middleton D, Vahidassr DM, Savage DA, Mawhinney H, Curran MD, Passmore PA. HLA-DR alleles are not associated with late-onset sporadic Alzheimer's disease. Alzheimer Rep 1999;2:147–149.

147. Aisen PS, Luddy A, Durner M, Reinhard JF Jr, Pasinetti GM. HLA-DR4 influences glial activity in Alzheimer's disease hippocampus. J Neurol Sci 1998;161:66–69.

Index